Controlled Substance Management in Chronic Pain

Peter S. Staats · Sanford M. Silverman
Editors

Controlled Substance Management in Chronic Pain

A Balanced Approach

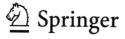 Springer

Editors
Peter S. Staats
American Society of Interventional Pain
  Physicians
Johns Hopkins University
Baltimore, MD
USA

and

Department of Anesthesiology and Critical
  Care
Premier Pain Centers
Shrewsbury, NJ
USA

and

Department of Oncology
Premier Pain Centers
Shrewsbury, NJ
USA

Sanford M. Silverman
Comprehensive Pain Medicine
Pompano Beach, FL
USA

and

Department of Integrated Medical Science
Charles E. Schmidt College of Medicine,
  Florida Atlantic University
Boca Raton, FL
USA

and

Department of Surgery
Boca Raton Regional Hospital
Boca Raton, FL
USA

and

Department of Surgery
Broward North Medical Center
Pompano Beach, FL
USA

ISBN 978-3-319-80930-4   ISBN 978-3-319-30964-4   (eBook)
DOI 10.1007/978-3-319-30964-4

Printed on acid-free paper

This Springer imprint is published by Springer Nature
The registered company is Springer International Publishing AG Switzerland

To my wife and kids.

To the healthcare workers who come to work each day attempting to help patients with chronic pain.

To the patients with chronic pain. Hopefully, this will help your doctors work with you to have a thoughtful and safe approach to managing your pain.

To the patients with addiction disorders, or who may develop problems with addiction in the future. We hope this book provides insight into minimizing the risks of addiction.

And to the families of patients with pain.

—Peter S. Staats

To my wife, children and office staff, who have all put up with me over the years and have seen what an interesting trip this has been.

To my patients with chronic pain and those with addiction; both are suffering, even the abusers and misusers.

To those families that have lost loved ones to prescription drug abuse, hopefully we can help prevent this from happening to others.

To the patients with chronic pain who have to deal with collateral damage of the new gauntlet of state and federal laws governing how we prescribe controlled substances which ultimately limit your access to them.

Hopefully we can right some of the wrongs and reduce the suffering and, most importantly, educate our fellow physicians to do the same.

—Sanford M. Silverman

Preface

Medicine is a forever changing field. The field of pain management is by some accounts the oldest field of medicine, while others would consider it quite new. Ancient Egyptian Kings are known to have been buried with poppy seeds. The use of controlled substances has waxed and waned over the decades, if not centuries. Prior to the controlled substance act of 1914 patients could freely use opioids for the treatment of a variety of maladies, from exhaustion and rheumatism to the management of pain. Undoubtedly, many patients were effectively treated for their pain using home remedies that included laudanum, or tincture of opium.

Unfortunately, problems with substance abuse did exist that required the passage of the Harrison controlled substance act. Between 1914 and 1970, 50 additional regulations were placed in the controlled substance act of 1970. In the 1970s there was grave concern with regard to opiates, leading to a great national restraint on their use. Nancy Reagan's well-intentioned campaign to stop the use of illicit drugs ("Just Say No") also led to the drive that no patients should receive opiates for the management of non-cancer-related pain.

In the 1980s, the pendulum began to swing back to pro opiates in certain settings. The cancer community noted that patients with cancer were dying with uncontrolled pain that could be potentially effectively managed with opiates, and encouraged the liberalization of their use of opiates. In the 1990s it was noted that patients with non-cancer pain may also benefit from the use of opiates. I heard questions like "Why should I have to get cancer in order to get control of my pain?" Studies were broadly quoted indicating that addiction was exceedingly rare. Prominent pain societies drafted guidelines indicating that it was appropriate to use opiates in certain settings. Physicians were told that the risk of addiction was extremely low in chronic pain patients. Pharmaceutical companies marketed the use of opiates as a means of controlling pain. Literally, hundreds of millions of dollars were spent on marketing to patients and physicians, and billions of dollars in profits were generated by sale of opiates for patients with non-cancer-related pain. However, we were all mistaken in underestimating the potential for abuse and misuse of prescription opioids.

In spite of the enormous costs, chronic pain remains one of the greatest healthcare crises affecting the world today. It costs the American people more than cancer and heart disease combined. The Joint Commission on Hospital Accreditation listed pain as the fifth vital sign. Hospitals are now reimbursed (among other things) on patient satisfaction, which includes the management of pain. Many employed physicians' salaries are also tied to patient satisfaction surveys. Poor pain control would potentially decrease reimbursement to hospitals and group practices. This in turn may have led to overprescribing of controlled substances by well-intentioned physicians who are improperly trained to manage pain. Unfortunately, clear guidelines on the management of pain do not clearly state how to manage the pain, or when to use opioids. In fact, quality evidence is lacking on the use of opioids in chronic non-cancer pain.

The combination of pressures from the government pushing pain control, pharmaceutical companies marketing opiates, the enormous size of the pain problem, and poor understanding of when to use opiates and how to use them safely has led to an explosion of deaths related to the use of prescription controlled substances.

In this text we have asked many world experts to contribute, specifically related to the area they have great expertise in. We hope to provide a balance and a framework for discussion on the appropriate use of opiates. Clearly, some patients require opiates for uncontrolled pain. But how do we do that safely? How do we keep both ourselves and our patients out of trouble? What are the limitations to the use of controlled substances, and what are some reasonable alternatives? We hope that this book and several others frame the discussion and where opiates fit in with pain management. It is our aim to help healthcare providers balance the discussion around appropriate opiate prescription, provide alternative strategies, minimize abuse diversion, addiction, and the unintentional deaths known to be associated with controlled substances.

Peter S. Staats
Sanford M. Silverman

Contents

Contributors

Gerald M. Aronoff Department of Pain Medicine, Carolina Pain Associates, PA, Charlotte, NC, USA

Jen Bolen The Legal Side of Pain, Lenoir City, TN, USA

Steven Chinn Department of Anesthesiology, Montefiore Medical Center, Bronx, NY, USA

Michael R. Clark Department of Psychiatry and Behavioral Sciences, Johns Hopkins Medicine, Baltimore, MD, USA

Timothy Furnish Department of Anesthesiology, UC San Diego Medical Center, San Diego, CA, USA

J. Gregory Hobelmann Department of Psychiatry and Behavioral Sciences, Johns Hopkins University, Baltimore, MD, USA

Karina Gritsenko Department of Anesthesiology, Montefiore Medical Center, Albert Einstein College of Medicine, Bronx, NY, USA

Hans Hansen Pain Relief Centers, Conover, NC, USA

Judith Holmes The Compliance Clinic, LLC, Golden, CO, USA

Kenneth L. Kirsh Clinical Research and Advocacy, Millennium Health, San Diego, CA, USA

Sean Li Premier Pain Centers, LLC, Shrewsbury, NJ, USA

Laxmaiah Manchikanti Anesthesiology and Perioperative Medicine, University of Louisville, Paducah, Louisville, KY, USA

Steven D. Passik Clinical Research and Advocacy, Millennium Health, San Diego, CA, USA

Joseph V. Pergolizzi Department of Medicine, Johns Hopkins University School of Medicine, Bonita Springs, FL, USA

Sanford M. Silverman Department of Integrated Medical Science, Clinical Biomedical Science, Charles E. Schmidt College of Medicine, Florida Atlantic University, Boca Raton, FL, USA; Comprehensive Pain Medicine, Pompano Beach, FL, USA; Department of Surgery, Boca Raton Regional Hospital, Broward North Medical Center, Pompano Beach, FL, USA

Peter S. Staats Department of Anesthesiology and Critical Care, Department of Oncology, Johns Hopkins University, Baltimore, MD, USA; President, American Society of Interventional Pain Physicians, Paducah, KY, USA; Department of Anesthesiology and Critical Care, Department of Oncology, Premier Pain Centers, Johns Hopkins University, Shrewsbury, NJ, USA

Andrea M. Trescot Pain and Headache Center, Wasilla, AK, USA

Alicia A. Trigeiro Clinical Research Associate, Millennium Health, San Diego, CA, USA

Mark Wallace Department of Anesthesiology, University of California San Diego, La Jolla, CA, USA

Lynn R. Webster Early Development Services, PRA Health Sciences, Salt Lake City, UT, USA

Chapter 1
Scope of the Pain Problem

Steven Chinn, Karina Gritsenko and Laxmaiah Manchikanti

"Pain" is an entity which can mean different things to different people. It is, at the same time, a subjective and objective sensation. For the patient experiencing the pain, it is an unpleasant sensation that causes undue suffering. For the diagnostician, pain is a *symptom* or *sign*, the characteristics of which may help to elucidate where in the body the disease process is taking place. For the surgeon, acute pain at the incision may be an untoward postoperative side effect of performing the surgery; and for the pain medicine physician, pain is a complex multidimensional problem. Therefore, "pain" exists along the full spectrum of a disease process, from diagnosis to treatment. But regardless of its many presentations and etiologies, *pain* has been defined as "an unpleasant sensory and emotional experience associated with actual or potential tissue damage, or described in terms of such damage," according to the International Association for the Study of Pain [1]. This definition is kept broad, so that it can encompass multiple sources, including (1) actual unpleasant sensory input (i.e., nociception) to pain receptors of the body, (2) but also the modulation of this input within the central and peripheral nervous systems by neurohumoral responses, (3) and the perception of the input by cognitive and psychological responses created by the brain. Just as a small amount of tissue damage may

S. Chinn
Department of Anesthesiology, Montefiore Medical Center, 111 East 210th Street, Bronx, NY 10467, USA
e-mail: schinn@montefiore.org

K. Gritsenko (✉)
Department of Anesthesiology, Montefiore Medical Center, Albert Einstein College of Medicine, Montefiore Pain Center, 3400 Bainbridge Ave, LL400, Bronx, NY 10467, USA
e-mail: karina.gritsenko@gmail.com

L. Manchikanti
Anesthesiology and Perioperative Medicine, University of Louisville, 2831 Lone Oak Road, Paducah, Louisville, KY 42003, USA
e-mail: drlm@thepainmd.com

© Springer International Publishing Switzerland 2016
P.S. Staats and S.M. Silverman (eds.), *Controlled Substance Management in Chronic Pain*, DOI 10.1007/978-3-319-30964-4_1

"snowball" into a massive response in one patient, it is equally plausible that massive tissue damage may elicit little more than a wince from another patient.

Consequently, chronic pain is a complex and multifactorial phenomenon characterized by persistent and/or long-lasting pain. Chronic pain has been described using multiple definitions, with pain persistent 6 months after an injury, pain beyond the usual course of an acute disease [2], or pain that extends beyond the expected period of healing [3]. A comprehensive definition has been provided by the American Society of Interventional Pain Physicians which defines chronic pain as, "a complex and multifactorial phenomenon with pain that persists 6 months after an acute injury and/or beyond the usual course of an acute disease or a reasonable time for a comparable injury to heal, that is associated with chronic pathologic processes that cause continuous of intermittent pain for months or years that may continue in the presence or absence of demonstrable pathology and may not be amenable to routine pain control methods with healing never occurring [4]."

Determining the prevalence and incidence in the USA and globally has been difficult, because of multiple factors, including the subjective nature of pain and the lack of consensus regarding diagnoses. Difficulty in recalling the first, true "episode" of a recurrent pain condition makes determining incidence difficult, as well as the inability to discern between pain conditions with constant, chronic pain and those states with recurrent, episodic courses. There is a continuum, rather than absolute states [5]. Historically, another hindrance had been the dearth of morbidity data prior to the 1980s. Until then, mortality data had driven research into the general health status of populations, which in turn drove research into more established conditions such as cardiovascular disease and cancer. However, chronic pain conditions such as musculoskeletal disease and lower back pain do not contribute much to mortality trends, and therefore, its trends and statistics have not been trended in the past [6]. Furthermore, the identification of pain conditions has been hampered by ambiguous case definitions and lack of population disease registries or other patient databases for pain statistics [5]. Luckily, there is evidence of increased reporting of chronic pain in the past few decades; this likely represents an increase in self-reported pain, taken from general health surveys and pain-focused studies [6].

Self-reported data from general health surveys provide important information about the frequency of chronic pain and the global burden of disease. According to the WHO World Mental Health Surveys, prevalence of chronic pain is 37 and 41 % for developed and developing countries, respectively [7]. This "composite" percentage falls within the range of other prevalence statistics for individual developed countries such as Denmark, Norway, the Netherlands, Sweden, Israel, and Scotland, with the range being 20–55 % [8]. Using the Population Reference Bureau's world population data from 2013, these prevalence numbers represent approximately 461 million and 2.42 billion people who have chronic pain in developed and developing countries, respectively [9].

The global burden of chronic pain is a very useful metric to measure, because it illustrates the need for the medical community to approach chronic pain from a public health perspective and apply epidemiological techniques to analyze it, just as with more well-defined diseases such as obesity, diabetes mellitus, and cardio-vascular disease. But from a clinical perspective, it serves to characterize chronic pain into more specific divisions and determine the individual prevalence and incidence statistics, because it may have diagnostic and prognostic value. Pain conditions can be stratified along numerous different lines: body site, adult versus pediatric, acute versus chronic, single site versus multisite, nociceptive pain versus neuropathic pain, and cancer versus non-cancer pain.

Among adults, spinal pain is extremely common with a lifetime prevalence of 51–84 % [5, 10]. The 1-year incidence of any lower back pain is reported from 1.5 to 38 % according to some estimates, with recurrence rates at 1 year of 24–80 % [11]. Again, the wide spread of estimates from multiple studies highlights the heterogeneity of authors' definition of "episodic" or "recurrent."

Looking into the pediatric and adolescent population, there have been few longitudinal studies following the trends and risk factors associated with the development of chronic pain. Again, the lack of data stems from a lack of con-sistency in case definitions for pain conditions, which preclude useful comparisons between different studies. However, in a large epidemiological review of 41 studies since 1991, the authors determined that headache was the most common single pain reported in studies with a 23 % prevalence rate. Back pain, abdominal pain, and musculoskeletal pain were also common. Subject risk factors included female sex, anxiety, depression, and low self-esteem, while environmental risk factors included parental education, mental health status, socioeconomic status, type of residence, and amount of time allowed watching television. From the earliest age through the later adolescent years, they found increasing prevalence for headache, back pain, and musculoskeletal pain, but interestingly, a decrease in recurrent abdominal pain [12]. Other studies have corroborated these rates. In Henschke et al., the 1-month prevalence of chronic lower back pain ranges from 18.0 to 24.0 %, while 1-year incidence rates for lower back pain ranges from 11.8 to 33 %. The 1-month prevalence of headaches and stomachaches are estimated as high as 69 and 49.8 %, respectively [5].

What about cancer pain? There are many similarities between cancer and non-malignant pain. Anatomically, physiologically, and biochemically speaking, there is no difference. The ultimate impact of pain is related to severity, which neg-atively affects function, but may have no relation to cause. Both cancer and non-cancer chronic pain patients can have comorbid anxiety and depression. But several important aspects differentiate them. Cancer patients will experience cachexia, dys-pnea, anorexia, or symptoms resulting from organ dysfunction [13]. Some estimates report 36 % of non-metastatic cancer patients with pain, while 59–67 % of metastatic cancer patients suffer from chronic pain [8].

On the individual level, the consequences of pain can affect multiple facets of a subject's life. For example, poorly treated acute pain following surgical procedures can reduce quality of life, increase recovery time, and increase cost of hospital stays and insurance expenditures. The most feared complication from acute pain is the development of chronic pain; subjects eventually suffer reduced mobility, loss of strength, disturbed sleep patterns, and immune impairment. These effects, again, reduce the quality of life and functional status even further, causing a downward spiral [14].

On an emotional level, feelings of anxiety, anger, and depression are commonplace. In a vicious cycle, negative emotions can increase the intensity and perception of chronic pain, which then begets more negative emotions. This leads to increased disability, loss of social functioning, and increased isolation. Parents, spouses, and caretakers are unable to fulfill their duties. In fact, 40–50 % of chronic pain patients have a concomitant mood disorder. Anger is also fairly common among chronic pain sufferers. In one study by Okifuji et al., 96 chronic pain patients were surveyed about the frequency and intensity of their anger. 62 % reported anger toward healthcare providers, while interestingly, 74 % of them expressed anger toward themselves, which was significantly associated with depression in a multivariable comparison [15].

A good illustration of the effects of chronic pain on disability is in the older adult and geriatric population. Among older adults, pain is the number one symptom underlying disability, which is the inability to complete basic and instrumental activities of daily living. Again, prevalence rates of chronic pain in the older population have wide distributions depending on the study, but have ranged from 24 to 72 %. In the National Health and Aging Trends Study (NHATS), over 8200 adults beyond the age of 65 were surveyed in regard to their health status; one of the aspects studied was the presence of pain. There was an approximate 52.9 % prevalence of any type of pain. Disability was 70 % more common in persons with pain than those without; and furthermore, this was magnified with subjects who reported multiple sites of pain [16]. Interestingly, this study and other studies have shown that as age increases, there is an increased prevalence of severe back pain, while that of mild severity lower back pain decreased [17].

Taking all of these studies into account, there seems to be several clear messages regarding chronic pain; that musculoskeletal pain, notably back and joint pain, is the dominant single type of chronic pain, but that most people with chronic pain have multiple sites of pain.

Economically speaking, the yearly cost of chronic pain in the United States is estimated to be at least $560–$635 billion per year. However, these data from the Institute of Medicine [14], based on Gaskin and Richard [18], have been shown to be inaccurate [19]. This also showed that approximately 100 million Americans suffer with chronic pain. This study, out of Johns Hopkins [18], defined persons with pain as follows:

- Persons who reported that they experienced pain limiting their ability to work, which is appropriate and includes 43.9 million of the total 100 million being estimated and discussed here with 21.3 million suffering with moderate pain and 22.6 million suffering with severe pain.
- However, the number 2 category is persons who were diagnosed with joint pain or arthritis, which is estimated to be 123.7 million.
- Finally, they also included 24.7 million persons who had a disability that limited their ability to work that had nothing to do with pain.

Consequently, multiple conditions, unrelated to chronic non-cancer pain were not only repeatedly counted, but also included, very costly arthritis and functional disability, which are not related to chronic non-cancer pain. A liberal estimate would be approximately 30 million requiring therapy for chronic non-cancer pain, either with interventional procedures, physical therapy, surgical interventions, or chronic opioid therapy. Two studies by Martin et al. [20, 21], in assessing the effect of chronic spinal pain on the US economy, found that costs were approximately $86 billion, with an increase of 65 % between 1997 and 2005, and a 49 % increase in the number of patients seeking spine-related care. In 2008, federal and state agencies, such as Medicare, Medicaid, and the Department of Veterans Affairs paid out approximately $99 billion in payments related to pain.

With the rising prevalence of chronic pain reaching epidemic proportions, as illustrated previously, the role of treating chronic pain began to take center stage. The public health management of pain reached the forefront of multiple regulatory agencies including the Joint Commission on Accreditation of Healthcare Organizations (JCAHO), the American Pain Society (APS), and the Center for Medicare/Medicaid Services. In 1995, the APS coined the term "pain: the fifth vital sign" and in 1999, JCAHO officially declared pain as "The Fifth Vital Sign," with the hope that monitoring and treating pain became as important as treating and monitoring high blood pressure. However, studies have been equivocal in determining how effective utilizing pain as a vital sign has been in improving the quality of pain management [22]. There have been multiple claims that this aspect in conjunction with multiple other liberalizations strategies has led to escalation of opioid use leading to the epidemic [23]. Nonetheless, this movement has spurred other agencies, such as the Veterans' Health Administration to adopt systematic practices to monitor and reduce pain.

From a treatment standpoint, there are different goals for each group. Rehabilitation and restoration are primary goals for non-cancer chronic pain, while relief and balance of side effects are goals for cancer patients. A cancer pain management plan will have more psychosocial support and increased polypharmacy. A more "liberal" use of opioids is acceptable in the cancer pain management arena, without addiction being a major issue. Why is it acceptable to give sedative doses of opioid medication to cancer patients? Yet, fear of addiction to opioids and other analgesics represents a huge barrier to treatment for non-malignant chronic pain patients; even if it may be warranted. In reality, the treatment of cancer versus non-cancer pain is along a continuum, utilizing the same medications in different dosages and for different indications [13]. Without a doubt, opioid medication prescribed by all physicians, not just pain medicine physicians, represents a major player in the armamentarium for pain of all types: acute, chronic, and cancer-related. Utilizing opioids for extended use in a chronic pain regimen represents a slippery slope with many potential benefits and risks inherent to the nature of opioids' mechanisms of action.

Clearly, this chapter is not meant as a review of the anatomy, physiology, and biochemistry of somatosensory or pain processing, but to fully understand pain as a disease, we must have a firm grasp of all these aforementioned principles and structures.

Somatosensation is a process where physical stimuli activate neural substrates leading to the perception of touch, pressure, and pain. Nociception is the process of activating receptors and neural loops by physical stimuli that may actually damage tissue. In contrast, the sensation of pain is a conscious response, which results from the addition of potential psychosocial factors to afferent neural activation. In turn, pain can lead to suffering, which takes into account a multitude of other considerations, including social isolation, disability, and comorbid mood disorders [24].

The recognition of stimuli as painful can be summarized in four stages: trans-duction, transmission, modulation, and perception. Transduction represents the conversion of physical "energy," in the form of heat or mechanical, to specific patterns of electrical energy at the terminus of an afferent neural pathway. Pain receptors represent the *vehicle* for this conversion. Next, transmission represents the conduction of the action potentials throughout the peripheral and central nervous systems. Usually, this course involves three orders of neurons. Dorsal root ganglion (DRG) cells transmit action potentials to the spinal neurons, which ascend the spinal cord in established tracts and pathways in order to transmit the electrical activity to the thalamus and brainstem nuclei. Lastly, neurons originating in the brainstem transmit the impulses to the somatosensory cortical areas. The third stage involves modulation of stimulus transmission anywhere along its path. The dorsal horn of the spinal cord is a major site, where weakening or enhancement of the pain signal occurs. The final stage represents cognition and the subjective sensation of pain, processed by the somatosensory cortical areas [24].

Where do opioids exert their effects? Opiates and opioid peptides exert their effects via a family of receptors. In the 1960s, clinical studies looking at the effects of nalorphine and morphine led to the discovery of distinct receptors and the classification of mu and delta opioid receptors. Delta opioid receptors are selective for enkephalins, which are endogenous opioid pentapeptides. Activation of delta receptors results in anxiolysis and analgesia, but not respiratory depression, as with the other types. Mu receptors have high selectivity for morphine and its related synthetic compounds. Furthermore, subtypes of the mu receptor, specifically mu_1 and mu_2, differentiate the analgesic effects of opiates and their major side effects, respiratory depression, and constipation. Kappa receptor activity results in modest analgesia, dysphoria, disorientation, miosis, and mild respiratory depression. Endogenous dynorphins show preferential affinity for kappa receptors [13, 25]. These receptors are located throughout the peripheral and central nervous systems. They can be found at nerve terminals, within the dorsal horn of the spinal cord. Immune cells may even produce endogenous opioids and possess opioid receptors themselves; this may explain the concept of stress-induced analgesia. Clinical applications include peripheral use of opioids in wounds and inflammatory con-ditions [26].

Within the spinal cord, opioid receptors are located mostly within lamina I and II; mu receptors account for over 70 %, followed by delta (24 %) and kappa receptors (6 %). Supraspinally, mu receptors are found within the amygdala, nucleus accumbens, thalamus, and limbic structures. Here, opioids modulate the emotional components of pain. Within the brainstem, high densities of mu receptors exist in the periaqueductal gray matter, locus coeruleus, and rostral ventromedial medulla. These structures orchestrate a descending modulatory system that inhibits dorsal horn pain signaling [13].

What is the history of opioid use? What is their historical reference and has their role been in modern Western medicine? Opium, a natural extract from the leaves and fruits of the *Papver somniferum* plant go all the back to third century B.C. in ancient Greece. It has also been described in use during the Middle Ages throughout Europe. The large-scale trade of opium into Europe and the Orient follows a course originating in the Middle East. The British traded opium for tea from China. When the Chinese realized the addictive properties of opium, they attempted to halt the trade, resulting in the Opium Wars of the 1840s. Ultimately, the British won and was ceded Hong Kong. The opium trade was legalized and eventually brought into the USA via Chinese laborers [25, 27].

Morphine was isolated from opium in 1804 for use as an analgesic by Friedrich Serturner, named after Morpheus, the God of Dreams, from Greek mythology. Codeine was isolated from opium in 1832 by Robiquet and used as an all-purpose tonic for multiple ailments and problems; and heroin was developed by the Bayer Company in 1898 as a cough suppressant [27].

"Opiates," including morphine and codeine, refer to any natural or semisynthetic derivative of opium with morphine-like effects. However, the term "opioid" has been used to define all drugs contain that morphine-like qualities and bind to opioid receptors, whether they are natural, semisynthetic, or synthetic. The term also includes the endogenous opioid peptides found in the body, such as enkephalins, dynorphins, and endorphins.

The World Health Organization issued its well-known 3-step "analgesic ladder" in 1986, to be used as guidelines for the treatment of cancer pain. Taking a significant role in this ladder are opioid medications. Step 1 involves the use of non-opioid medications, such as acetaminophen and nonsteroidal anti-inflammatory medications to treat mild pain. Subsequently, step 2 adds a "weak" opioid, such as codeine or oxycodone, to the regimen for treating moderate pain. Finally, step 3 involves adding a "strong" opioid, such as morphine or hydromorphone for severe pain. In all 3 steps, the WHO also advocates for the possible inclusion of other adjuvant therapies, which may include corticosteroids, anti-epileptics, tricyclic antidepressants, and neuroleptic medications [25]. Though it was created specifically for the management of cancer pain, the WHO analgesic ladder has found significant applicability to other types of pain, namely acute pain and chronic non-cancer pain. Proposed modifications have been made to reflect advancements since 1986, including newer opioid agents and new treatment modalities (i.e., neuromodulation), to keep the ladder valid; but the essence of the original ladder remains [28]. Opioids are part of an established armamentarium for the treatment of cancer pain and chronic non-cancer pain.

The WHO analgesic ladder represents a set of guidelines, but not a "one-size-fits-all" set of rules. The extent to which chronic pain responds to opioid analgesics varies depending on patient characteristics and the etiology of the pain.

The patient receiving opioids for chronic pain must be monitored closely, in order that dosages can be titrated quickly and appropriately to address the pain. If the patient presents with severe enough pain levels, then starting at step 2 or step 3 may be warranted.

The anatomy of pain processing and neurochemistry of opioid action was briefly illustrated previously, but how does the binding of an opioid to its receptor translate into its behavioral mechanism of action? Each type of opioid has different behavioral effects that relieve pain and suffering. Opioids also relieve emotional pain, which make them one of the classic drugs of addiction, because of their actions in lessening the threatening effects of rage and aggression [29].

Non-medical use of opioids has been described in 3 modes: controlled users, marginal abusers, and compulsive users with addiction predilections. Controlled users limit their use of the drug to amounts that do not interfere with social functioning; their pattern of use would not be defined as addictive. At the other end of this spectrum, compulsive users may exhibit the classic signs and symptoms of addiction, including withdrawal and craving. They will likely meet the criteria for substance use disorder as defined by the Diagnostic and Statistical Manual of Mental Disorders, 5th edition (DSM-5). Marginal users exhibit behavior somewhere in between that of controlled users ad compulsive users [29].

What is addiction? According to the previous edition of the DSM, the DSM-IV, addiction encompassed two separate, but related constructs, drug *abuse* and drug *dependence*. The DSM-IV actually avoids the use of the term *addiction* because of its negative connotations. The meet the criteria for addiction, a patient must have had to manifest at least 3 of the 7 criteria for "dependence" and at least 1 of the 4 listed criteria for "abuse," both within a 12-month period. However, this choice of semantics has created confusion among clinicians, because of dual use of the term *dependence* to refer to both the physiological sequelae and compulsive behavior aspects, when in fact, these two are separate entities [30]. The DSM-5, which was published in 2013, merges the concepts of "abuse" and "dependence" into a general continuum of "substance use disorders." The new definition for addiction now requires meeting at least 2 of the newly categorized 11 criteria on the "substance use disorder" scale.

As pertains to the addiction cycle, opioid addiction can remain remarkably stable over decades, despite repeated cycles of remission and resumption of use. A prior longitudinal study of heroin addicts in an addiction treatment program followed 581 users over the course of 33 years from 1962 through 1997. During 1995 through 1997, 21 % of subjects tested positive for heroin, while another cumulative 24 % either refused testing or were incarcerated [31].

According to the National Survey on Drug Use and Health (NSDUH) from 2012, enough opioids were prescribed to medicate every American every 4 h for an entire year. Approximately 23.9 million subjects, aged 12 years or older, were current illicit drug users, representing 9.2 % of the US population in that year. In 2001–2002, the 12-month and lifetime prevalence rates of an opioid-use disorder were 0.4 and 1.4 %, respectively [30].

Opioid intoxication for an addicted individual has been described in 4 stages: "rush," "nod," "high," and "being straight." The "rush" describes a short period of intense pleasure and euphoria, which is resistant to tolerance. Next, the "nod" represents a detached state of consciousness, when subjects are detached and calm. Third, the "high" is a general feeling of well-being that may last several hours; but this state is vulnerable to tolerance. Lastly, "being straight" represents the time until withdrawal symptoms appear [27].

Opioid withdrawal syndrome consists of a constellation of symptoms and signs, including yawning, lacrimation, rhinorrhea, perspiration, pupillary dilation, tremors, restlessness, insomnia, weight loss, elevated blood pressure and tachycardia, just to name a few. Piloerection, or "goose bumps" are common, and interestingly, is the origin of the term "quitting cold turkey." Accompanying these somatic and autonomic changes is a characteristic negative emotional state with depressive-like symptoms. Purposeful symptoms, such as craving, pleading, and complaining, start to appear; these actions are goal-oriented toward obtaining more opioid medication. As far as a time course for withdrawal is concerned, purposeful behavior begins 6–8 h after the last dose of heroin, peaking at 36–72 h. The aforementioned autonomic signs also appear 8–12 h after the last dose, peaking at 72 h. The physical withdrawal syndrome can carry on for 7–10 days further, which then marks the end of the acute withdrawal syndrome. The time course for methadone is somewhat longer, while the time course for meperidine withdrawal is significantly shorter. Generally, shorter acting drugs produce a withdrawal syndrome that is shorter onset and of shorter duration.

Lastly, tolerance can be defined as a "state of adaption in which exposure to a drug induces changes that result in a diminution of one or more of the drug's effects over time," according to Freye and Levy [25]. Tolerance to opioids develops to the analgesic, euphorogenic, and depressant effects, although certain autonomic effects, such as constipation or miosis, may be resistant to tolerance. Tolerance develops from pharmacodynamic changes that are neuroadaptive in nature. There are extensive mechanisms for tolerance, involving changes in the receptors, transduction systems, and neuroplasticity. Desensitization of opioid receptor activity and internalization of receptors occurs [13].

Opioid-induced hyperalgesia has been observed in previously addicted opioid users. They display a heightened sensitivity toward pain for up to 6 months after they begin their abstinence. This pain leads to recurrent craving, leading to more relapses to addiction. Therefore, poor pain tolerance may be a significant risk factor for opioid addiction. What are some other risk factors? Genetic factors certainly play a significant role in predisposing certain individuals toward addiction to opioids; they may have increased pain sensitivity because of up-regulation nociception or down-regulated inhibitory modulation pathways. Environmental factors allowing for the subject to gain access to the drugs are another important risk factors. Personality plays a huge role in addiction; risk takers and "adrenaline junkies" may be more apt to experiment with opioids thinking they have enough self-control to stop whenever they simply choose to. However, once they get on the slippery slope of "controlled" drug use, momentum might carry them into addiction. "Allosteric load" is another theoretical construct that may explain how childhood experiences predispose an individual toward drug abuse. People who have had to adapt to multiple stresses during childhood, such as those who are poor, uneducated, or are abused, have exhausted their coping mechanisms by adulthood. This leads to increased overall morbidity, including painful conditions such as arthritis, musculoskeletal disease, and angina [14].

Despite all of these dangers and pitfalls of prescribing opioids for chronic pain, they still remain one of the most commonly prescribed analgesic medications, with enough opioids prescribed in 2012 to medicate every American every 4 h. So, they represent a double-edged sword for chronic pain patients and their healthcare providers. As detailed in the Institute of Medicine's blueprint for relieving pain in America, they declared the overall effectiveness of opioids as analgesic medication was found to be, surprisingly, inconclusive [14]. The report cites a meta-analysis looking at short-term opioid use in older adults; there were reductions in pain intensity and improvements in functioning, but decreased mental health. In another meta-analysis, looking at studies treating non-cancer pain in over 6000 patients, "weak" opioids were found to be equivalent to other drugs in relieving pain. Only "strong" opioids were outperformed the two other groups [32].

At the same time, chronic pain patients and healthcare providers should not fall prey to the multitude of misconceptions and myths surrounding the utilization of opioids, which is that they always lead to significant cognitive impairment; that doses require continual escalation; and most prominently, that a person in pain must be "drug seeking" if the "standard" dosage of a opioid they are receiving is not enough to control the pain [25]. As all the evidence seems to point toward, pain is not only a symptom that is just linearly associated with the severity of some underlying disease. Chronic pain has multiple components including the physical, cognitive, and the emotional, which make it much more complex than any one simple number on a numerical rating scale can adequately describe. Pain truly is a "condition in itself."

References

1. Merskey H, Bogduk N. Classification of chronic pain: descriptions of chronic pain syndromes and definition of pain terms. 2nd ed. Seattle: IASP Press; 1994.
2. Bonica JJ. Definitions and taxonomy of pain. In: Bonica JJ, Loesser JD, Chapman CR, et al., editors. The management of pain. 2nd ed. Philadelphia: Lea & Febiger; 1990. p. 18–27.
3. Turk DC, Okifuji A. Pain terms and taxonomies. In: Loesser JD, Butler SH, Chapman CR, Turk DC, editors. Bonica's management of pain. 3rd ed. Baltimore: Lippincott Williams & Wilkin; 2001. p. 18–25.
4. Manchikanti L, Abdi S, Atluri S, Benyamin RM, Boswell MV, Buenaventura RM, Bryce DA, Burks PA, Caraway DL, Calodney AK, Cash KA, Christo PJ, Cohen SP, Colson J, Conn A, Cordner HJ, Coubarous S, Datta S, Deer TR, Diwan SA, Falco FJE, Fellows B, Geffert SC, Grider JS, Gupta S, Hameed H, Hameed M, Hansen H, Helm S II, Janata JW, Justiz R, Kaye AD, Lee M, Manchikanti KN, McManus CD, Onyewu O, Parr AT, Patel VB, Racz GB,

Sehgal N, Sharma M, Simopoulos TT, Singh V, Smith HS, Snook LT, Swicegood J, Vallejo R, Ward SP, Wargo BW, Zhu J, Hirsch JA. An update of comprehensive evidence-based guidelines for interventional techniques of chronic spinal pain: part II: guidance and recommendations. Pain Physician. 2013;16:S49–283.

5. Henschke N, Kamper SJ, Maher CG. The epidemiology and economics consequences of pain. Mayo Clin Proc. 2015;90(1):139–47.

6. Blyth FM, van der Windt D, Croft P. The global occurrence of chronic pain: an introduction. In: Croft P, Blyth FM, van der Windt D, editors. Chronic pain epidemiology: from aetiology to public health. Oxford: Oxford University Press; 2010. p. 1–14.

7. Tsang A, Von Korff M, Lee S, Alonso J, Karan E, Angermeyer MC, et al. Common chronic pain conditions in developed and developing countries: gender and age differences and comorbidity with depression-anxiety disorders. J Pain. 2008;9:883–91.

8. Blyth FM, van der Windt D, Croft P. Introduction to chronic pain as a public health problem. In: Croft P, Blyth FM, van der Windt D, editors. Chronic pain epidemiology: from aetiology to public health. Oxford: Oxford University Press; 2010. p. 279–87.

9. Population Reference Bureau: 2013 World Population Data Sheet. http://www.prb.org/pdf13/2013-population-data-sheet_eng.pdf (2013). Accessed 15 Apr 2015.

10. McBeth J, Jones K. Epidemiology of chronic musculoskeletal pain. Best Pract Res Clin Rheumatol. 2007;21:403–25.

11. Hoy D, Brook P, Blyth FM, Buchbinder R. The epidemiology of loew back pain. Best Pract Res Clin Rheumatol. 2010;24:769–81.

12. King S, Chambers CT, Huguet A, MacNevin RC, McGrath PJ, Parker L, MacDonald AJ. The epidemiology of chronic pain in children and adolescents revisited: a systematic review. Pain. 2011;152:2729–38.

13. Davis M, Glare P, Hardy J. Opioids in cancer pain. 1st ed. Oxford: Oxford University Press; 2005.

14. Institute of Medicine (IOM). Relieving pain in America: a blueprint for transforming prevention, care, education, and research. Washington, DC: The National Academies Press; 2011.

15. Okifuji A, Turk DC, Curran SL. Anger in chronic pain: investigation of anger targets and intensity. J Psychosom Res. 1999;47(1):1–12.

16. Patel KV, et al. Prevalence and impact of pain among older adults in the United States: findings from the 2011 national health and aging trends study. Pain. 2013;154:2649–57.

17. Dionne CE, Dunn KM, Croft PR. Does back pain prevalence really decrease with increasing age? A systematic review. Age Aging. 2007;35:229–34.

18. Gaskin DJ, Richard P. The economic costs of pain in the United States. J Pain. 2012;13:715–24.

19. Manchikanti L, Candido KD, Singh V, Gharibo CG, Boswell MV, Benyamin RM, Falco FJE, Grider JS, Diwan S, Staats PS, Hirsch JA. Epidural steroid warning controversy still dogging FDA. Pain Physician. 2014;17:E451–74.

20. Martin BI, Deyo RA, Mirza SK, Turner JA, Comstock BA, Hollingworth W, Sullivan SD. Expenditures and health status among adults with back and neck problems. JAMA. 2008; 299: 656–64. (Erratum in: JAMA. 2008; 299: 2630).

21. Martin BI, Turner JA, Mirza SK, Lee MJ, Comstock BA, Deyo RA. Trends in health care expenditures, utilization, and health status among US adults with spine problems, 1997–2006. Spine. 2009;34:2077–84.

22. Walid MS, Donahue SN, Darmohray DM, Hyer LA, Robinson JS Jr. The fifth vital sign—what does it mean? Pain Practice. 2008;8:417–22.

23. Manchikanti L, Atluri S, Hansen H, Benyamin RM, Falco FJE, Helm S II, Kaye AD, Hirsch JA. Opioids in chronic noncancer pain: have we reached a boiling point yet? Pain Physician. 2014;17:E1–10.

24. Raja SN, Hoot MR, Dougherty PM. Anatomy and physiology of somatosensory and pain processing. In: Benzon HT, Raja SN, Molly RE, Liu SS, Fishman SM, editors. Essentials of pain medicine. 3rd ed. Philadelphia: Elsevier; 2011. p. 1–7.

25. Freye E, Levy JV. Opioids in medicine: a comprehensive review on the mode of action and the use of analgesics in different clinical pain states. 1st ed. Netherlands: Springer; 2008.

26. Stein C, Schafer M, Hansen AHS. Peripheral opioids receptors. Ann Med. 1995;27:219–21.

27. Koob GF. Opioids. In: Koob GF, Arends MA, Moal ML, editors. Drugs, addiction, and the brain. Amsterdam: Elsevier; 2014. p. 133–71.

28. Vargas-Schaffer G. Is the WHO analgesic ladder still valid? Twenty four years of experience. Can Fam Physician. 2010;56:514–7.

29. Koob GF. What is Addiction? In: Koob GF, Arends MA, Moal ML, editors. Drugs, addiction, and the brain. Amsterdam: Elsevier; 2014. p. 1–27.

30. Sdrulla AD, Chen G, Mauer K. Definition and demographics of addiction. In: Kaye AD, Vadivelu N, Urman RD, editors. Substance abuse. New York: Springer Science and Business; 2015. p. 1–15.

31. Hser YI, Hoffman V, Grella CE, Anglin MD. A 33-year follow-up of narcotic addicts. Arch Gen Psychiatry. 2001;58:503–8.

32. Furlan AD, Sandoval JA, Mailis-Gagnon A, Tunks E. Opioids for chronic non-cancer pain: a meta-analysis of effectiveness and side effects. CMAJ. 2006;174:1589–94.

Chapter 2
Scope of the Problem: Intersection of Chronic Pain and Addiction

Alicia A. Trigeiro, Kenneth L. Kirsh and Steven D. Passik

Introduction

The prevailing medical and societal view of opioids is a pendulum, swinging between opiophobia and opiophilia. Like this image, the intersection between pain and addiction is a moving target. Various stakeholders have attempted to find a balance between addressing the crisis of chronic pain in society, while not exacerbating the problem of substance abuse. We need to balance the benefits and harms of opioids and other controlled substances with the risks of addiction.

Over the past 15–20 years, there has been a call to re-evaluate the role of opioids in the management of chronic, non-cancer pain. This has led to a dramatic expansion in legitimate prescribing of opiates. The rhetoric that accompanied this expansion tended to overstate the benefits and trivialize the risks of improving access to prescription opioids. As a result of improved availability, prescription drug abuse has been amplified. This appropriate concern makes physicians and caregivers much more cautious about opioid prescribing. The pendulum thus appears to be swinging from opiophilia back to opiophobia.

Physicians are concerned that opioids have long-term limited efficacy, that hyperalgesia may occur for those taking long-term opioids, and that addiction and abuse are real concerns that physicians need to be concerned with. On the other

A.A. Trigeiro
Clinical Research Associate, Millennium Health,
16981 via Tazon, San Diego, CA 92127, USA
e-mail: alicia.trigeiro@millenniumhealth.com

K.L. Kirsh · S.D. Passik (✉)
Clinical Research and Advocacy, Millennium Health,
16981 via Tazon, San Diego, CA 92127, USA
e-mail: steven.passik@millenniumhealth.com

K.L. Kirsh
e-mail: Kenneth.kirsh@millenniumhealth.com

© Springer International Publishing Switzerland 2016
P.S. Staats and S.M. Silverman (eds.), *Controlled Substance Management in Chronic Pain*, DOI 10.1007/978-3-319-30964-4_2

hand, some practitioners believe that these drugs, like many other classes of drugs, have benefits as well as risks. To derive the benefits and contain the risks takes time, expertise, assessment and reassessment, along with open, honest and detailed doctor–patient communication. Opioids cannot be used in a one-size-fits-all fashion. Patients who are treated with opioids need to be adequately assessed and triaged to the appropriate level of care. Significant time and decision making are required to safely prescribe opiates.

There is a general agreement that opioids are only first-line in certain situations (postoperative; severe acute; end-of-life care). However, the risk–benefit ratio is relatively low for an older person with arthritis or other medical comorbidities that contraindicate the use of nonsteroidal anti-inflammatory drugs. It is reasonable to prescribe opioids in some settings, as long as coordinated and monitored care is provided.

While opioid medications do have potential abuse, the risk of addiction shows significant patient variability. This depends upon the patient's history of addiction, psychiatric comorbidities, environmental stressors, and the way in which opioid therapy is delivered (with or without the appropriate level of safeguards for their level of risk). The epidemic of prescription drug abuse is not simply the result of the drugs being "powerful and highly addictive" but is also related to a failure to assess risk, match the use of appropriate safeguards, and then employ the safeguards and monitor the patients in a manner necessary to ensure safety. When a high-risk patient is treated as if they have a low risk, this can lead to abuse diversion or addiction.

There are several risk factors for addiction delineated below:
The agent must be

- Readily available;
- Relatively low cost;
- Rapidly enter the CNS;
- Demonstrate efficacy as a rewarding agent.

Environment must be

- Occupation;
- Peer group;
- Culture;
- Social instability.

Host must be

- Genetic predisposition;
- Familial problems;
- Coexisting psychiatric disorder.

Opioid pain therapy means there will be such an exposure. Identifying the latter two issues requires time and assessment.

People with pain are almost inevitably evaluated at a vulnerable time. Frequently a person with chronic pain begins medical treatment after a prolonged period of time, and the pain may be considered chronic in nature (6–12 months). During this time, they start to relinquish pleasurable activities, restorative sleep is disrupted, libido is reduced, depression develops, they cannot work, and there may be financial stressors.

If there is an exposure at a vulnerable time and the person has any of the known vulnerabilities—younger age (85 % of the addictions in the world are manifested by the age of 35, so an exposure in a young person is results in greater risk than in an older person), male gender, personal or family history of addiction, current psychiatric problems such as major depression, post-traumatic stress disorder (PTSD), panic disorder etc., history of sexual trauma, and a history of smoking. When these vulnerabilities are unassessed or unaccounted for in the context of an opioid exposure, this may lead to problematic behavior. However, when appropriate safeguards are instituted, these treatments can be successful. There are settings in which monitoring can be less frequent or intense. For example, the older person with arthritis, no personal or family history of addiction, and no current psychological problems (and not surrounded by friends, family members, or others who might "borrow" some of their medicines) can probably be seen monthly and manage a 30-day supply of opioids without problem. On the other hand, a traumatized, 27-year-old coal miner in southeastern Kentucky with a history of PTSD, depression, marijuana use, and cigarette smoking will be more complicated. He may need treatment for his psychological problems, an alteration in the medical regimen (our team might well have used a long-acting opioid such as a 24-h, once-per-day morphine preparation doled out in small supplies, such as 7 tablets, and see the person weekly), and the provision of tools to help in coping. He will need tools to safeguard his medication supply, and we may also choose to employ certain longer-acting medications, perhaps even one that has an abuse deterrent formulation to deter crushing or altering the formulation so as to help deter misuse. A 30-day supply of short-acting opioids (possibly 120–240 tablets) prescribed to this man without safeguards and monitoring is likely to be problematic.

Key Definitions

Unfortunately, the intersection of pain and addiction is clouded by several overlapping, poorly defined terms and phenomenologically difficult to separate concepts. Thus, we start with a definition of terms.

Addiction

Addiction is a relapsing brain disease characterized by compulsive and overwhelming involvement with the use of a drug, despite harmful consequences [1]. It begins with a voluntary decision to use a drug; however, control over usage decreases radically over time due to recurrent drug use. The behavioral pattern of substance abuse is generally thought to be chronic, and recovery is possible but is a lifelong process. The transition from voluntary user to addict happens through changes to the structure or wiring of the brain from repeated drug exposure. An individual who continues to use the drug despite physical, psychological, and social harm is considered to have an addiction problem. Addiction implies loss of control and is often confused with physical dependence, which is actually a different phenomenon [2].

If a physician believes that their patient is suffering from addiction, they should evaluate the 4 Cs—compulsive use, continued use despite harm, loss of control, and cravings. These must be assessed as part of an evaluation of addiction.

Physical Dependence

Physical dependence is characterized by the manifestation of physical withdrawal symptoms when a drug is discontinued or the dose is reduced. It can also lead to pseudo-addictive behaviors when a patient requires a drug in order to function normally [3]. Behaviors such as aggressively complaining about the need for higher doses or occasional unilateral drug escalations, which appear to be addicted on the surface, may be indications that the patient's pain is not well managed [4].

Tolerance and physical dependence on a drug can develop for both pain relief and the euphoric effects of a drug and can be produced by psychological and pharmacological factors. Withdrawal symptoms, such as sweating, anxiety, and insomnia, can occur when a patient has developed dependence on an opioid, and the drug is discontinued. It is thought to be caused by rebound at the central adrenergic nuclei [5]. Withdrawal symptoms can lead patients to seek opioids from both legitimate and illegitimate sources. While the current DSM-5 excludes tolerance and withdrawal from the diagnostic criteria for substance-use disorder during medical drug treatment, it should be noted that pain patients who are treated continuously with opioids may not manifest any aberrant behaviors.

A law in the state of Washington came into effect in 2012 that attempts to limit the amount of opioids that can be prescribed for those with chronic pain without consultation from an expert. This law was passed in response to high death rates from prescription opioid overdoses in the state. In some cases, some physicians began to taper patients who were using high-dose opioids who had for years. Several patients experienced reemergence of anhedonia and severe pain, both of which were likely to be effects of withdrawal. In this setting, tapering patients' high opioid doses may have destabilized them, leaving them with constant cravings and aberrant behavior [5].

Many clinicians confuse physical dependence with addiction. Physical dependence has been suggested to be a component of addiction, and it has been proposed that patients who seek to avoid withdrawal symptoms construct behaviors that reinforce drug-seeking behavior. However, these assumptions are not supported by experience acquired during opioid therapy for chronic pain. Animal models have provided indirect evidence for a fundamental distinction between physical dependence and addiction through opioid self-administration. This demonstrates that in the absence of physical dependence, drug-taking behavior is allowed to persist. However, clinical observation also fails to support the conclusions that analgesic tolerance plays a significant part in the development of addiction [2].

Tolerance

Tolerance occurs when an individual becomes habituated to a drug and needs the dose increased to maintain the same effect as an earlier dose. There has been a long-standing basic definition of tolerance as a pharmacologic property highlighted by the need for increasing doses to maintain effects. Tolerance and physical dependence are both common occurrences among patients taking opioids for chronic pain and are unrelated to true addiction [1].

The widely accepted 2001 definition by the American Academy of Pain Medicine, the American Pain Society, and the American Society of Addiction Medicine makes it clear that such a definition is too narrow. Their consensus document states that tolerance "is a state of adaptation in which exposure to a drug induces changes that result in a diminution of one or more of the drug's effects over time" [6]. Opioids are usually begun at a low dose in order to minimize side effects, and are increased as tolerance develops to the side effects. Early upward dosing is therefore expected. In addition, pain relief is often accompanied by an increase in physical activity, and the increased activity in itself often requires additional medication to provide adequate pain relief. This in itself can explain why early dose escalation is so frequently found. Delayed dose escalation may also herald the appearance of a progressive painful lesion or the development of new pains. In the absence of tolerance, the greatest need for opioid titration occurs during the first 3 months for most patients, and thereafter, further dose escalation may be gradual and minimal unless a mitigating event like disease progression or new injury occurs [2].

Withdrawal

Withdrawal symptoms occur due to the cessation or decrease in the amount of drug that an individual has been taking. The individual must first have developed a physical dependence to the drug in order to experience withdrawal symptoms. Withdrawal symptoms such as nausea, muscle aches, diarrhea, and insomnia can develop within minutes to several days after the reduction in opioid use that had previously been heavy or prolonged [7].

Opioid-Induced Hyperalgesia

Opioid-induced hyperalgesia (OIH) has been suggested as an explanation for the decreased analgesic efficacy of opioids in some patients requiring high doses. Chronic opioid use may increase sensitivity to specific pain stimuli but not others and does not produce allodynia [2]. It has been shown that opioids can cause nociceptive sensitization, can aggravate existing pain, or potentially cause new pains [8, 9]. The mechanisms and signal transduction pathways that mediate OIH are very similar to those of neuropathic pain and opioid tolerance. Hyperalgesia should be considered when patients have unexplained pain that is unassociated with the original pain or increasing levels of pain when their dosage of opioids has also increased. Treatment of hyperalgesia generally includes reducing the opioid dosage or utilizing NMDA receptor antagonists [9, 10].

While hyperalgesia clearly exists in animal models, there is inconsistent evidence to support or refute the existence of opioid-induced hyperalgesia in humans in clinical settings. However, animal models have limitations for accurately predicting human opioid pharmacology [11]. There is significant evidence in the animal literature to suggest that rodents exposed to very low doses of opioids showed signs of hyperalgesia, whereas those exposed to larger doses resulted in a reduction in sensitivity to painful stimuli. There are no animal studies, however, that examine hyperalgesia in chronic pain, so one should be careful in attributing increased sensitivity to pain to hyperalgesia since the evidence supporting it is somewhat thin [12].

Hyperalgesia, or at least decreased opioid effectiveness, also might be explained by low testosterone (hypogonadism) caused by long-term opioid use. Passik and colleagues [13] have recently shown that low testosterone lowers the pain threshold and triggers decreased pain tolerance in men undergoing androgen ablation. Perhaps treating these patients with hormone replacement therapy could help treat their pain sensitivity and restore efficacy of their regimen in the absence of opioid dose escalation or taper. Certain types of people also could be predisposed to this problem as well, such as those with a personal or family history of addiction [14].

Chemical Coping

Chemical copers occasionally use their medications in non-prescribed ways to cope with stress. A major hallmark of chemical coping is the fixation on the procurement of drugs for pain and the inflexibility about non-drug components of care. Medication use becomes central to life, while other interests become less important, and as a result, chemical copers in treatment often fail to move forward toward stated psychosocial goals. They are typically uninterested in treating pain or coping with pain non-pharmacologically. It should be noted, however, that while all addicts are chemical copers, not all chemical copers have addiction disorders.

Chemical copers also occasionally self-escalate their medication dosage in times of stress and sometimes need to have prescriptions refilled early [15]. The treatment approach for these types of patients might rely mainly on the use of long-acting opioids with a de-emphasis on drug-taking as a way of managing pain throughout the day. Psychotherapy and rehabilitative approaches are particularly important for this group of patients. Motivation for multiple lifestyle changes should be introduced so that the patients can regain the desire to live full lives despite having the disease of chronic pain [16].

Risks of Death and Other Comorbidities

Opioid prescribing has increased dramatically in North America from the time when opioids were mainly being prescribed to cancer patients. The population of non-cancer opioid users is much more diverse in terms of age, psychiatric and addiction histories and comorbidities, and duration of exposure [17]. The results of this change, however, have been mixed. Rather than the self-titration model based on the assumption that risk of misuse and addiction was uniformly minimal across patients (generally a cancer pain model), a specific type of risk stratification model was created for these types of patients. Some of the risk factors include younger age, personal or family history of addiction, a history of sexual trauma, and active mental health comorbidity. These types of risks were seen as indicators in a poor outcome in opioid therapy, unless the delivery of this therapy was tailored to the needs of the individual with the implementation of safeguards such as urine drug testing and prescription monitoring programs [3]. In 2013, for example, an estimated 7.7 million adults aged 18 or older (3.2 % of adults) had co-occurring mental illness and substance-use disorders in the previous year. The percentage of adults who had co-occurring mental illness and substance-use disorders in the past year was highest among adults aged 18–25 (6.0 %), followed by those aged 26–49 (4.5 %) and then by those aged 50 or older (1.1 %). Co-occurring mental illness and substance-use disorders were higher among males than females (3.6 % vs. 2.8 %) [18].

A co-occurring mental illness is one of the stronger risk factors for abuse for patients on opioid therapy. An estimated 2.3 million adults aged 18 or older (1.0 % of adults) had co-occurring serious mental illnesses (SMI) and substance-use disorders in the past year in 2013. Percentages were similar for adults aged 18–25 (1.7 %) and those aged 26–49 (1.4 %), both of which were higher than among adults aged 50 or older (0.4 %). Adults with major depressive orders also had a high use of substance abuse disorder in the past year at an estimated 3.3 million adults in the USA [19]. About half of adults with those comorbidities received either mental health care or substance-use treatment (47.8 %), including 7.7 % who received both types of care.

Another example of the risks patients involved who use opioids was documented in a survey in Denmark that revealed that 22.5 % of men and 27.8 % of women aged 65 and older reported chronic pain [20]. Out of these men and women, 35 %

of them were not satisfied with the type of pain treatment that was offered. Patients who are dissatisfied with their care could possibly seek out other types of pain relievers, such as non-prescribed medication. In one study of 100 patients with chronic pain (average age near 50), 23 tested positive for illegal drugs and 12 tested positive for opioids even though they had no prescription and denied taking opioids [21]. In another study of primary care patients in a Veterans Affairs facility who were receiving opioids for the treatment of chronic pain (average age 59), 78 % reported at least one indicator of medication misuse during the prior year, with significantly more of those who misused pain medications reporting comorbid substance-use disorder [22]. This is consistent with a more recent examination of a subset of data from the Researched Abuse, Diversion and Addiction-Related Surveillance system (RADARS) that found that though severe chronic pain is common in adults entering treatment for prescription opioid abuse, it is exponentially more prevalent in adults older than 45 years (70 %) relative to adults aged 18–24 (45 %) [23]. Older adults represent a particularly vulnerable population based on the fact that chronic pain and severe mental illness are comorbid problems [3].

Pill Mills

In the past ten years, prescription drug abuse has exploded around the country. There have been stories of pain clinics being opened up in Florida and Georgia by former auto-traders and twenty somethings, none of whom had medical degrees. In other states, only individuals with medical licenses may own and operate pain clinics. The pill mill epidemic became a national problem in 2010, and lax laws in Florida allowed it to become the nation's hot spot to easily buy prescription drugs. Many individuals came from out of state to buy prescription drugs from Florida, and the state became colloquially known as the "OxyContin Express." However, in the last several years, many "pill mills" have been shuttered and their owners and doctors arrested due, in part, to new prescription drug monitoring programs (PDMPs) that have been put into place. Missouri is currently the only state without a PDMP as of 2015. This increase in states with PDMPs is not surprising after states with the largest problems, such as Florida, enacted laws to curb the tide of overdose deaths and misuse of painkillers. After Florida enacted laws requiring legitimate pain clinics to register with the state and dispensers to report state's PDMP, they were able to shut down 250 rogue pain clinics and the number of high-volume oxycodone prescribers dropped from 98 in 2010 to 13 in 2012. The policy changes in Florida were followed by a decline in the prescribing of drugs but an increase in deaths associated with heroin, hydromorphone, and morphine after 2010, which might be a sign of a switch to the use of street drugs and alternative opioids [24].

Organized crime also has ties to the pill mill industry and helped to fuel the growing problem of prescription pill abuse. In 2013, the New Jersey State Commission of Investigation found that corrupt doctors had been charging Medicare for prescriptions and were funneling the reimbursements into bank accounts linked to the Russian mafia. New Jersey is working on a series of reforms that would help combat this type of drug problem and prevent future pill mills from being able to set up shop so easily. The plan involves imposing prescription standards for physicians, establishing harsher penalties for prescription drug diversion and oversight of medical practice and ownership, and enhancing New Jersey's prescription monitoring program [25].

Problems with Diversion

Diversion is one of the many problems that can occur with opioid prescription use. In 2013, there were 6.5 million current (past month usage) non-medical users of prescription-type drugs, including 4.5 million non-medical users of prescription pain relievers aged 12 and older. In 2013 as well, 2.2 % of adolescents aged 12–17 were current non-medical users of prescription-type drugs, including 1.7 % who used pain relievers. Of the 22.4 million adults aged 18 or older who used illicit drugs in 2013, 2.5 % of those used non-medical prescription-type drugs including 1.7 % who used pain relievers [18].

Signs to watch for that could indicate that patients are diverting their opioid medications include: [26]

1. Strange stories—Be wary of new patients with stories that do not seem right or make sense. Some may deliberately request appointments at the end of office hours or ask to be seen right away because they have to "catch a plane" or "need to get to an important appointment."
2. Reluctance to cooperate—Diverters will often refuse a physical examination or deny you permission to access previous medical records. These patients might leave the office suddenly if things are not going their way.
3. Unusual high or low understanding of medications—many diverters may request specific medication brands and may resist any attempts to prescribe them generic forms or substitutes.
4. Strange symptoms—Diverters might fake or exaggerate symptoms.

Problems with Opioids with Muscle Relaxants and Anxiolytics

Prescribing both benzodiazepines and opioids for a patient can potentiate respiratory depression, leading to serious consequences if they are not monitored correctly. Of the 22,767 deaths relating to pharmaceutical overdose in 2013, 16,235 (71.3 %) involved opioid analgesics, and 6973 (30.6 %) involved benzodiazepines [27]. Patients with chronic pain who use opioids alongside benzodiazepines (BZD) are at a higher risk for overdosing and demonstrate more aberrant behaviors.

Combining BZD and opioids increases the euphoric effects of the opioids. For example, it appears as though the addition of a BZD drug to methadone or buprenorphine may allow one to achieve a more powerful opioid effect often described as "heroin-like" [28]. To improve patient outcomes, clinicians should monitor for treatment compliance, screen for aberrant behavior, document medical necessity, and adjust treatment to clinical changes when necessary. Regardless of the risk that patients might possess for aberrant behaviors, patients on chronic opioid therapy should periodically undergo urine drug testing to confirm that the patients remain adherent to their prescribed treatment [29].

Opioid Risk Stratification

It is essential that proper assessments be completed to take reasonable steps to guard against abuse and diversion and to ensure that patients will be treated safely and effectively. A chronic pain assessment should include a detailed assessment of the pain itself, including intensity, quality, location, and radiation of pain. It also should ask about the identification of factors that increase and decrease the pain as well as a review of the effectiveness of various interventions that have been tried to relieve the pain. Clinicians should also assess the impact of pain on sleep, mood, level of stress, and function in work, relationships, and recreational activities since improvement in these areas may be a goal of pain treatment and a measure of the efficacy of interventions. If an individual has a predilection toward recreational drug use, prescription of opioids could lead to the abuse and/or diversion of the drugs and at worst, addiction. Several patient factors have been found to be predictive of a patient's risk for opioid misuse or abuse. A mental health disorder is a moderately strong predictor of opioid abuse, while a history of illicit drug and alcohol abuse or legal problems is also predictive of future aberrant drug behaviors. Tobacco use is highly prevalent among substance misusers, and the Screening Instrument for Substance Abuse Potential (SISAP) and the Screener and Opioid Assessment for Patients with Pain (SOAPP) include tobacco use as a factor in determining risk [3, 30, 31].

Assessment

There are several methods of assessment that the clinician can use to obtain details about the type of pain that a patient has and also as a tool to evaluate the best pain management strategy to employ.

Pain Assessment and Documentation Tool (PADT)—This type of assessment is a two-sided chart note that assesses pain relief, side effects, and aspects of functioning as well as potential aberrant drug behavior. It consists of 41 items and takes about 10 min to administer and score. It helps to assess the long-term patient progress on opioid therapy for chronic pain. PADT is a chart note intended to help clinicians to assess and document their observations when treating chronic pain patients on opioid therapy. The tool is based on the assumption that systematic pain assessment and documentation can assist in improving patient care [32].

Numerical Opioid Side Effect (NOSE) assessment tool—One available tool for the quantification of adverse effects is the NOSE assessment tool. The NOSE instrument is a simple, rapid, self-administered tool which has the potential to be utilized in a busy clinical setting to document and longitudinally follow trends of opioid adverse effects. The NOSE assessment tool is easy to administer as well as easy to interpret and may provide clinicians with important clinical information which could potentially impact various therapeutic decisions [33].

Opioid Risk Tool—This tool has 5 items that cover questions about family history of drug abuse, personal history of drug abuse, age, history of sexual abuse, and psychological disease. It takes less than a minute to administer and score, and it assesses the risk of aberrant behaviors when patients are prescribed opioids for chronic pain. One of its features is that it provides excellent discrimination between high- and low-risk patients. It also has the advantage of having brief and simple scoring [34].

Screening Tools

Screener and Opioid Assessment for Patients with Pain—Revised (SOAPP-R)— SOAPP-R is a 24-item self-administered screening tool developed and validated for those persons with chronic pain who are being considered for long-term opioid therapy. It takes less than 10 min to complete it, a quick and easy way to predict aberrant drug-related behaviors. This questionnaire includes subtle items that encourage the patient to admit to certain factors that are positively correlated with opioid misuse yet outwardly are not perceived to lead to reprisals. Any individual who scores more than 18 on the SOAPPR is rated as being at risk for opioid misuse [31].

Urine drug test (UDT)—UDT is one of the most widely available methods for monitoring opioid use in pain and addiction patients. It is a valuable tool that can help physicians in the clinical setting. Most evidence suggests that UDT is best used in concert with other clinical monitoring tools, such as continuous assessments of a patient's pain levels, quality of life, risk stratification for possible misuse, checks of the state prescription database, and psychosocial indicators [35]. The value of urine drug testing to pain clinicians has grown considerably as laboratories offering more accurate, sensitive, and specific forms of testing are now capable of providing these results in clinically actionable time frames.

There are two different testing methodologies that can be used in UDT, immunoassay and chromatographic; the latter category can be further subdivided into gas chromatography mass spectrometry (GC-MS) and liquid chromatography tandem mass spectrometry (LC-MS/MS). Immunoassay tests, also called point-of-care testing (POCT), are primarily used for on-site testing as the method is inexpensive, convenient, and less accurate and is the preferred initial test for screening. The immunoassay test (IA) uses antibodies to detect the presence of numerous drugs or drug classes and can determine whether a class of a substrate is present or absent [36]. It uses antibodies that are designed to bind to a specific type of drug without binding to the other substrates in the sample. This type of test exhibits adequate sensitivity for many purposes such as the forensic or vocational or screening in pain management. However, it typically does not identify specific metabolites and often does not distinguish between different drugs of the same class (e.g., opioids) and thus not able to function as the definitive testing method for pain management clinicians. Cross-relativities with other substances also are very common with this type of test, and this can produce many false positives, such as quinolone antibiotics and opiates or poppy seeds and opiates. The observed interference from cross-reactivity with substances other than the drug of interest may vary from assay to assay [37]. POCT also has higher cutoff levels than laboratory testing which can produce a high rate of false negatives (i.e., missed opportunities for clinicians to be informed about and intervene in cases of illicit drug use or the use of non-prescribed legal drugs).

Urine drug testing also is performed in laboratories that use GS-MS or LC-MS/MS technology which is a more highly sensitive and definitive method of testing than immunoassay tests. In many instances, this type of technology is used in confirmation testing as a second test positively identify a drug or metabolite from a positive specimen but this also approach it has been shown should not be limited to confirmation of positives alone given the high rate of false negatives in the pain management setting. This type of testing is often used as the sole testing method since it provides more accurate information as it typically measures the concentrations of all drugs, metabolites, and illicit substances ordered. One of the key clinical differences between LC-MS/MS and GC-MS is that LC-MS/MS can function more independently from IA; LC-MS/MS does not depend on and thus is not subject to the inaccuracies of the IA method, as it can test for many drugs at the same time. This is unlike GC-MS which depends on the IA result to guide the preparation for subsequent testing as the specimen must be volatilized individually for all individual drugs; thus, it is less versatile functioning outside of the confirmation of positive mode.

Pharmacogenetic testing—Numerous genes are involved in the pharmacokinetics and pharmacodynamics of opioid analgesia, the discussion of which is beyond the scope of this chapter. Here, we will discuss the ways in which genotyping can be used, in part, to predict pain responses for patients and to help avoid adverse drug reactions and thus are related to improving adherence to prescribed medication. The two genetic profiles that can greatly affect drug metabolism are ultrarapid metabolizers (Have 1 or more alleles which result in increased enzyme activity) or poor metabolizers (Have 2 non-functional alleles with little to no enzyme activity). The impact on each genetic profile on the opioid depends on the role of the enzyme in the metabolism of the drug.

Successful implementation of pharmacogenetic testing in a clinical practice can assist patients and clinicians with therapeutic decisions, risk communication, and reduce healthcare costs [38]. Choosing medications to which a given patient is more likely to respond might very well be a way in which clinicians can avoid poorly treated pain that might lead to overuse of medication or pseudo-addiction like behaviors on the part of the patient.

Another example of how genetics can affect the drug metabolism of chronic pain patients is the occurrence of withdrawal symptoms between scheduled doses of a drug in users with a specific genotype that could lead to overuse of opioids. In our clinical experience, we saw this not infrequently; patients on short-acting medications would begin to feel unwell at the end of a dosing interval, and this in turn was often a cue for taking the next dose (and not necessarily increasing pain). Perhaps particular genetic phenotypes might be even more vulnerable to withdrawal symptoms between opioid doses, such as a CYP2D6 ultrarapid metabolizer. A number of opioids are metabolized by the CYP450 system, which includes the CYP2D6-specific enzyme. Some of the opioids that are metabolized by this enzyme are broken down into metabolites for analgesic effectiveness and for elimination from the body. CYP enzyme expression and function can vary greatly between patients and they can be categorized as a poor metabolizer (inactive or minimally active enzyme), as an intermediate metabolizer (underactive enzyme), as an extensive metabolizer (normal enzymatic function), or as a rapid or ultrarapid metabolizer (overactive enzyme). The ultrarapid metabolizers will metabolize the opioids much more quickly than the extensive and intermediate metabolizers, while the poor metabolizers have little or no enzymatic functionality. If a CYP2D6 ultrarapid metabolizer takes short-acting hydrocodone, they might go into withdrawal between doses, prompting them to take the medication more frequently, which could lead to loss of control. Switching to a long-acting medication or one targeting an alternate metabolic pathway would potentially avoid this issue and could lead to a resolution of this problem [39].

Conclusion

Opioid prescribing has increased dramatically in the last several years. Some have benefited, but others have been harmed. With nearly 70 million people in the USA reporting chronic pain, any argument that one particular therapy is right or wrong for all or nearly all of them is not worth pursuing. It is clear that there are risks and benefits that can be balanced with time, expertise, and the use of the tools and strategies that have emerged over the past few turbulent years. What people suffering with pain need is neither a blank check for opioids nor a complete avoidance of them on the part of their providers. Pain physicians need to balance the treatment of pain with concerns of addiction. Healthcare providers need to be careful and open-minded so that they can artfully derive a treatment program—with or without opioids—that can help them live a full and meaningful life. Our humanity is not manifest in our willingness to provide opioids or protect people from them; our humanity is manifest in maximizing what we can do to help and minimizing harming those who trust in us.

References

1. Jamison R, Serraillier J, Michna E. Assessment and treatment of abuse risk in opioid prescribing for chronic pain. Pain Res Treat. 2011;2011:1–12.
2. Schneider J, Kirsh K. Defining clinical issues around tolerance, hyperalgesia, and addiction: a quantitative and qualitative outcome study of long-term opioid dosing in a chronic pain practice. J Opioid Manage. 2010;6(6):385–95.
3. Passik S, Miller N, Ruehle M, Kirsh K. Substance abuse in oncology. In: Grassi L, Riba M, editors. Psychopharmacology in oncology and palliative care. 1st ed. Springer: Berlin; 2014. p. 267–93.
4. Passik S, Kirsh K. Assessing aberrant drug-taking behaviors in the patient with chronic pain. Curr Pain Headache Rep. 2004;8(4):289–94.
5. Ballantyne J, Sullivan M, Kolodny A. Opioid dependence vs addiction. Arch Intern Med. 2012;172(17):1342.
6. American Society of Addiction Medicine (ASAM) Definitions related to the use of opioids for the treatment of pain. 2001. Available from: http://www.asam.org/docs/publicy-policy-statements/1opioid-definitions-consensus-2-011.pdf?sfvrsn=0 (cited 26 Feb 2015).
7. American Psychiatric Association. Diagnostic and statistical manual of mental disorders. 4th ed. Washington, DC: American Psychiatric Publishing; 2000.
8. Lee M, Silverman S, Hansen H, Patel V, Manchikanti L. A comprehensive review of opioid-induced hyperalgesia. Pain Physician. 2011;14:145–61.
9. Ruscheweyh R, Sandkuhler J. Opioids and central sensitisation: II. Induction and reversal of hyperalgesia. Eur J Pain. 2005;9(2):149–52.
10. Silverman S. Opioid induced hyperalgesia: clinical implications for the pain practitioner. Pain Physician. 2009;12:679–84.
11. Fishbain D, Cole B, Lewis J, Gao J, Rosomoff R. Do opioids induce hyperalgesia in humans? An evidence-based structured review. Pain Med. 2009;10(5):829–39.
12. Angst M, Clark J. Opioid-induced hyperalgesia: a qualitative systematic review. Acute Pain. 2006;8(4):191.
13. Jones C, Bruehl S, Passik S. Androgen ablation is associated with increased pain sensitivity and lowered pain threshold in men with prostate cancer. In preparation.
14. Basaria S, Travison T, Alford D, Knapp P, Teeter K, Cahalan C, et al. Effects of testosterone replacement in men with opioid-induced androgen deficiency. Pain. 2015;156(2):280–8.
15. Kwon J, Tanco K, Hui D, Reddy A, Bruera E. Chemical coping versus pseudoaddiction in patients with cancer pain. Pall Supp Care. 2014;12(05):413–7.
16. Passik S, Kirsh K. Chemical coping: the clinical middle ground. In: Smith H, Passik S, editors. Pain and chemical dependency. 1st ed. New York: Oxford University Press; 2008. p. 299–302.
17. Kirsh K, Peppin J, Coleman J. Characterization of prescription opioid abuse in the United States: focus on route of administration. J Pain Palliat Care Pharmacother. 2012;26(4):348–61.
18. Substance Abuse and Mental Health Services Administration. The NSDUH Report: Substance Use and Mental Health Estimates from the 2013 National Survey on Drug Use and Health: Overview of Findings. Rockville, MD: SAMHSA Substance Abuse and Mental Health Services Administration, Center for Behavioral Health Statistics and Quality; 2014.
19. Substance Abuse and Mental Health Services Administration. Results from the 2013 National Survey on Drug Use and Health: Mental Health Findings. Rockville, MD: NSDUH Series H-49, HHS Publication No. (SMA) 14-4887; 2014.
20. Sjogren P, Ekholm O, Peuckmann V, Gronbaek M. Epidemiology of chronic pain in Denmark: an update. Eur J Pain. 2009;13(3):287–92.
21. Manchikanti L, Singh A. Therapeutic opioids: a ten-year perspective on the complexities and complications of the escalating use, abuse, and nonmedical use of opioids. Pain Physician. 2008;11(2S):S63–88.
22. Morasco B, Dobscha S. Prescription medication misuse and substance use disorder in VA primary care patients with chronic pain. Gen Hosp Psychiatry. 2008;30(2):93–9.

23. Cicero T, Surratt H, Kurtz S, Ellis M, Inciardi J. Patterns of prescription opioid abuse and comorbidity in an aging treatment population. J Subst Abuse Treat. 2012;42(1):87–94.
24. Johnson H, Paulozzi L, Porucznik C, Mack K, Herter B. Centers for Disease Control and Prevention. Decline in drug overdose deaths after state policy changes—Florida, 2010–2012. Morb Mortal Wkly Rep (MMWR). 2014;63(26):569–74.
25. State of New Jersey Commission of Investigation. Scenes from an epidemic: a report on the SCI's investigation of prescription pill and heroin abuse. NJ: Trenton; 2013.
26. Cole B. Recognizing and preventing medication diversion. Fam Pract Manage. 2001;8(9):37–41.
27. Cdc.gov. CDC—Facts—Drug Overdose—Home and Recreational Safety—Injury Center [Internet]. 2015. Available from: http://www.cdc.gov/homeandrecreationalsafety/overdose/facts.html (cited 24 Feb 2015).
28. Jones J, Mogali S, Comer S. Polydrug abuse: a review of opioid and benzodiazepine combination use. Drug Alcohol Depend. 2012;125(1–2):8–18.
29. Gudin J, Mogali S, Jones J, Comer S. Risks, management, and monitoring of combination opioid, benzodiazepines, and/or alcohol use. Postgrad Med. 2013;125(4):115–30.
30. Coambs R, Jarry J. The SISAP: a new screening instrument for identifying potential opioid abusers in the management of chronic nonmalignant pain within general medical practice. Pain Res Manage. 1996;1(3):155–62.
31. Butler S, Budman S, Fernandez K, Jamison R. Validation of a screener and opioid assessment measure for patients with chronic pain. Pain. 2004;112(1):65–75.
32. Passik S, Kirsh K, Whitcomb L, Portenoy R, Katz N, Kleinman L, Dodd S, Schein J. A new tool to assess and document pain outcomes in chronic pain patients receiving opioid therapy. Clin Ther. 2004;26(4):552–61.
33. Smith H, Kirsh K. Documentation and potential tools in long-term opioid therapy for pain. Anesthesiol Clin. 2007;25(4):809–23.
34. Webster L, Webster R. Predicting aberrant behaviors in opioid-treated patients: preliminary validation of the opioid risk tool. Pain Med. 2005;6(6):432–42.
35. Webster L. the role of urine drug testing in chronic pain management: 2013 update. Pain Med News. 2013;11:45–50.
36. Nafziger A, Bertino J. Utility and application of urine drug testing in chronic pain management with opioids. Clin J Pain. 2009;25(1):73–9.
37. Lum G, Mushlin B. Urine drug testing: approaches to screening and confirmation testing. Lab Med. 2004;35(6):368–73.
38. Haga S, LaPointe N. The potential impact of pharmacogenetic testing on medication adherence. Pharmacogenomics J. 2013;13(6):481–3.
39. Tennant F. Cytochrome P450 testing in high-dose opioid patients. Practical Pain Management [Internet]. 2012;12(7). Available from: http://www.practicalpainmanagement.com/treatments/pharmacological/opioids/cytochrome-p450-testing-high-dose-opioid-patients (cited 24 Feb 2015).

Chapter 3
Evidence-Based Treatment for Chronic Pain with Opioids

Sean Li and Peter S. Staats

Introduction

It was the Sumerians, back in 3000 BC who first cultivated the poppy plant for its opium content. In human civilization, the earliest recorded use of opiates was described by Homer in 300 BC when it was given to Helen, the daughter of Zeus to treat her grief over the absence of Odysseus [1]. In 1804, the semi-synthetic morphine was discovered by Friedrich Sertürner. It was named morphine, after Morpheus, the God of Dreams. Morphine became commercially made available by the pharmaceutical giant, Merck in 1827. Prior to the Harrison Controlled Substance Act of 1914, opioids could be purchased over the counter and were used for a variety of maladies. Recognizing the concerns for addiction, the federal government placed greater controls on opioids. By the 1970s and early 1980s, the use of opioids in non-cancer pain was considered heresy and even malpractice by many medical boards. Increased awareness for pain relief by patient advocate groups in the early 1990s, followed by new pain management guidelines by the Joint Commission on the Accreditation of Health Care Organizations (JACHO) in 2000, and later by aggressive marketing strategies of opioid manufacturers, cultivated a culture of opioid use and subsequent over utilization [2]. Opioids have become the most commonly prescribed class of medications in the USA [3]. The prevalence of chronic pain has steadily increased to 25 % of the adult population

S. Li (✉)
Premier Pain Centers, LLC 170 Avenue at the Common, Suite 6,
Shrewsbury, NJ 07702, USA
e-mail: sli@premierpain.com

P.S. Staats
President, American Society of Interventional Pain Physicians, Paducah, KY, USA

P.S. Staats
Department of Anesthesiology, Critical Care and Department of Oncology,
Johns Hopkins University, 167 Avenue at the Common, Shrewsbury, NJ 07702, USA

© Springer International Publishing Switzerland 2016
P.S. Staats and S.M. Silverman (eds.), *Controlled Substance Management in Chronic Pain*, DOI 10.1007/978-3-319-30964-4_3

and fueling the explosive healthcare costs and the opioid epidemic [2, 4]. The use of opioids for the treatment of chronic non-cancer pain has been contentious, controversial, and confusing. This discrepancy is founded by the unequal balance between the amount of opioids being prescribed (both nationally and to given individuals with chronic pain) and the paucity of strong clinical evidence supporting its use. The challenge lies in the difficult balance between a clinician's commitment to treat chronic pain and the terrifying realities of the opioid epidemic. This chapter will attempt to review the available evidence behind the use of opioids in the treatment of chronic non-cancer pain.

When to Start Opioid Therapy

Much of the previous opioid therapy strategies have been adapted from the treatment of cancer pain. The World Health Organization's (WHO) analgesic ladder served as the foundation to current guidelines. However, the chronic non-cancer pain syndrome is complicated by a unique multifactorial process that includes physical and psychosocial dimensions that are distinct from terminal illnesses including cancer pain. For example, there has been little evidence to support the concept of breakthrough pain in non-cancer patients. The practice of supplementing long-acting opioids with additional short-acting opioids for breakthrough pain has contributed to the unnecessary use and possible abuse of prescription opioid medications [5]. Despite the lack of robust evidence supporting long-term opioids in chronic non-cancer pain, clinicians must achieve a delicate balance between patient accesses to safe compassionate care while mitigating the known risks of opioid medications. As part of a multidisciplinary treatment plan, chronic opioid use should be considered when conservative non-pharmacologic care, non-opioid analgesics, and appropriate interventional therapy have been considered or failed. A careful differential diagnosis (see Staats Li Silverman, Chap. 15) must be made and the decision to move to chronic opiate therapy should not be undertaken lightly. Initiation of opioid therapy must be goal oriented and carefully addressed with the patient. The provider and patient must identify specific functional goals of opioid therapy, understand the necessary monitoring process, and discuss the endpoints of therapy. Various professional societies have published recommendation guidelines. Table 3.1 illustrates recommended steps from the American Society of Interventional Pain Physicians (ASIPP) to help ensure safer administration of opioids and attempts to minimize the inherent risks associated with opioid therapy. This comprehensive list outlines key concepts such as establishing treatment goals, initiating opioid therapy, evaluating efficacy, monitoring, managing side effects, and opioid rotation along with the level of evidence supporting its role [6]. Specific topics such as opioid monitoring, urine drug screening, opioid rotation will be addressed in other chapters of this book.

Table 3.1 Recommendations from the American Society of Interventional Pain Physicians ASIPP

Step	Recommendation	Evidence
Initial steps of opioid therapy	Comprehensive assessment and documentation before initiating opioid therapy	Good
	Screening for opioid use	Limited
	Implementation of prescription drug monitoring programs (PDMPs)	Good to fair
	Implementation of urine drug testing (UDT) along with subsequent adherence monitoring	Good
Establish diagnosis	Establishment of appropriate physical diagnosis and psychological diagnosis if available prior to initiating opioid therapy	Good
	Caution in ordering imaging and other evaluations, and providing patients only with appropriate relevant clinical information when there is correlation of the symptoms with findings	Good
	Pain management consultation, for non-pain physicians, if high-dose opioid therapy is being utilized	Fair
Establishing medical necessity	Establishment of medical necessity prior to initiation or maintenance of opioid therapy	Good
Establishing treatment goals	Establishment of treatment goals of opioid therapy with regard to pain relief and improvement in function	Good
Assessment of effectiveness of opioid therapy	Understanding the effectiveness and adverse consequences of long-term opioid therapy in chronic non-cancer pain and its limitations	Fair for short-term, limited for long-term
	Use of high doses of long-acting opioids only in specific circumstances with severe intractable pain that is not amenable to short-acting or moderate doses of long-acting opioids	Fair
	Trial of opioid rotation tor patients requiring escalating doses	Limited
	Evaluation of contraindications to opioid use in chronic non-cancer pain	Fair to limited
Informed decision-making	Development of a robust agreement which is followed by all parties for initiating and maintaining opioid therapy	Fair
Initial treatment	Once medical necessity is established, initiation of opioid therapy with low doses and short-acting drugs with appropriate monitoring to provide effective relief and avoid side effects	Fair for short-term, limited for long-term effectiveness

(continued)

Table 3.1 (continued)

Step	Recommendation	Evidence
	Recommended doses of up to 40 mg of morphine equivalent doses as low dose, 41–90 mg of morphine equivalent dose as a moderate dose, and greater than 91 mg of morphine equivalence as high dose	Fair
	Caution in titration of long-acting opioids	Good
	Use of methadone in late stages after failure of other opioid therapy and only by clinicians with specific training in the risks and uses	Limited
Adherence monitoring	Obtaining an electrocardiogram prior to initiation, at 30 days and yearly thereafter for monitoring methadone prescription	Fair
	Adherence monitoring by UDT and PDMPs to identify non-compliant patients or prescription drugs or illicit drug abuse	Fair
Monitoring and managing side effects	Monitoring for and appropriate management of side effects, including discontinuation of opioids if indicated	Fair
	Close monitoring for constipation and initiation of a bowel regimen as soon as deemed necessary	Good
	Development and monitoring of a policy for driving under the influence of drugs during initiation of therapy, changes in the dosages, and addition of other centrally acting agents	Good
The final phase	Continuation of chronic opioid therapy with continuous adherence monitoring, modified at any time during this phase, in conjunction with or after failure of other modalities of treatments with improvement in physical and functional status and minimal adverse effects	Fair
	Use of methadone and buprenorphine in late stages after failure of other opioid therapy and only by clinicians with specific training in the risks and uses	Limited
	A trial of opioid rotation for patients requiring escalating doses	Limited
	Monitoring of chronic opioid therapy for adverse effects, with appropriate management	Good

PDMP prescription drug monitoring program
UDT urine drug testing
From Cheung et al. [6]

Efficacy of Opioids

Many patients are placed and maintained on opioids for many years. The scarcity of scientific evidence and realities of the opioid epidemic are two major driving forces behind responsible opioid prescribing and the paradigm shift away from opioids for treating chronic non-cancer pain. Long-term effectiveness of opioids is limited by the lack of quality double-blind controlled studies and the lack of outcomes data beyond 1 year. The current body of evidence does not include controlled trials with long-term follow-up [7, 8].

The American Society of Interventional Pain Physicians (ASIPP) latest opioid prescribing guidelines for the treatment of non-cancer pain has extensively reviewed the literature for original manuscripts and systematic reviews evaluating the efficacy of opioids in the treatment of non-cancer pain (ASIPP 2012, part I). Table 3.2 shows a summary of these studies.

Potential Risks of Long-term Opioid Therapy

The long-term effects and potential risks of opioid therapy must be considered separately from the physiologic effects of long-term use and the detrimental effects of opioid overuse, misuse, and abuse. The medical side effects of long-term opioid use include addiction, tolerance, physical dependence cognitive impairment, respiratory depression, constipation, immunosuppression, neuroendocrine dysfunction, hypogonadism, loss of libido, osteoporosis, peripheral edema, and cardiovascular dysfunction. As the use of opioids for treating chronic pain disproportionately increases, despite weak evidence there is an alarming rise in opioid abuse and related mortality. Opioids have been linked to increased mortality in patients receiving higher doses of opioids or when used with other agents [8].

Specific Drug Formulations

Tramadol

Once considered a weak atypical opioid agonist, tramadol is often misrepresented as a "non-narcotic" analgesic. Because of known abuse potential, tramadol has been rescheduled as a Schedule IV drug as of August 14, 2014, by the United State Drug Enforcement Agency. Tramadol does have multiple known mechanisms of action. It has weak binding affinity at the Mu-opioid receptor and inhibits the reuptake of both norepinephrine and serotonin. The evidence for tramadol in the treatment of chronic osteoarthritis pain is fair [7]. Tramadol was also shown to be effective in the treatment of chronic pain due to diabetic neuropathy [9]. In comparison with other

Table 3.2 Summary of studies evaluating the efficacy of opioids in the treatment of chronic non-cancer pain

Study/methods	Participants	Opioids studied	Outcomes	Conclusions
Fulan et al. [35] meta-analysis 28 studies average duration 5 weeks	$n = 6019$ various chronic pain (80 % nociceptive, 12 % neuropathic, 7 % fibromyalgia, 1 % mixed)	Codeine, morphine, oxycodone, tramadol, propoxyphene	Pain and functional status	Opioids were more effective than placebo, 1/3 of patients discontinued treatment
Kalso et al. [36] meta-analysis 15 studies 7–24 month study duration	$n = 388$	Various opioids, not including tramadol or codeine	Short-term effectiveness, 30 % pain reduction, effectiveness comparable for neuropathic and musculoskeletal pain	High drop-out rate. Only 44 % remained in the study between 7 and 24 months
Martell et al. [37] meta-analysis 2378 studies screened 5 studies compared opioid versus opioid, 4 studies compared opioid vs placebo	n/a	Various opioids	Effectiveness of opioids in treating low back pain, prevalence, and associated addiction	Opioids are common prescribed for low back pain, efficacious for short-term, efficacy beyond 16 weeks is unclear, 24 % aberrant behavior observed
Eisenberg et al. [38] cochrane database review of 22 trials	$n = 14$, less than 24 h $n = 8$, 8–70 days	Various opioids	Effectiveness of opioids in short-term and intermediate-term	Opioids are effective in the intermediate-term for treating neuropathic pain compared to placebo; short-term evidence was equivocal

(continued)

Table 3.2 (continued)

Study/methods	Participants	Opioids studied	Outcomes	Conclusions
Deshpande et al. [39] cochrane database review of 4 trials	n/a	3 trials studied tramadol	Efficacy of opioids in treating chronic low back pain	Trials achieved high validity scores, questionable long-term efficacy
Cepeda et al. [40] meta-analysis of 11 RCTs	n = 1019 Patient with osteoarthritis	Tramadol	12 % reduction in pain with tramadol compared to placebo	Decreased pain and improved functioning
Chou et al. [41] meta-analysis of 34 RCTs	n = 3608 Patient with chronic non-cancer pain 5 days-24 weeks	Various short and long-acting opioids	No sufficient evidence to show superiority of one long-acting opioid versus short-acting opioid	All trials were of short duration
Kalso et al. [42] meta-analysis of 15 RCTs	n = 1145 11 RCTs focused on oral opioids with n = 1025, 4 days and 8 weeks	Various oral and intravenous opioids including oxycodone	30 % improvement of neuropathic and nociceptive pain compared to placebo; 7 studies showed improvement of sleep	Evidence supports short-term use of opioids. 80 % experience at least 1 adverse event
Manchikanti et al. [43] systematic review of 111 trials	318 trials screened, 111 RCTs evaluated	Various oral opioids	4 studies evaluated results beyond 6 months	One study (12) reported positive evidence for tapentadol at 12 months with comparable efficacy to oxycodone at reduced GI side effects
Taylor et al. [44] 11 studies reviewed	n = 167, 3 placebo-controlled trials, 6 comparative studies, 1 pharmacokinetic study, 1 long-term safety study	Various opioids and controlled release formulations	Controlled release oxycodone was effective and safe compared to immediate release formulations	This study only focused on patient with moderate-to-severe chronic non-cancer pain due to osteoarthritis

(continued)

Table 3.2 (continued)

Study/methods	Participants	Opioids studied	Outcomes	Conclusions
Smith et al. [45] contemporary opinion	Pathophysiology of neuropathic pain	Various opioids	Peripheral neuropathic pain may be more responsive to opioids compared to central neuropathic pain states	Overall neuropathic pain less responsive to opioids than nociceptive pain. Variable response requires individualized management
Krashin et al. [46] meta-analysis of 324 articles over 10 year period	Review of medical management of HIV-related pain	Various opioids and non-opioids	Higher risk profile with greater psychosocial impact. Patient often have comorbid psychiatric illness and substance abuse history	Challenging treatment population. HIV-related chronic pain often undertreated. Proceed with caution and follow current opioid prescribing guidelines
Pergolizzi et al. [10] meta-analysis of 3 double-blinded, randomized, placebo-controlled trials	$n = 981$, $n = 2020$, $n- = 588$ chronic low back pain or osteoarthritis. 3-week titration followed by 12-week maintenance phase	Tapentadol CR, oxycodone CR	Controlled release tapentadol was non-inferior to oxycodone CR. Associate with reduced side effects	Tapentadol CR may be as effective for treatment of chronic low back and osteoarthritis pain compared to oxycodone CR

opioid analgesics, tramadol is a relatively weak analgesic that is well tolerated in the elderly.

Tapentadol

A relatively new opioid analgesic, tapentadol has gained increased interest for the treatment of chronic non-cancer pain. Several studies have shown comparable efficacy to oxycodone but with less associated side effect. In a meta-analysis of 3 double-blind randomized placebo-controlled multicenter trials by Pergolizzi et al. in 2012, tapentadol was shown to have equal efficacy as oxycodone for the treatment of chronic low back or osteoarthritis pain [10]. In a larger randomized, controlled study of 1117 subjects, Wild et al. showed comparable efficacy of extended release tapentadol and oxycodone in the treatment of chronic low back or osteoarthritic knee/hip pain for up to 1 year. The tapentadol group reported better gastrointestinal tolerability and less overall adverse effects [11]. More recently, a meta-analysis of chronic pain patients with osteoarthritis ($n = 2010$), low back pain ($n = 965$), and diabetic peripheral neuropathy ($n = 389$) by Afilalo and Morlion showed comparable analgesic efficacy of extended release tapentadol and oxycodone. Tapentadol was associated with less side effects and improved compliance in the treatment of moderate-to-severe chronic pain conditions with both nociceptive and neuropathic etiologies [12].

Morphine

Morphine is the prototypic opioid in the treatment of pain and remains the most studied in its class. There are several studies that support its efficacy but all fail to show long-term benefit beyond 12 months. Maier and colleagues utilized a phone survey study to determine the efficacy of long-term opioids 5 years after the initiation of opioid therapy. Of the 433 patients involved, 3-year data were collected from 121 patients. Patients undergoing long-term opioid treatment reported significant pain relief and improved quality of life. Noticeably, there was a large reported number of high-dose increases along with inconsistent dose adjustments. This was dependent on who was managing the patient (pain specialist vs. general practitioner). Pain specialists tended to write higher doses of opioids than primary care physicians [13]. Tassain et al. reported on the neuropsychological performance of chronic non-cancer pain patients receiving sustained release oral morphine. At 12 months, 18 of the 28 patients enrolled showed improvement in pain, function, and mood without significant disruption in cognitive function [14]. Compared to other opioids, sustained release morphine has also been shown to be more effective than other sustained release formulations. Rauck et al. [15] compared twice a day sustained release oxycodone with once daily sustained release morphine in a randomized, open-label, multicenter trial consisting of 266 patients and noted improved function and quality of life in the group receiving systemic morphine. In a double-blind placebo by Moulin published in the Lancet, there was minimal separation from placebo at forty weeks.

Hydrocodone

As a morphine derivative, hydrocodone was the most prescribed drug in the USA up until 2014 when it was reclassified as a Schedule II medication. Despite its popularity among healthcare providers, there have not been any studies on its long-term effectiveness. In a large observational study among 11,352 patients who were prescribed the combinations of tramadol, non-steroidal anti-inflammatory (NSAID), and hydrocodone, the 12-month abuse rates were 2.7, 2.5, and 4.9 %, respectively. There was no significant improvement of pain when hydrocodone was compared to tramadol or NSAID [16].

Oxycodone

There are several studies that evaluate the efficacy of oxycodone despite its negative portrayal in the public and media. Similar to all other opioids, quality studies to supports oxycodone's long-term efficacy for the treatment of chronic non-cancer pain are limited. Portenoy et al. reviewed the efficacy of sustained release oxycodone in 233 chronic non-cancer pain patients over a period of 3 years. He noted that 70–80 % of the patients were unchanged or improved with sustained release morphine. Interestingly, the adverse effects were reported in 88 % of the patients [17]. Hermos et al. noted in a large observational study of veterans that oxycodone had significant treatment problems when there is concurrent treatment involving benzodiazepines, psychogenic pain, alcohol abuse, and HIV [18].

Fentanyl

Fentanyl is a highly potent synthetic opioid first introduced to treat acute pain. Sustained release transdermal formulations have made fentanyl available for chronic pain applications. In a multicenter trial, Allan et al. reviewed the efficacy of transdermal fentanyl in 338 strong opioid naïve chronic non-cancer pain patients over 13 months. Primary end point was 50 % reduction of pain complaints. Of the 338 patients, this improvement was observed in 40 % who rested, 47 % who were active during the day, and 53 % of patients who were active during night. The study results were confounded by the concomitant usage of strong short-acting opioids in

80 % of the participants [18]. In a prospective open-labeled study, Mystakidou et al. compared transdermal fentanyl with oral codeine or morphine in the treatment of chronic non-cancer pain over a period of 10 months. This study found significant improvement of quality of life within 28 days and effective pain relief within 48 h with the use of transdermal fentanyl [19]. Transdermal fentanyl was compared to various oral opioid formulations by Milligan et al. in an international, multicenter, open-label trial including 524 patients over 12-month period. Of the 57 % who completed this trial, 86 % preferred transdermal fentanyl and 67 % reported good to moderate pain relief. There was a 25 % attrition rate due to adverse effects [20].

Hydromorphone

Hydromorphone is a semi-synthetic derivative of morphine. Its high potency and water solubility has been utilized for quick onset relief of acute pain. Extended release formulations have been applied in the treatment of chronic non-cancer pain. The extended release formulation was approved for commercial use by the Federal Drug Administration in 2010. The short service record of this drug is reflected in the paucity of research data. In a 90-day study of 197 patients, 70 are with cancer-related pain and 127 are with non-cancer-related chronic pain. In both groups, hydromorphone was shown to have a statistically significant improvement in their average pain scores and quality of life. Specifically, the average pain score reduction was from 8.1 to 3.3 [21].

In addition, as extended-release hydromorphone was approved by the FDA, the final separation between placebo and active drug from a 12-week study was less than one point.

Methadone

The unique pharmacokinetics and molecular properties of methadone allow it to be both very effective as an analgesic in treating chronic pain but also potentially dangerous if abused or inappropriately prescribed. Once regarded as a common treatment for opioid addiction maintenance because of its extremely long 5-day half-life, the use of methadone in the treatment of chronic pain as increased but has been followed by a disproportionately large spike in overdose deaths [22]. Due to its long pharmacokinetic half-life, active metabolites of methadone may build up to toxic levels before the patient reports pain relief. The accumulation of these metabolites may result in lethal respiratory depression after the patient has taken additional doses when pain relief is not obtained. To this date, there have not been any randomized controlled trials studying the short or long term efficacies of methadone. Sandoval et al. reviewed 21 articles with 545 patients taking oral methadone for non-cancer pain. This systematic review included both short and long term methadone patients. Of the 526 participants, 59 % reported pain relief and 50 % reported side effects. These results were measured in observational studies without control groups [23].

Codeine

There is one retrospective study focused on codeine and oxycodone in treating chronic pain associated with rheumatic disease. This study reported 50 % side effects, with constipation being most common. Effective pain relief from codeine was reported among 644 patients with rheumatic disease [24].

Buprenorphine

Buprenorphine is unique molecule with opioid agonist/antagonist properties. Transdermal formulations of buprenorphine have been used for analgesia. The efficacy of buprenorphine for the treatment of chronic pain has been limited. A Polish study of 4030 cancer and 764 non-cancer pain patients showed effective pain relief with buprenorphine patch [25]. In a randomized, active-control, double-blind trial of 1160 patients, buprenorphine patch was found with similar efficacy to immediate release oxycodone 40 mg/day. Within the same study, adverse reactions from the two opioids were 77 % for buprenorphine and 73 % for oxycodone [26].

Special Populations

High-risk Patient Population

Chronic non-cancer pain is heavily co-diagnosed with behavioral and psychiatric disorders [27]. The added complexity and increased potential for opioid-related complications require additional care in patient risk assessment and mitigation. Opioid dosing, drug monitoring, and abuse prevention will be addressed in separate chapters. In addition, there are several pain conditions that are considered contraindicated due to the poor evidence for efficacy [28]. These conditions include primary headache, functional disorders, fibromyalgia, mental health disorder with chronic pain as the major manifestation, chronic pancreatitis, chronic inflammatory bowel disease, concurrent substance abuse, and current/planned pregnancy.

Opioids and Driving

Driving while under the influence of prescription opioids poses a unique dilemma to those who take the medication for legitimate pain relief and the potential risk to the general public. We know cognitive impairment is associated with opioid use in the opioid naive population. Patients are advised not to drive for 24 h after receiving anesthesia comprising sedative and opioids. There are no specific guidelines for patients on chronic opioids and driving. Fishbain et al [29] showed no impairment of driving skills in opioid-dependent or tolerant patients. Wilhelmi and Cohen later described the term "driving under the influence of drugs" to designate the action of operating an automobile after consuming prescription medications other than alcohol. Interestingly, this study found a significant percentage of the driving public with detectable levels of opioids. They concluded psychomotor impairment following acute opioid administration or dose escalation. These effects are diminished over time with stable dose [30].

Elderly

When considering any medications for the elderly population, one has to take into account the physiologic changes in hepatic and renal function, comorbidities, and potential drug–drug or drug–disease interactions [31]. The provider must understand the unique challenges and needs of the older patients. For example, most elderly patients take between 2 and 5 scheduled medications and have a fixed income. Thus, special consideration must be given to dosing schedules, drug–drug interaction, and cost [32]. There are no specific clinical trials of opioid medications targeting older patients, and our current recommendations rely on available evidence collected from the general chronic pain population. American Geriatric Society concluded that patients with moderate-to-severe chronic pain should be considered for opioid therapy [33].

Conclusion

From a global perspective, nearly 25 % of adults have moderate-to-severe chronic pain, and about 10 % have incapacitating chronic pain that limits work and daily activities [34]. The treatment of chronic non-cancer pain with opioids has been challenged by the explosive overutilization of opioids, the alarming number of casualties from the opioid epidemic, superimposed with public awareness and governmental pressures. Healthcare providers are caught between the need to offer compassionate care and keeping patients safe from the deadly complications of opioid overdose. The lack of strong clinical evidence for the use of opioids in treating chronic non-cancer pain compounds this dilemma. There should be balance between access to necessary pain relieving opioids and patient safety. Education of both patients and physicians must remain at the forefront of this effort. Physicians and providers must work together in cooperation. They must identify clear treatment goals and start/end points. Opioid contracts, prescription monitoring, and urine drug screening should be incorporated into foster trust. Common goal must be focused on patient safety, function, and quality of life.

References

1. Brownstein MJ. A brief history of opiates opioid peptide, and opioid receptors. Proc Nat Acad Sci. 1993;90:5391–3.
2. Manchikanti L, Helm S, Fellws B, et al. Opioid epidemic in the United States. Pain Physician. 2012;15: ES9–38.
3. Kuehn BM. Prescription drug abuse rises globally. JAMA. 2007;297–306.
4. Von Korff, et al. Long-term opioid therapy reconsidered. Ann of Intern Med. 2011;155:325–8.
5. Manchikanti L, et al. Breakthrough pain in chronic non-cancer pain: fact, fiction, abuse. Pain Physician. 2011;14:E103–17.
6. Cheung C, et al. Chronic opioid therapy for chronic non-cancer pain: a review and comparison of treatment guidelines. Pain Physician. 2014;17:401–14.
7. Manchikanti L, et al. American society of interventional pain physicians (ASIPP) guidelines for responsible opioid prescribing in chronic non-cancer pain: part I-evidence assessment. Pain Physician. 2012;15:S1–66.
8. Chou R, et al. The effectiveness and risks of long-term opioid therapy for chronic pain: a systematic review for a National Insitutes of Health Pathways to Prevention Workshop. Ann of Int Med. 2015;162:276–86.
9. Harati Y, et al. Maintenance of the long-term effectiveness of tramadol in treatment of the pain of diabetic neuropathy. J Diabetes Complications. 2000;14:65–70.
10. Pergolizzi J, et al. Current consideration for the treatment of severe chronic pain: the potential for tapentadol. Pain Pract. 2012;12:290–306.
11. Wild J, et al. Long-term safety and toleraibility of tapentadol extended release for the management of chronic low back pain or osteoarthritis pain. Pain Pract. 2010;10:416–27.
12. Afilalo M, Marlion B. Efficacy of tapentadol ER for managing moderate to severe pain. Pain Physician. 2013;16:27–40.
13. Maier C, et al. Long-term efficacy of opioid medication in the patients with chronic non-cancer-associated pain. Results of a survey 5 years after onset of medical treatment. Schmerz. 2005;19:410–7.
14. Tassain V, et al. Long term effects of oral sustained release morpine on the europsychological performance in patients with chronic non-cancer pain. Pain. 2003;104:389–400.
15. Rauck R, et al. A randomized, open-label, multicenter trial comparing once-a-day Avinza (morphine sulfate extended-release capsules) versus twice-a-day OxyContin (oxycodone hydrochloride controlled release tablets) for the treatment of chronic, moderate to severe low back pain; improved physical function in the ACTION trial. J Opioid Manage. 2007;3:35–43.
16. Adams E, et al. A comparison of the abuse liability of tramadol, NSAIDs, and hydrocodone in patients with chronic pain. J Pain Symptom Manage. 2006;31:465–76.
17. Portenoy R, et al. Long-term use of controlled-release oxycodone for non-cancer pain: results of a 3-year registry study. Clin J Pain. 2007;23:287–99.
18. Hermos J, et al. Characterization of long-term oxycodone/acetaminophen prescriptions in veteran patients. Arch Intern Med. 2004;164:2361–6.

19. Mytakidou K, et al. Long-term management of non-cancer pain with transdermal therapeutic system-fentanyl. J Pain. 2003;4:298–306.
20. Milligan K, et al. Evaluation of long-term efficacy and safety of transdermal fentanyl in the treatment of chronic non-cancer pain. J pain. 2001;2:197–204.
21. Stepanovi A, et al. Clinical efficacy of OROS® hydromorphone in patients suffering from severe chonric pain: a study undertaken in routine clinical practice. Wien Klin Wochenschr. 2011;123:531–5.
22. Centers for Disease Control and Prevention (CDC). Vital signs: risk for overdose from methadone used for pain relief-United States, 1999–2011. MMWR Morb Mortal Wkly Rep. 2012;61:493.
23. Sandoval J, et al. Oral methadone for chronic non-cancer pain: a systemic literature review of reasons for administration, prescription patterns, effectiveness, and side effects. Clin J Pain. 2005;21:503–12.
24. Ytterber S, et al. Codeine and oxycodone use in patients with chronic rheumatic disease pain. Arthritis Rheum. 1998;41:1603–12.
25. Przeklasa-Muszyska A, et al. Transdermal buprenorphine in the treatment of cancer and non-cancer pain-the results of a multicenter studies in Poland. Pharmacol Rep. 2011;63:935–48.
26. Steiner D, et al. Efficacy and safety of Buprenorphine Transdermal System (BTDS) for chronic moderate to severe low back pain: a randomized, double-blinded study. J Pain. 2011;12:1163–73.
27. Manchikanti L, et al. Psychological factors as predictors of opioid abuse and illicit drug use in chronic pain patients. J Opioid Manage. 2007;3:89–100.
28. Hauser W, et al. Long-term opioid use in non-cancer pain. Dtsch Arztebl Int. 2014;111:732–40.
29. Fishbain, et al. Are opioid-dependent/tolerant patients impaired in driving-related skills? A structured evidence-based review. J Pain Symptom Manage. 2003;25:559–77.
30. Wilhelmi B, Cohen S. Creating balanced driving under the influence of drugs policy for the opioid using driver. Pain Physician 2012;15:ES215–30.
31. Christo P, et al. Effective treatment for pain in the older patient. Curr Pain Headache Rep. 2011;15:22–34.
32. Mclean A, et al. Aging biology and geriatric clinical pharmacology. Pharmacol Rev. 2004;56:163–84.
33. American Geriatrics Society Panel on Pharmacological Management of Persistent Pain in Older Persons. Pharmacological management of persistent pain in older persons. J Am Geriatr Soc. 2009;57:1331–46.
34. Croft P, et al. Chronic pain epidemiology: from aetiology to public health. Oxford: Oxford University Press. 2010;9–18.
35. Furlan A, et al. Opioids for chronic noncancer pain: a meta-analysis of effectiveness and side effects. Can Med Assoc J. 2006;174:1589–94.
36. Kalso E, et al. Opioids in chronic non-cancer pain: systematic review of efficacy and safety. Pain. 2004;112:372–80.
37. Martell B, et al. Systematic review: opioid treatment for chronic back pain: prevalence, efficacy, and association with addiction. Ann Intern Med 2007;146:116–127.
38. Eisenberg E, et al. Opioids for neuropathic pain (review). Cochrane Database Syst Rev 2006; 3:CD006146.
39. Deshpande A, et al. Opioids for chronic low back pain (review). Cochrane Database Syst Rev 2007;3:CD004959.
40. Cepeda M, et al. Tramadol for osteoarthritis: a systematic review and meta-analysis. J Rheumatol. 2007;34:543–55.
41. Chou R, et al. Drug class review on long-acting opioid analgesics. Oregon Evidence-based Practice Center. 2008; 04.
42. Kalso E, et al. Opioids in chronic non-cancer pain: systematic review of efficacy and safety. Pain. 2004;112:372–80.

43. Manchikanti L, et al. A systematic review of randomized trials of long-term opioid management for chronic non-cancer pain. Pain Physician. 2011;14:91–121.
44. Taylor R, et al. Controlled release formulation of oxycodone in patients with moderate to severe chronic osteoarthritis: a critical review of the literature. J Pain Res. 2012;5:77–87.
45. Smith H. Opioids and neuropathic pain. Pain Physician. 2012;15:ES93–110.
46. Krashin D, et al. Opioids in the management of HIV-related pain. Pain Physician. 2012;15: ES159–98.

Chapter 4
Opioid Pharmacology and Pharmacokinetics

Andrea M. Trescot

Introduction

Opioids are compounds that work at specific receptors in the brain to provide analgesia. Originally derived from the sap of the poppy plant (*Papaver somniferum*), opioids may be naturally occurring, semi-synthetic, or synthetic, and their clinical activity is a function of their affinity for the various opioid receptors in the brain. Opioids are useful for a wide variety of painful conditions, including acute pain, cancer pain, and chronic pain, and cough suppression and air hunger. However, opioid use is associated with a significant misuse, has legal ramifications, and carries the potential for addiction, which limits their use and contributes to the current "opioid-phobia."

Opioid Receptor Pharmacology

"*Opiates*" are naturally occurring compounds derived from the poppy and would include morphine and codeine. The term "*opioid*" is now used broadly to describe any compound that exerts activity at an opioid receptor [1]. The opioid receptors were first discovered in 1972 by Candice Pert as a graduate student [2], and the first endogenous opioid, "*endorphin*," was identified in 1975 [3]. Multiple opioid receptors have now been identified, including **mu, kappa,** and **delta receptors** (Table 4.1), and opioids can work at one or several of these receptors. **Mu receptors** (where morphine molecules attach) are found primarily in the brain stem, ventricles, and medial thalamus; activation of these receptors can result in supraspinal analgesia, respiratory depression, euphoria, sedation, decreased

A.M. Trescot (✉)
Pain and Headache Center, 5431 Mayflower Lane, Suite 4, Wasilla, AK 99654, USA
e-mail: DrTrescot@gmail.com

© Springer International Publishing Switzerland 2016
P.S. Staats and S.M. Silverman (eds.), *Controlled Substance Management in Chronic Pain*, DOI 10.1007/978-3-319-30964-4_4

45

Table 4.1 Analgesic effects at opioid receptors

	Mu	Kappa	Delta
Endorphins			
Enkephalin	Agonist		Agonist
Beta endorphin	Agonist		Agonist
Dynorphin	Agonist	Agonist	
Opioids			
Morphine	Agonist	Weak agonist	
Codeine	Weak agonist		Weak agonist
Fentanyl	Agonist		
Methadone	Agonist		
Oxycodone	Agonist	Agonist	
Buprenorphine	Partial agonist	Antagonist	
Pentazocine	Partial agonist	Agonist	
Nalbuphine	Antagonist	Agonist	
Butorphanol	Partial agonist	Strong agonist	
Antagonists			
Naloxone	Antagonist	Weak antagonist	Antagonist
Naltrexone	Antagonist	Weak antagonist	Antagonist

Modified from Trescot et al. [1]

gastrointestinal motility, and physical dependence. They are now recognized to be at least 3 mu receptors—Mu_1, Mu_2, and Mu_3. Mu_1 is responsible for analgesia, euphoria, and serenity, while Mu_2 is related to respiratory depression, pruritus, prolactin release, dependence, anorexia, and sedation [4]; Mu_3 is proposed to be an important immune link [5]. **Kappa receptors** (named for ketocyclazocine that was used to find the receptor) are found in the limbic system, brain stem, and spinal cord and are felt to be responsible for spinal analgesia, sedation, dyspnea, dependence, dysphoria, and respiratory depression [4]. **Delta receptors** (found using delta-alanine-delta-leucine-enkephalin) are located largely in the brain itself and are thought to be responsible for psychotomimetic and dysphoric effects [4], as well as the development of tolerance.

Mechanism of Action in Pain Relief

Opioid receptors are found throughout the body, but primarily in the brain, spinal cord, and intestinal tract. These receptors are complex structures made up of 7 amino acid chains, each of which bridges the membrane, forming a channel which can allow calcium ions to pass in or out of the neuron. Opioid receptors are G-linked proteins within the membranes of cells; when activated, the receptor releases a protein, which migrates within the cell, activating Na/K channels or influencing enzymes within the cell, or influencing nuclear gene transcription

(Fig. 4.1) [6]. These opioid receptors can be presynaptic or postsynaptic. Presynaptic opioid receptors inhibit neurotransmitter release of compounds such as acetylcholine, norepinephrine, serotonin, and substance P. It is important to remember that the inhibition of an inhibitory neuron may then result in excitation [6].

The natural reward centers of the brain reside in the dopaminergic system of the ventral tegmental area (VTA), and GABA neurons usually inhibit these dopaminergic systems. Opioids inhibit the presynaptic receptors on the GABA neurons, which increases the release of dopamine, which is intensely pleasurable. Other drugs of abuse such as alcohol, nicotine, and benzodiazepines have their activity in the same areas of the brain [7] (Fig. 4.2).

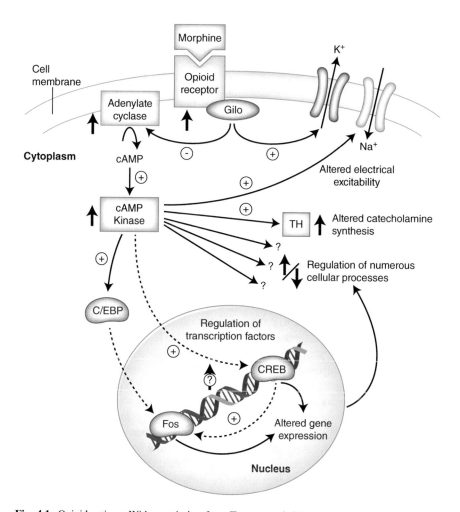

Fig. 4.1 Opioid actions. With permission from Trescot et al. [1]

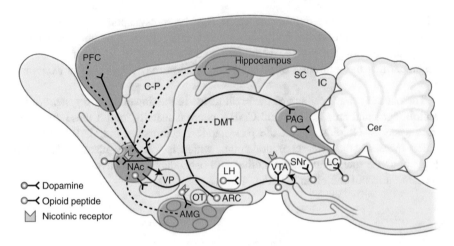

Fig. 4.2 Site of action of opioids and other drugs of abuse. *AMG* amydala; *ARC* arcuate nucleus; *CER* cerebellum; *C-P* caudate putamen; *DMT* dorsomedial thalamus; *IC* inferior colliculus; *LC* locus coeruleus; *LH* lateral hypothalamus; *Nac* nucleus accumbens; *OT* olfactory tubercle; *PAG* periaqueductal gray; *PFC* frontal cortex; *SC* superior colliculus; *SNr* substantia nigra; *VP* ventral pallidum; *VTA* ventral tegmental area. With permission from Trescot et al. [1]

Opioid Routes of Administration

Major advances in the pharmacotherapy of chronic pain have led to the development of extended-release opioid delivery systems, thereby allowing less frequent dosing than the classic short-acting formulas. It is the patterns in serum drug levels that define the difference between short-acting opioids (SAO) and long-acting opioids (LAO); with SAOs, serum opioid levels rise rapidly following administration and then decline rapidly, while LAO administration allows for less fluctuation in serum opioid levels and an extended period within the therapeutic range [8]. The assumption that plasma levels of opioids correspond to analgesia has led to the additional concept of minimum effective concentration (MEC), the plasma level of an opioid below which there is ineffective analgesia. Long-acting opioids can have a true intrinsic long-acting effect (i.e., methadone) or could be made in a sustained-release preparation. For the purposes of this discussion, we are including short-acting opiates prepared in a sustained-release preparation as "long-acting opioids."

There are many proposed advantages of the long-acting opioid formulas compared to the short-acting formulas. Because of the longer duration of action, there is a lessening of the frequency and severity of end-of-dose pain [9]. Furthermore, it has been suggested that less frequent dosing leads to increased compliance and improved efficacy [10]. Sustained analgesia and uninterrupted sleep are other potential advantages of the extended-release formulation compared to the short-acting variety. However, in a recent systematic review of long-acting versus short-acting opioids, Rauck [11] noted that, while it was clear that long-acting opioids achieved more stable drug levels, there was no clear evidence from appropriately designed comparative trials to make a case for the use of one type of formulation over the other on the basis of clinical efficacy.

Opioid Formulations

Oral

The standard and mainstay route of opioid administration, especially for chronic pain, is the oral route. Short- and long-acting opioids (see above) are available for many of the opioids described below, with and without adjuvant medications such as acetaminophen or NSAIDs. Oral absorption and onset of action depend on stomach pH, GI motility, and formulation.

Transmucosal

Oral transmucosal fentanyl citrate (OTFC) has become a mainstay in the treatment of breakthrough cancer pain, because it provides faster absorption of the lipophilic fentanyl than any other oral opioid formulation [12]. This "fentanyl lollipop" consists of medication on the end of a stick, which is applied to the buccal membrane. A newer formulation of fentanyl, the fentanyl buccal tablet (FBT), was designed to provide an even faster relief. Additional delivery systems for intranasal [13, 14] and inhaled fentanyl [15] have been developed.

Intravenous

Intravenous delivery of opioids allows for rapid and reliable delivery of medicine, but accessing a vein for administration of drugs is not always viable. In general, the IV dose is approximately 1/3rd of the oral dose, since IV medications do not have a first pass effect. Opioids can be delivered intermittently or continuously; patient-controlled analgesia (PCA) is now available for outpatient use, so that small doses of opioid are delivered when the patient pushes a button, with or without a continuous infusion of opioid.

Subcutaneous

Subcutaneous opioid injections can be an option for the patient unable to tolerate oral medications but without IV access. The medication is administered through a butterfly needle and can be given intermittently or continuously. Onset is slower and lower peak effect than IV, but this may be a better option for acute or escalating pain than transdermal fentanyl, which has an even slower onset and prolonged effect [16]. Subcutaneous infusions up to 10 cc/h can be usually absorbed, but patients are usually more comfortable with 2–3 cc/h.

Rectal

The rectal mucosa absorbs many medications easily, including most opioids, and the blood flow from the rectum bypasses the liver, so that rectal morphine results in blood levels that are almost 90 % of the oral dose [17]. A double-blind, double-dummy, crossover study in 1995 compared oral versus rectal morphine, which was shown to be effective, easy to manage, and inexpensive, with a rapid onset of action [18].

Transdermal

The skin is the largest organ in the body, with a surface area of one to two square meters. It can be used to deliver typically lipophilic medications, which makes it appealing as a drug absorbtion modality. However, the skin functions as a barrier to the elements, and those same properties limit its effectiveness as a drug delivery site. Medications must have a small molecular weight with high lipid solubility to pass across the skin barrier, and fentanyl is one of the most effective opioids for transdermal delivery [19]. Although all opioids have similar side effects (see opioid side effects), transdermal fentanyl appears to have less constipation, but did show skin reactions in 1–3 % of the 153 cancer pain patients studied [20].

Intrathecal/Epidural

Oral and parenteral opioids work by dulling the brain so that it does not recognize the pain signals as easily. Intrathecal and epidural opioids attach to opioid receptors at the spinal level, blocking pain signals from reaching the brain. The medications are more potent when administered intrathecally as opposed to systemically. There are several conversion tables that have been suggested, but one needs to use great caution in moving from a systemic to intrathecal administration. As an example, in the past, 300 mg of morphine orally (systemically) has been felt to be equivalent to 5 mg in the epidural space or 1 mg in the spinal fluid (intrathecal space). However, there is significant variability in patients' response, and one needs to use significant caution in using these kinds of conversion tables. These dramatically lower doses result in less sedation and mental clouding. Single-dose administration of intrathecal opioids has been used for acute pain, such as post postoperative pain. Continuous infusions for cancer pain and chronic noncancer pain utilized implanted subcutaneous pumps connected to intrathecal catheters. However, because these systems require specialist's placement and care, they are often not considered until very late in the course of the cancer, and hematologic abnormalities such as chemotherapy-induced thrombocytopenia may severely limit the ability to safely access the spinal canal. Although intrathecal opioid pain relief can be dramatic, procedural complications remain high, including infection, pump and catheter failures, drug errors, and post-dural puncture headaches [21]. Pruritus is seen more commonly with neural axial opioids than systemic opioids, with an incidence between 30 and 100 %, effectively reversed by opioid antagonists. Although respiratory depression is the dreaded complication of intrathecal opioids, its incidence is low (0.09–0.4 %) [22].

Common Opiates in Clinical Practice

Codeine

It is believed that the analgesic activity from codeine occurs from metabolism of codeine to morphine by CYP2D6. Because of the great heterogeneity in the CYP2D6 enzyme, with both fast metabolizers and slow metabolizers, codeine may not be an effective drug in all populations. In 2007, the FDA issued a Public Health Advisory [23] regarding a serious side effect in nursing infants whose mothers are apparent CYP2D6 ultra-rapid metabolizers, who, while taking codeine, had rapid and higher levels of morphine in the breast milk, with subsequent potentially fatal neonate respiratory depression.

Although codeine is often referred to as a "weak" analgesic, in a cancer pain study comparing 25 mg of hydrocodone (a "strong" analgesic) to 150 mg of codeine (a "weak" analgesic), 58 % of the codeine patients obtained relief compared to 57 % of the hydrocodone patients [24].

Hydrocodone

Hydrocodone is similar in structure to codeine and is a weak mu receptor agonist, but the CYP2D6 enzyme demethylates it into hydromorphone (see below), which has much stronger mu binding and therefore stronger opioid activity [25]. Like codeine, it has been proposed that hydrocodone is a pro-drug. In other words, patients who are CYP2D6 deficient, or patients who are on CYP2D6 inhibitors, may not produce the hydromorphone metabolites and therefore may have less than expected analgesia.

Until recently, hydrocodone was only available in a short-acting medication, containing either ibuprofen or acetaminophen; however, hydrocodone is now available as an extended release.

Hydromorphone

Hydromorphone is a hydrogenated ketone of morphine [26]. Like morphine, it acts primarily on mu-opioid receptors and to a lesser degree on delta receptors. While hydromorphone is 7–10 times more potent than morphine in single-dose studies [27], the oral and parenteral steady-state equivalence is 1:5, while the equivalence of chronic infusions may be as little as 1:3:5 [28]. It is highly water-soluble, which allows for very concentrated formulations, and in patients with renal failure, it may be preferred over morphine. Hydromorphone is metabolized primarily to hydromorphone-3-glucuronide (H3G), which, similar to the corresponding M3G, is not only devoid of analgesic activity but also evokes a range of dose-dependent excited behaviors including allodynia, myoclonus, and seizures in animal models [29]. Hydromorphone is available in an immediate-release as well as extended-release formulation [30].

Oxycodone

Oxycodone has activity at multiple opiate receptors including the kappa receptor, which gives it a unique antisedative effect ("perky Percocet"). It undergoes extensive hepatic metabolism, by glucuronidation to noroxycodone (which has less than 1 % of the analgesia potency of oxycodone), and by CYP2D6 to oxymorphone [31], which is about 50 % more potent [32]. Because oxycodone is dependent on the CYP2D6 pathway for clearance, it is possible that drug–drug interactions can occur with 2D6 inhibitors, and genetic issues may also interfere with metabolism. Oxycodone is available as a combination product with acetaminophen, in a short-acting formulation without acetaminophen, and in an extended-release formulation without acetaminophen.

Morphine

Morphine is metabolized by glucuronidation, producing morphine-6-glucuronide (M6G) and morphine-3-glucuronide (M3G) in a ratio of 6:1. M6G is believed to be responsible for some additional analgesic effects of morphine [33]. M3G, on the other hand, is believed to potentially lead to hyperalgesia [34], with increased pain, agitation, and myoclonus. Morphine is also metabolized in small amounts to codeine and hydromorphone. For instance, in one study, hydromorphone was present in 66 % of morphine consumers without aberrant drug behavior [35]; this usually occurs with doses higher than 100 mg/day.

Methadone

Methadone is a synthetic mu-agonist medication. It is a racemic mixture of 2 enantiomers; the R-methadone form is more potent, with a 10-fold higher affinity for opioid receptors (which accounts for virtually all of its analgesic effect), while S-methadone is the NMDA antagonist. The NMDA antagonistic effect makes it potentially useful in neuropathic and "opioid-resistant" pain conditions. The S-isomer also inhibits reuptake of serotonin and norepinephrine, which should be recognized when using methadone in combination with SSRIs and TCAs. Although it has traditionally been used to treat heroin addicts, its flexibility in dosing, use in neuropathic pain, and cheap price have led to a recent increase in its use. Unfortunately, a lack of awareness of its metabolism and potential drug interactions, its cardiac effects, and its long half-life has led to a dramatic increase in the deaths associated with this medication [36].

Methadone is unrelated to standard opioids, leading to its usefulness in patients with "true" morphine allergies. Methadone is metabolized in the liver and intestines and excreted almost exclusively in feces, an advantage in patients with renal insufficiency or failure.

The metabolism of methadone is always variable [37]. Methadone is metabolized by CYP3A4 primarily and CYP2D6 secondarily; CYP2D6 preferentially metabolizes the R-methadone, while CYP3A4 and CYP1A2 metabolize both enantiomers. CYP1B2 and CYP2C19 are possibly involved, and a newly proposed enzyme CYP2B6 may be emerging as an important intermediary metabolic transformation [38]. CYP3A4 expression can vary up to 30-fold, and there can be genetic polymorphism of CYP2D6, ranging from poor to rapid metabolism. The initiation of methadone therapy can induce the CYP3A4 enzyme for 5–7 days, leading to low blood levels initially, but unexpectedly high levels may follow about a week later if the medication has been rapidly titrated upward. A wide variety of substances can also induce or inhibit these enzymes [39]. The potential differences in enzymatic metabolic conversion of methadone may explain the inconsistency of observed half-life.

Methadone has no active metabolites and therefore may result in less hyperalgesia, myoclonus, and neurotoxicity than morphine. It may be unique in its lack of profound euphoria, but its analgesic action (4–8 h) is significantly shorter than its elimination half-life (up to 150 h), and patient's self-directed redosing and a long half-life may lead to the potential of respiratory depression and death.

Methadone also has the potential to cause cardiac arrhythmias, specifically prolonged QTc intervals and/or torsade de pointes under certain circumstances [40–44]. Congenital QT prolongation, high methadone levels (usually over 60 mg per day), drug–drug interaction (such as some antidepressants, antiarrhythmics, chloroquine, quinolone, macrolide antibiotics), and conditions that increase QT prolongation (such as hypokalemia and hypomagnesemia) or IV methadone [45] (because it contains chlorobutanol, which prolongs QTc intervals) may increase that risk [46]. Combining methadone with a CYP3A4 inhibitor such as ciprofloxacin [47] potentially can increase that risk. Therefore, several experts recommend that pretreatment and possibly periodic cardiograms be obtained in patients starting or increasing methadone [48, 49].

It is recommended that a switch to methadone from another opioid be accompanied by a large (50–90 %) decrease in the calculated equipotent dose [50]. It cannot be too strongly emphasized that the dosing of methadone can be potentially lethal and must be done with knowledge and caution.

In addition, there have been several tragic deaths, when patients were identified with respiratory depression and then treated with naloxone; unfortunately, because methadone has such a long half-life, these patients were discharged from the ER, only to die from respiratory depression when the naloxone wore off before the methadone sedation resolved [51].

Fentanyl

Fentanyl is approximately 80 times more potent than morphine, is highly lipophilic, and binds strongly to plasma proteins. Fentanyl undergoes extensive metabolism in the liver. Fentanyl is metabolized by CYP3A4, but to inactive and nontoxic metabolites [52]; however, CYP3A4 inhibitors may lead to increased fentanyl blood levels. It is available in an intravenous formulation, and is commonly used for anesthesia and procedure analgesia. The transdermal formulation has a lag time of 6–12 h to onset of action after application and typically reaches steady state in 3–6 days. When a patch is removed, a subcutaneous reservoir remains, and drug clearance may take up to 24 h. Because fentanyl is highly lipophilic, it can also be absorbed sublingually/transbuccally as well intranasally or inhaled.

The usual recommendation for calculating the equipotent dose of different opioids involves calculating the 24-hour dose as "morphine equivalents." However, Hanks and Fallon [53] instead suggest relating the starting doses to 4-hour doses of morphine rather than 24-hour doses. For example, in patients receiving 5–20 mg oral morphine every 4 hours (or the equivalent in controlled-release morphine), start with 25 mcg/hour fentanyl patches that are changed every 72 hours; patients on 25–35 mg oral morphine every 4 hours would start with 50 mcg/hour fentanyl patches; 40–50 mg oral morphine every 4 hours would be equivalent to 75 mcg/hour fentanyl patches, and 55–65 mg oral morphine every 4 hours would convert to 100 mcg/hour fentanyl patches. They feel that the controversies over appropriate morphine to fentanyl potency ratio calculations miss the point that fentanyl transdermally behaves differently and cannot be equated with oral routes when calculating relative potency.

Buprenorphine

Buprenorphine is a mu-opioid partial agonist with strong affinity but low efficacy at the mu receptor as well as kappa-antagonist activity [54]. It has been used for acute pain for many years and more recently has been used as well for treatment of opioid dependence and now for chronic pain. It is metabolized via CYP3A4 to an active metabolite and also by CYP2C8. Both the drug and its metabolite are also metabolized by glucuronidation, which reduces the risk of clinically significant medication interaction [55].

As a partial agonist, buprenorphine can be used to treat withdrawal, stimulating the opioid receptors without significant euphoria. Because buprenorphine has such a strong affinity for the mu receptor, it prevents the activity of illicit mu-receptor agonists such as heroin, which makes it an excellent medication for opioid maintenance therapy. However, it is also a useful medication for acute and chronic pain, particularly as an initial medication before escalating to full mu agonists, as well as treatment for opioid hyperalgesia (OIH). OIH is a condition where the opioid appears to cause more pain, which results in an escalation in opioid use without improvement in analgesia. Spinal dynorphin (a known kappa agonist) increases during opioid administration [56], and the kappa-antagonist effect of buprenorphine appears to be related to its positive effect on OIH. Buprenorphine is available for intravenous, transdermal, and sublingual use.

There are multiple opioid conversion tables that have been used to rotate the patient from one opioid to another. Unfortunately, most of these tables were developed based on acute levels of opioid dosing, not chronic usage, which can lead to relative overdose. Similarly, morphine to methadone conversions need to take into account the effect of opioid-induced hyperalgia from morphine, so that the

Table 4.2 Oral morphine to methadone conversion

Oral morphine dose (mg)	MS: methadone ratio
30–90	4:1
90–300	8:1
300–800	12:1
800–1000	15:1
>1000	20:1

Modified from Ripamonti et al. [77]

higher the dose of morphine, the smaller the equivalent methadone dose (see Table 4.2). Webster and Fine [57] have recently suggested that standard opioid conversion tables have contributed to fatal and near-fatal opioid overdoses.

Opioid Side Effects

Opioids are well known to cause a variety of side effects, most commonly nausea and vomiting, constipation, sedation, and respiratory depression [58]. These side effects can be significant, and some patients avoid opioids even in the face of significant pain, in an effect to limit such side effects, which may act as a significant barrier to adequate pain relief [59].

Constipation

Constipation is the most common adverse effect from opioids, occurring in 40–95 % of patients treated with opioids [60], and is caused by opioid receptor stimulation in the gut. The subsequent decrease in GI motility results in increased fecal fluid absorption, decreased peristalsis, as well as increased pyloric and anal sphincter tone, all resulting in hard, dry stools and reduced spontaneous bowel movements. It is essential that prophylactic treatment be instituted on the initiation of opioid treatment, since this, of all the side effects of opioids, does not resolve over time.

Nausea

Nausea has been reported to occur in up to 25 % of patients treated with opioids [61]. Mechanism for this nausea may include direct stimulation of the chemotactic trigger zone (CTZ), reduced gastrointestinal motility leading to gastric distention, and increased vestibular sensitivity [62].

Pruritus

Two to ten percent of patients on opioids will develop pruritus [63], which results from a direct release of histamine, and not usually an antigen/antibody reaction. It is therefore better considered an adverse reaction than an allergic reaction and is usually treated symptomatically with antihistamines such as diphenhydramine.

Sedation and Cognitive Dysfunction

The incidence of sedation can vary from 20 to 60 % [64], is usually associated with an initiation or increase in opioids, and is usually transient. Cognitive dysfunction can be compounded by the presence of infection, dehydration, metabolic abnormalities, or advanced disease [65].

Respiratory Depression and Sleep Apnea

A significant proportion of patients taking long-term opioids develop central apnea during sleep. Teichtahl and colleagues [66] examined 10 patients in a methadone maintenance program and performed a clinical assessment and overnight polysomnography. They found that all 10 patients had evidence of central sleep apnea, with 6 patients having a central apnea index (CAI) [the number of central apnea events per hour] [67] greater than 5 and 4 patients with a CAI greater than 10. In a larger follow-up study of 50 patients taking long-term methadone, 30 % of the patients had a CAI greater than 5, and 20 % had a CAI greater than 10 [68].

Endocrine Effects

Endorphins appear to be primarily involved in the regulation of gonadotropins and ACTH release [69]. Amenorrhea developed in the 52 % female patients on opioids for chronic pain [70], while the testosterone levels were subnormal in 74 % of males on sustained-release oral opioids [71]. These effects are more profound with IV or intrathecal opioids than oral opioids [72].

Immunologic Effects

Acute and chronic opioid administration can cause inhibitory effects on antibody and cellular immune responses, natural killer cell activity, cytokine expression, and phagocytic activity. Chronic administration of opioids decreases the proliferative capacity of macrophage progenitor cells and lymphocytes [73].

Relationship Between Side Effects and Sex or Ethnicity

Several studies suggest that sex and ethnic differences exist to explain the differences seen in side effect profiles. Women have, for instance, been found to be more sensitive to the respiratory effects of morphine [74] and more often have nausea and emesis with opioids [75, 76].

Future Directions

Opioids of lower addictive potential, such as tamper resistant extended-release opioids, are coming on the market, in an effort to expand the use of opioids while decreasing the addiction and diversion potential. Opioid abuse screening tools (such as the Opioid Risk Tool—ORT), genetic testing, and fMRIs to look at brain areas associated with addiction and pain perception may also help identify those patients at risk for opioid abuse, while maintaining access for those patients in whom opioids are appropriate management for their painful condition.

Conclusion

Opioids are broad-spectrum analgesics, with multiple effects and side effects. When used wisely and with appropriate caution and knowledge of metabolism and interactions, opioids can offer significant relief from soul-draining pain.

> Few things a doctor does are more important than relieving pain...Pain is soul destroying. No patient should have to endure intense pain unnecessarily. The quality of mercy is essential to the practice of medicine; here, of all places, it should not be strained.
> Marcia Angell, MD

References

1. Trescot AM, Datta S, Lee M, Hansen H. Opioid pharmacology. Pain Physician. 2008; 11(opioid special issue):S133–53.
2. Pert CB, Snyder SH. Opiate receptor: demonstration in nervous tissue. Science. 1973;179 (4077):1011–4.
3. Hughes J, Smith TW, Kosterlitz HW, Fothergill LA, Morgan BA, Morris HR. Identification of two related pentapeptides from the brain with potent opiate agonist activity. Nature. 1975;258 (5536):577–80.
4. Trescot AM, Boswell MV, Atluri SL, Hansen HC, Deer TR, Abdi S, et al. Opioid guidelines in the management of chronic non-cancer pain. Pain Physician. 2006;9(1):1–39.

5. Makman MH. Morphine receptors in immunocytes and neurons. Adv Neuroimmunol. 1994;4 (2):69–82.
6. Chahl LA. Opioids—mechanism of action. Aust Prescr. 1996;19:63–5.
7. Nestler EJ. Molecular basis of long-term plasticity underlying addiction. Nat Rev Neurosci. 2001;2(2):119–28.
8. McCarberg B, Barkin R. Long-acting opioids for chronic pain; pharmacotherapeutic opportunities to enhance compliance, quality of life, and analgesia. Am J Ther. 2001;8:181–6.
9. Kaplan R, Parris WC, Citron ML, Zhukovsky D, Reder RF, Buckley BJ, et al. Comparison of controlled-release and immediate-release oxycodone tablets in patients with cancer pain. J Clin Oncol. 1998;16(10):3230–7.
10. American Pain Society. Principles of analgesic use in the treatment of acute pain and cancer pain. Glenview, IL: American Pain Society; 2003.
11. Rauck RL. What is the case for prescribing long-acting opioids over short-acting opioids for patients with chronic pain? A critical review. Pain Pract. 2009;9(6):468–79.
12. Coluzzi PH, Schwartzberg L, Conroy JD, Charapata S, Gay M, Busch MA, et al. Breakthrough cancer pain: a randomized trial comparing oral transmucosal fentanyl citrate (OTFC) and morphine sulfate immediate release (MSIR). Pain. 2001;91(1–2):123–30.
13. Karlsen AP, Pedersen DM, Trautner S, Dahl JB, Hansen MS. Safety of intranasal fentanyl in the out-of-hospital setting: a prospective observational study. Ann Emerg Med. 2014;63 (6):699–703.
14. Mercadante S, Radbruch L, Popper L, Korsholm L, Davies A. Efficacy of intranasal fentanyl spray (INFS) versus oral transmucosal fentanyl citrate (OTFC) for breakthrough cancer pain: open-label crossover trial. Eur J Pain. 2009;13:S198.
15. Bausewein C, Simon ST. Inhaled nebulized and intranasal opioids for the relief of breathlessness. Curr Opin Support Palliat Care. 2014;8(3):208–12.
16. Ripamonti C, Fagnoni E, Campa T, Brunelli C, De Conno F. Is the use of transdermal fentanyl inappropriate according to the WHO guidelines and the EAPC recommendations? A study of cancer patients in Italy. Support Care Cancer. 2006;14(5):400–7.
17. McCaffery M, Martin L, Ferrell BR. Analgesic administration via rectum or stoma. J ET Nurs (official publication, International Association for Enterostomal Therapy). 1992;19(4):114–21.
18. De Conno F, Ripamonti C, Saita L, MacEachern T, Hanson J, Bruera E. Role of rectal route in treating cancer pain: a randomized crossover clinical trial of oral versus rectal morphine administration in opioid-naive cancer patients with pain. J Clin Oncol. 1995;13(4):1004–8.
19. Jeal W, Benfield P. Transdermal fentanyl. A review of its pharmacological properties and therapeutic efficacy in pain control. Drugs. 1997;53(1):109–38.
20. Muijsers RB, Wagstaff AJ. Transdermal fentanyl: an updated review of its pharmacological properties and therapeutic efficacy in chronic cancer pain control. Drugs. 2001;61(15): 2289–307.
21. Rathmell JP, Lair TR, Nauman B. The role of intrathecal drugs in the treatment of acute pain. Anesth Analg. 2005;101(5 Suppl):S30–43.
22. Gustafsson LL, Schildt B, Jacobsen K. Adverse effects of extradural and intrathecal opiates: report of a nationwide survey in Sweden. 1982. Br J Anaesth. 1998;81(1):86–93; discussion 85.
23. Food and Drug Administration. Public Health Advisory: use of codeine by some breastfeeding mothers may lead to life-threatening side effects in nursing babies 2007 [1/1/15]. Available from: http://www.fda.gov/drugs/drugsafety/postmarketdrugsafetyinformationforpatientsand providers/ucm054717.htm.
24. Rodriguez RF, Castillo JM, Del Pilar Castillo M, Nunez PD, Rodriguez MF, Restrepo JM, et al. Codeine/acetaminophen and hydrocodone/acetaminophen combination tablets for the management of chronic cancer pain in adults: a 23-day, prospective, double-blind, randomized, parallel-group study. Clin Ther. 2007;29(4):581–7.

25. Otton SV, Schadel M, Cheung SW, Kaplan HL, Busto UE, Sellers EM. CYP2D6 phenotype determines the metabolic conversion of hydrocodone to hydromorphone. Clin Pharmacol Ther. 1993;54(5):463–72.
26. Murray A, Hagen NA. Hydrocodone. J Pain Symptom Manage. 2005;29:S57–66.
27. Vallner JJ, Stewart JT, Kotzan JA, Kirsten EB, Honigberg IL. Pharmacokinetics and bioavailability of hydromorphone following intravenous and oral administration to human subjects. J Clin Pharmacol. 1981;21(4):152–6.
28. Davis MP, McPherson ML. Tabling hydromorphone: do we have it right? J Palliat Med. 2010.
29. Wright AW, Mather LE, Smith MT. Hydromorphone-3-glucuronide: a more potent neuro-excitant than its structural analogue, morphine-3-glucuronide. Life Sci. 2001;69 (4):409–20.
30. Coluzzi F, Mattia C. OROS(R) hydromorphone in chronic pain management: when drug delivery technology matches clinical needs. Minerva Anestesiol. 2010;76(12):1072–84.
31. Poyhia R, Seppala T, Olkkola KT, Kalso E. The pharmacokinetics and metabolism of oxycodone after intramuscular and oral administration to healthy subjects. Br J Clin Pharmacol. 1992;33(6):617–21.
32. Gabrail NY, Dvergsten C, Ahdieh H. Establishing the dosage equivalency of oxymorphone extended release and oxycodone controlled release in patients with cancer pain: a randomized controlled study. Curr Med Res Opin. 2004;20(6):911–8.
33. Lotsch J, Geisslinger G. Morphine-6-glucuronide: an analgesic of the future? Clin Pharmacokinet. 2001;40(7):485–99.
34. Smith MT. Neuroexcitatory effects of morphine and hydromorphone: evidence implicating the 3-glucuronide metabolites. Clin Exp Pharmacol Physiol. 2000;27(7):524–8.
35. Wasan AD, Michna E, Janfaza D, Greenfield S, Teter CJ, Jamison RN. Interpreting urine drug tests: prevalence of morphine metabolism to hydromorphone in chronic pain patients treated with morphine. Pain Med. 2008;9(7):918–23.
36. Mercadante S. Switching methadone: a 10-year experience of 345 patients in an acute palliative care unit. Pain Med. 2012;13(3):399–404.
37. Li Y, Kantelip JP, Gerritsen-van Schieveen P, Davani S. Interindividual variability of methadone response: impact of genetic polymorphism. Mol Diagn Ther. 2008;12(2):109–24.
38. Reddy S, Hui D, El Osta B, de la Cruz M, Walker P, Palmer JL, et al. The effect of oral methadone on the QTc interval in advanced cancer patients: a prospective pilot study. J Palliat Med. 2009;13(1):33–8.
39. Leavitt SB, Bruce RD, Eap CB, Kharasch E, Kral L, McCance-Katz E, et al. Addiction treatment forum: methadone-drug interactions 2009. Available from: http://www.atforum. com/SiteRoot/pages/rxmethadone/methadone.shtml.
40. De Bels D, Staroukine M, Devriendt J. Torsades de pointes due to methadone. Ann Intern Med. 2003;139:58.
41. Gil M, Sala M, Anguera I, Chapinal O, Cervantes M, Guma JR, et al. QT prolongation and Torsades de Pointes in patients infected with human immunodeficiency virus and treated with methadone. Am J Cardiol. 2003;92(8):995–7.
42. Hanon S, Seewald RM, Yang F, Schweitzer P, Rosman J. Ventricular arrhythmias in patients treated with methadone for opioid dependence. J Interv Card Electrophysiol. 2010;28(1): 19–22.
43. Krantz MJ, Lewkowiez L, Hays H, Woodroffe MA, Robertson AD, Mehler PS. Torsade de pointes associated with very high dose methadone. Ann Int Med. 2002;137:501–4.
44. Latowsky M. Methadone death, dosage and torsade de pointes: risk-benefit policy implications. J Psychoactive Drugs. 2006;38(4):513–9.
45. Kornick CA, Kilborn MJ, Santiago-Palma J, Schulman G, Thaler HT, Keefe DL, et al. QTc interval prolongation associated with intravenous methadone. Pain. 2003;105(3):499–506.
46. Chugh SS, Socoteanu C, Reinier K, Waltz J, Jui J, Gunson K. A community-based evaluation of sudden death associated with therapeutic levels of methadone. Am J Med. 2008;121(1): 66–71.

47. Herrlin K, Segerdahl M, Gustafsson LL, Kalso E. Methadone, ciprofloxacin, and adverse drug reactions. Lancet. 2000;356(9247):2069–70.
48. Cruciani RA. Methadone: to ECG or not to ECG…That is still the question. J Pain Symptom Manage. 2008;36(5):545–52.
49. Krantz MJ, Martin J, Stimmel B, Mehta D, Haigney MC. QTc interval screening in methadone treatment. Ann Intern Med. 2009;150(6):387–95.
50. Gazelle G, Fine PG. Methadone for the treatment of pain. Palliat Med. 2003;6:621–2.
51. Aghabiklooei A, Hassanian-Moghaddam H, Zamani N, Shadnia S, Mashayekhian M, Rahimi M, et al. Effectiveness of naltrexone in the prevention of delayed respiratory arrest in opioid-naive methadone-intoxicated patients. BioMed Res Int. 2013;2013:903172.
52. Feierman DE, Lasker JM. Metabolism of fentanyl, a synthetic opioid analgesic, by human liver microsomes. Role of CYP3A4. Drug Metab Dispos. 1996;24(9):932–9.
53. Hanks GW, Fallon MT. Transdermal fentanyl in cancer pain: conversion from oral morphine. J Pain Symptom Manage. 1995;10(2):87.
54. Helm S, Trescot AM, Colson J, Sehgal N, Silverman S. Opioid antagonists, partial agonists, and agonists/antagonists: the role of office-based detoxification. Pain Physician. 2008; 11(2):225–35.
55. Gruber VA, McCance-Katz EF. Methadone, buprenorphine, and street drug interactions with antiretroviral medications. Curr HIV/AIDS Rep. 2010;7(3):152–60.
56. Silverman SM. Opioid induced hyperalgesia: clinical implications for the pain practitioner. Pain Physician. 2009;12(3):679–84.
57. Webster LR, Fine PG. Review and critique of opioid rotation practices and associated risks of toxicity. Pain Med. 2012;13(4):562–70.
58. Benyamin R, Trescot AM, Datta S, Buenaventura R, Adlaka R, Sehgal N, et al. Opioid complications and side effects. Pain Physician. 2008;11(2 Suppl):S105–20.
59. McNicol E, Horowicz-Mehler N, Fisk RA, Bennett K, Gialeli-Goudas M, Chew PW, et al. Management of opioid side effects in cancer-related and chronic noncancer pain: a systematic review. J Pain. 2003;4(5):231–56.
60. Swegle JM, Logemann C. Opioid-induced adverse effects. Am Fam Physician. 2006; 74(8):1347–52.
61. Meuser T, Pietruck C, Radbruch L, Stute P, Lehmann KA, Grond S. Symptoms during cancer pain treatment following WHO-guidelines: a longitudinal follow-up study of symptom prevalence, severity and etiology. Pain. 2001;93(3):247–57.
62. Flake ZA, Scalley RD, Bailey AG. Practical selection of antiemetics. Am Fam Physician. 2004;69(5):1169–74.
63. McNicol E, Horowicz-Mehler N, Fisk RA, Bennett K, Gialeli-Goudas M, Chew PW, et al. Management of opioid side effects in cancer-related and chronic noncancer pain: a systematic review. J Pain. 2003;231–256.
64. Cherny NI, Ripamonti C, Pereira J, Davis C, Fallon M, McQuay H, et al. Strategies to manage the adverse effects of oral morphine: an evidence-based report. J Clin Oncol. 2001;19: 2542–54.
65. Cherny NI. The management of cancer pain. CA: Cancer J Clin. 2000;50(2):70–116; quiz 7–20.
66. Teichtahl H, Prodromidis A, Miller B, Cherry G, Kronborg I. Sleep-disordered breathing in stable methadone programme patients: a pilot study. Addiction. 2001;96(3):395–403.
67. Downey R, Gold PM. Obstructive sleep apnea 2014 [12/15/14]. Available from: http://emedicine.medscape.com/article/295807-print.
68. Wang D, Teichtahl H, Drummer O, Goodman C, Cherry G, Cunnington D, et al. Central sleep apnea in stable methadone maintenance treatment patients. Chest. 2005;128(3):1348–56.
69. Howlett TA, Rees LH. Endogenous opioid peptides and hypothalamo-pituitary function. Annu Rev Physiol. 1986;48:527–36.
70. Daniell HW. Opioid endocrinopathy in women consuming prescribed sustained action opioids for control of nonmalignant pain. J Pain. 2008;9:28–36.
71. Daniell HW. Hypogonadism in men consuming sustained-action oral opioids. J Pain. 2002;3:377–84.

72. Merza Z. Chronic use of opioids and the endocrine system. Horm Metab Res. 2010 (epublish):1–6.
73. Roy S, Loh HH. Effects of opioids on the immune system. Neurochem Res. 1996; 21(11):1375–86.
74. Zacny JP. Morphine responses in humans: a retrospective analysis of sex differences. Drug Alcohol Depend. 2001;63:23–8.
75. Zun LS, Downey LV, Gossman W, Rosenbaumdagger J, Sussman G. Gender differences in narcotic-induced emesis in the ED. Am J Emerg Med. 2002;20(3):151–4.
76. Cepeda MS, Farrar JT, Roa JH, Boston R, Meng QC, Ruiz F, et al. Ethnicity influences morphine pharmacokinetics and pharmacodynamics. Clin Pharmacol Ther. 2001;70(4):351–61.
77. Ripamonti C, Conno FD, Groff L, et al. Equianalgesic dose/ratio between methadone and other opioid agonists in cancer pain: comparison of two clinical experiences. Ann Oncol. 1998;9(1):79–83.

Chapter 5
Pharmacogenetics

Andrea M. Trescot

Introduction

Although opioids have been used for thousands of years, it has only been recently that the genetics of analgesia have been studied, with a resultant improved understanding of the variability of response to medications. This chapter discusses the role of pharmacogenetics in clinical practice.

Genetics of Pain

When we administer an opioid for pain relief, there is a continuum of responses, from good analgesia and an improvement in function, to poor analgesia, to tolerance, to physical dependence, and addiction [1]. There are several ways that genetics can influence analgesic response, including drug metabolism enzymes, drug transporters, activity at opioid or other pain medication receptors, and structures involved in the perception and processing of pain. There are two specific genetic issues involving analgesia:

- The genetic contribution of a variety of different pain types, including the varying mechanisms of nociceptive, neuropathic, and visceral pain.
- The genetic influence on drug effectiveness and safety [2].

A.M. Trescot (✉)
Pain and Headache Center, 5431 Mayflower Lane, Suite 4, Wasilla, AK 99654, USA
e-mail: DrTrescot@gmail.com

© Springer International Publishing Switzerland 2016
P.S. Staats and S.M. Silverman (eds.), *Controlled Substance Management in Chronic Pain*, DOI 10.1007/978-3-319-30964-4_5

Primer of Metabolism Issues

Drug Actions

Drug *pharmacokinetics* describes a patient's metabolic status, or their ability to metabolize certain drugs. As an example, a patient with impaired metabolism may be unable to activate a prodrug such as codeine into the active morphine metabolite. *Pharmacodynamics* describes a patient's ability to respond to a drug at the level of the drug target or receptor. Here, an example would be a patient who has a non-functional receptor for a certain drug who will be unable to respond to that drug regardless of the dosage.

Pharmacogenetics describes the genetic influence on both the pharmacokinetics and pharmacodynamics. Polymorphic genes (also called polymorphism) that encode the drug-metabolizing enzymes, drug transporters, drug receptors, and other proteins can serve as valuable markers, predictive of the efficacy and adverse responses in human subjects. *Pharmacogenomics* is the science that examines the inherited variations in genes that dictate drug response, predicting whether a patient will have a good response to a drug, a bad response to a drug, or no response at all. So, *pharmacogenetics* refers to the study of inherited differences in drug metabolism and response, while *pharmacogenomics* refers to the general study of the many genes that determine drug behavior. The distinction between the two terms is considered arbitrary and they can be used interchangeably.

Drug Interactions

There are 3 major types of enzyme interactions. A *substrate* is any medication metabolized by that enzyme. An *inhibitor* is a medication that slows the metabolism of another medication, which may result in excessively high blood levels, extended effect, and related toxicity; however, if this is a drug that has to be activated (a *prodrug*), there may be decreased effect. An *inducer* is a medication that boosts the metabolism of another medication, which may result in accelerated breakdown, increase clearance, shortened duration, subtherapeutic levels, or withdrawal; it may also cause increased activity in a prodrug.

Cytochrome P450 Enzymes (CYP450)

The CYP450 enzyme system is a heme-containing, microsomal drug metabolism superfamily involved in biosynthesis and degradation of endogenous compounds, chemicals, toxins, and medications. More than 90 % of current therapeutic drugs are metabolized by this system. There have been 57 enzymes identified in humans, and they are divided into family, subfamily, isoenzymes, and allele variants [3]. However, metabolism of most of the currently used drugs occurs using about 8 clinically relevant enzymes: CYP1A2, CYP2B6, CYP2C8, CYP2C9, CYP2C19, CYP2D6, CYP2E1, and CYP3A4/5, all of which have different (but partially overlapping) catalytic activities.

Many medicines are substrates (Table 5.1), inhibitors (Table 5.2), or inducers (Table 5.3) of medicines used in pain treatments.

Table 5.1 Common substrates of CYP enzymes

1A2	2B6	2C19	2D6	3A4/5
Amitriptyline	Bupropion	Barbiturates	Codeine	Alprazolam
Nabumetone	Methadone	Topiramate	Tramadol	Midazolam
Desipramine	Ketamine	Diazepam	Meperidine	Cyclosporine
Tizanidine	Testosterone	Amitriptyline	Oxycodone	Sildenafil
Imipramine		Imipramine	Hydrocodone	Indinavir
Acetaminophen	2C9	Clomipramine	Dextromethorphan	Verapamil
Cyclobenzaprine	Valproic acid	Sertraline	Amitriptyline	Atorvastatin
Clozapine	Piroxicam	Citalopram	Nortriptyline	Lovastatin
Fluvoxamine	Celecoxib	Phenytoin	Doxepin	Digoxin
Theophylline	Ibuprofen	Carisoprodol	Tamoxifen	Amiodarone
Melatonin	Warfarin	Clopidogrel	Amphetamines	Methadone
Duloxetine			Duloxetine	Erythromycin
Caffeine			Metoclopramide	Trazodone
Lidocaine			Propranolol	Fentanyl
Warfarin			Venlafaxine	Buprenorphine
Methadone			Methadone	Risperidone
				Zolpidem

Modified from Indiana University Web site [http://medicine.iupui.edu/clinpharm/DDIs/ClinicalTable.aspx] and Genelex Web site [http://youscript.com/healthcare-professionals/why-youscript/cytochrome-p450-drug-table/], and among others

Table 5.2 Common inducers of CYP enzymes

1A2	2C9	2C19	2D6	3A4
Carbamazepine	Rifampin	Carbamazepine	Carbamazepine	Carbamazepine
Griseofulvin	Ritonavir	Rifampin	Phenobarbital	Phenytoin
Lansprazole	Barbiturates	Ginko	Phenytoin	Nevirapine
Omeprazole	St. John's Wort		Rifampin	Modafinil
Ritonavir			Dexamethasone	Topiramate
Tobacco				Butabutal
St. John's Wort				St. John's Wort
				Rifampin

Table 5.3 Common inhibitors of CYP enzymes

1A2	2C9	2C19	2D6	3A4/5
Fluvoxamine	Fluvoxamine	Fluoxetine	Duloxine	Ketoconazole
Ciprofloxin	Paroxetine	Fluvoxamine	Cimetidine	Erythromycin
Mexiletine	Amiodarone	Paroxetine	Sertraline	Mifepristone
Verapamil	Modafinil	Topiramate	Fluoxetine	Nefazodone
Caffeine	Tamoxifen	Modafinil	Haloperidol	Grapefruit
Grapefruit		Birth control pill	Methadone	Indinavir
			Paroxetine	Ritonavir
			Quinidine	Verapamil
			Celecoxib	Diltiazem
			Bupropion	Clarithromycin
			Ritonavir	
			Amiodarone	
			Metoclopramide	
			Chlorpromazine	
			Ropivicaine	

Types of Metabolizers

Patients can be classified by how effectively they metabolize a medication, which is based on how many copies of normal or abnormal alleles they inherited. An *extensive metabolizer* (EM) or normal metabolizer (NM) has 2 normal or "wild-type" alleles and is considered "normal." An *intermediate metabolizer* (IM) has one normal and one reduced allele or 2 partially deficient alleles. A *poor metabolizer* (PM) has 2 mutant alleles leading to a very limited or complete loss of activity, while the *ultrarapid metabolizer* (UM) has multiple copies of functional alleles leading to excess activity.

These alternate genes, known as SNPs (single nucleotide polymorphisms), are identified by letters or numbers. For example, normal functional activity alleles of the CYP2D6 gene are designated CYP2D6*1 and CYP2D6*2. Although there are more than 75 CYP2D6 variants, the four most common mutant alleles are CYP2D6*3, CYP2D6*4, CYP2D6*5, and CYP2D6*6 and account for 93–97 % of the PM phenotypes in the Caucasian population [4].

There is also an ethnic distribution of this polymorphism. Approximately 7–10 % of Caucasians are CYP2D6 deficient (PM), but 2–7 % of African American and only 0–0.5 % of Asians are PMs. Approximately 30 % of Asians and African Americans have intermediate metabolism of CYP2D6. On the other hand, approximately 29 % of Ethiopians, 20 % of Saudi Arabians, 10 % of Southern Europeans, 8–10 % of Turks and Spaniards, 5 % of African Americans, 1–2 % of Northern Europeans, and only 1 % of Chinese are ultrametabolizers [4, 5]. In psychiatry, 52 % of the psychiatric and 62 % antidepressant or antipsychotic drugs are metabolized by CYP2D6 [6]. A prospective 1-year clinical study of 100 psychiatric inpatients suggested a trend toward longer hospital stays and higher treatment costs for UMs and PMs of CYP2D6 [7]. As another example, tamoxifen must be metabolized via CYP2D6 to endoxifen to be effective; a PM might therefore be at risk for failure of breast cancer treatment [8]. And, as we will see shortly, CYP2D6 activity can have substantial influence on the opioids that are commonly used in pain management.

Receptors and Transporters

Medicines exert their activity through a variety of ways, one of which is through interactions at a specific receptor, either as an *agonist* (stimulating the receptor) or as an *antagonist* (blocking the receptors). There are receptors for opioids (see below) as well as for a variety of psychoactive compounds, such as GABA, serotonin, and dopamine. Each receptor is genetically controlled.

Transporters are necessary to carry medications across membranes, such as from the gut into the blood stream, or across the blood–brain barrier. Many compounds, such as dopamine, require specific transporters, which are also genetically controlled.

Opioid Genetics

Each of the opioid receptors (mu, kappa, and delta) has a different receptor affinity, which is genetically controlled. For example, OPRM1, the gene that encodes the mu receptor, is polymorphic, and approximately 20–30 % of the population have changes in the alleles associated with altered sensitivities to pain and opioids [9]. Morphine concentrations at the mu receptor are at least partially dependent on the "ATP binding cassette subfamily B membrane 1" (ABCB1) gene, also known as the "multidrug resistance 1" (MDR1) gene, which controls how much opioid enters the central nervous system. Different opioids also have different relative affinity for each receptor (Table 5.4), so that the same opioid may have very different effects on different people, and the same person might have different effects from different opioids, depending on their genetic makeup.

All opioids are substantially metabolized, mainly by the cytochrome P450 system as well as to a lesser degree the UDP-glucuronosyltransferase (UGT) system. Activity of these enzymes depends on whether patient is homozygous for nonfunctioning alleles (PM), or has a least one functioning allele (IM), 2 normal alleles (NM) or has multiple copies of a functional allele (UM) [10].

Approximately 60 % of *morphine* is glucuronidated by UGT2B7 to morphine-3-glucuronide (M3G), while 5–10 % is glucuronidated to morphine-6-glucuronide (M6G). M6G adds to the analgesic effect of morphine, but M3G is

Table 5.4 Analgesic effects at opioid receptors

	Mu	Kappa	Delta
Endorphins			
Enkephalin	Agonist		Agonist
Beta endorphin	Agonist		Agonist
Dynorphin	Agonist	Agonist	
Opioids			
Morphine	Agonist	Weak agonist	
Codeine	Weak agonist		Weak agonist
Fentanyl	Agonist		
Methadone	Agonist		
Oxycodone	Agonist	Agonist	
Buprenorphine	Partial agonist	Antagonist	
Pentazocine	Partial agonist	Agonist	
Nalbuphine	Antagonist	Agonist	
Butorphanol	Partial agonist	Strong agonist	
Antagonists			
Naloxone	Antagonist	Weak antagonist	Antagonist
Naltrexone	Antagonist	Weak antagonist	Antagonist

hyperalgic, which causes more pain [11]. Since the activity of UGT2B7 is genetically controlled, the morphine dose needed for postoperative pain relief after similar surgeries may vary fivefold between individuals, and the dose needed at a defined stage of cancer pain varies threefold [12], depending on the activity of the morphine metabolism system (UGT).

As another example, CYP2D6 is a critical enzyme involved in the metabolism of a variety of opioids (such as codeine, tramadol, hydrocodone, and oxycodone); activity of this enzyme is highly variable, and there may be as much as a 10,000 fold difference among individuals [13].

Codeine is an inactive compound (a prodrug), metabolized by CYP2D6 into its active form, *morphine*. It has only a weak affinity for the mu receptor, 300 times less than morphine [14]. Therefore, CYP2D6 PM patients and patients taking CYP2D6 inhibitors who are given Tylenol#3® are really being given only Tylenol, while UM patients may have dangerously high levels of morphine after standard doses [15].

Tramadol is metabolized by CYP2D6 to its M1 metabolite, which is at least 6 times more potent than the parent compound [16]. *Hydrocodone* is metabolized to *hydromorphone* via CYP2D6; in one study [17], the metabolism of hydrocodone to hydromorphone was 8 times faster in EMs than in PMs. Medications may also interfere with enzyme activity; in this same study, quinidine, a potent CYP2D6 inhibitor, reduced the excretion of hydromorphone, resulting in plasma levels 5 times higher in EMs than PMs.

Oxycodone is metabolized by glucuronidation to noroxycodone (which has less than 1 % of the analgesia potency of oxycodone), and by CYP2D6 to *oxymorphone*. Oxycodone is an analgesic, not a prodrug; however, oxymorphone is an active metabolite of oxycodone and may have significant impact on analgesia. Because oxycodone is dependent on the CYP2D6 pathway for excretion, it is possible that toxicity and overdose can occur with CYP2D6 inhibitors [18].

Significance

Drug Effectiveness

Amitriptyline (AT) a tricyclic antidepressant, widely used for its low price. AT is metabolized by CYP2C19 to nortriptyline (NT), the active form, which is then metabolized by CYP2D6 to 10-OH-NT, which is inactive. Both CYP2C19 and CYP2D6 are widely polymorphic. Because side effects are primarily associated with NT levels, Steimer et al. [19] identified that slow CYP2D6 metabolizers who are also fast CYP2C19 metabolizers had a low risk of side effects from AT, while slow CYP2C19/fast CYP2D6 metabolizers had a high risk of cardiac arrhythmias, orthostatic hypotension, and urinary obstruction.

Jannetto and Bratanow [20] looked at the steady-state blood levels of methadone, oxycodone, hydrocodone, and tramadol compared to CYP2D6 genotyping. PMs in general had the highest steady-state drug concentrations. Eighty percentage of the patients reporting adverse drug reactions also had impaired CYP2D6 metabolism.

Clinical Significance

Figure 5.1 shows an actual genetic analysis report. There are a few notable issues with this genetic analysis. Because of an altered response of the dopamine D_2 receptor (DRD2), antidepressants such as bupropion, which stimulate the dopamine receptor, would be expected to be less effective. Interestingly, smokers using bupropion for smoking cessation are 3 times more likely to be abstinent with the normal DRD2 gene than when they have this variant [21], so smokers with this variant may do better with nicotine replacement therapies. There may be some issues with difficulty getting a "dopamine reward" from pleasurable activities, leading to depressive-like "anhedonism" feeling [22]. Combined with this patient's low catecholamine-O-methyl-transferase (COMT) activity (which prevents the body from making noradrenaline, dopamine, and serotonin), this genetic profile suggests an increased risk for depression [23] as well as potential risk of addiction from medications (such as amphetamines) or illegal drugs (such as cocaine) as well as risky behavior (such as gambling) that stimulate the dopamine receptor.

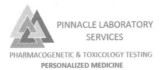
PINNACLE LABORATORY
SERVICES

PHARMACOGENETIC & TOXICOLOGY TESTING
PERSONALIZED MEDICINE

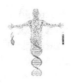

1410 NE 8th Ave, Ocala FL 34470
Phone: 877.736.4347 | Fax: 352.236.4240
Web: www.pinnaclelabservices.com
Medical Director: Andrea Trescot, MD
PGx Senior Geneticist: Sharon Norton, MS, MT (AAB)

Test Results

Gene	Genotype	Phenotype	Clinical Consequences
ANKK1/DRD2	DRD2:Taq1A AG	Altered DRD2 function	Consistent with a reduced dopamine receptor D2 function.
Apolipoprotein E	ε3/ε3	No Increased Risk of Hyperlipidemia/Atherosclerotic Vascular Disease	No Increased Risk of Cardiovascular Diseas
COMT	Val158Met AA	Low COMT Activity	Consistent with a significantly reduced catechol O-methyltransferase (COMT) function.
CYP1A2	*1F/*1F	Normal Metabolizer - Higher Inducibility	Consistent with a typical CYP1A2 activity in absence of inducing substances. Rapid Metabolism occurs in presence of inducers such as barbiturates, cruciferous vegetables, carbamazepine, rifampin and smoking.
CYP2B6	*1/*1	Normal Metabolizer	Consistent with a typical CYP2B6 activity. This test did not identify risks for side effects or loss of efficacy with drug substrates.
CYP2C19	*1/*1	Normal Metabolizer	Consistent with a typical CYP2C19 activity. This test did not identify risks for side effects or loss of efficacy with drug substrates.
CYP2C9	*1/*2	Intermediate Metabolizer	Consistent with a moderate deficiency in CYP2C9 activity. Potential risk for side effects or loss of efficacy with drug substrates.
CYP2D6	*1/*4	Normal Metabolizer	Consistent with a typical CYP2D6 activity. This test did not identify risks for side effects or loss of efficacy with drug substrates.
CYP3A4	*1/*1	Normal Metabolizer	Consistent with a typical CYP3A4 activity. Caution is advised when prescribing narrow therapeutic index drugs. Alternative drugs or dose adjustment may be required if CYP3A inhibitors or inducers are co-prescribed.
CYP3A5	*3/*3	Poor Metabolizer	Consistent with a poor CYP3A5 activity. Caution is advised when prescribing narrow therapeutic index drugs. Alternative drugs or dose adjustment may be required if CYP3A inhibitors or inducers are co-prescribed.
Factor II Factor V Leiden	20210G>A GG 1691G>A CC	No Increased Risk of Thrombosis	The patient's risk of thrombosis is not increased (average risk of clotting is about 1 in 1000 for anyone in a year). However, because this test cannot find all of the inherited reasons for abnormal clotting, other factors may affect this risk assessement.
MTHFR	1298A>C AA 677C>T CT	No Increased Risk of Hyperhomocysteinemia	The patient's small reduction in MTHFR activity is not a risk factor for hyperhomocysteinemia. Unless other risk factors are present, the patient is not expected to have an increased risk for venous thromboembolism (VTE).
OPRM1	A118G AA	Normal OPRM1 Function	Consistent with a normal OPRM1 receptor signaling efficiency induced by exogenous opioids. This is associated with a good analgesia following standard opioid doses and a poor response to naltrexone.
SLCO1B1	521T>C TT	Normal Transporter Function	Consistent with a typical SLCO1B1 transporter function. The patient's risk for statin-induced myopathy is not increased.
UGT2B15	*1/*2	Intermediate Metabolizer	Consistent with a moderately decreased UGT2B15 glucuronidation function. Potential risk for side effects with drug substrates.
VKORC1	-1639G>A G/A	Intermediate Warfarin Sensitivity	VKORC1 is the site of action of warfarin. The patient may require a decrease in warfarin dosage.

Fig. 5.1 Test results

CYP1A2 metabolizes medications such as TCAs, acetaminophen, duloxetine as well as caffeine. Genetic mutations in CYP1A2 have been associated with an increased risk of lung cancer [24], colorectal cancer [25], and gastric cancer [26].

Methadone metabolism, especially the R-enantiomer (associated with analgesia), is mediated by CYP2B6 [27] as well as CYP3A4 and CYP2D6. Caution should be used when using methadone in CYP2B6-deficient patients, or combining methadone with CYP2B6-inducing agents, such as carbamazepine, phenytoin, rifampin, and phenobarbital, or with CYP2B6-inhibiting agents, such as paroxetine, sertraline, and desipramine [28].

This patient also has the poor activity of CYP3A5 (present in 7 % of Caucasians). The metabolism of antipsychotic drugs such as risperidone may be delayed, leading to increased blood levels and adverse drug reactions [29]. More concerning, the combination of poor CYP3A5 and poor DRD_2 has been associated with an increased risk of tardive dyskinesia [30], a potentially permanent movement disorder associated with antipsychotic medications.

UGT is involved in the metabolism of many drugs (such as morphine and acetaminophen) as well as the biotransformation of important endogenous substrates (e.g., bilirubin, estrogen, and testosterone). UGT2B metabolizes morphine into 2 different compounds—morphine-6-glucuronide (M6G), which is analgesic, and morphine-3-glucuronide (M3G), which actually causes pain and may account for some of the opioid-induced hyperalgesia (OIH) seen with high levels of morphine. Poor UGT2B activity can influence the levels of M3G compared to M6G, making morphine less effective.

Also noted is a low VKORC1 activity; this patient should be started on lower than normal doses of warfarin and monitored carefully with frequent INR testing until stable.

Conclusion

Although there is still only limited evidence that genetic testing changes clinical outcomes, understanding the potential interactions between medication and genetics continues to provide insights into the individual response to medications, predicting effects and side effects.

> If it were not for the great variability among individuals, medicine might as well be a science and not an art—William Ostler (1892).

References

1. Reynolds KK, Ramey-Hartung B, Jortani SA. The value of CYP2D6 and OPRM1 pharmacogenetic testing for opioid therapy. Clin Lab Med. 2008;28(4):581–98.
2. Webster LR. Pharmacogenetics in pain management: the clinical need. Clin Lab Med. 2008;28 (4):569–79.
3. Linder MW, Valdes R. Fundamentals and applications of pharmacogenetics for the clinical laboratory. Ann Clin Lab Sci. 1999;29(2):140–9.

4. Bernard S, Neville KA, Nguyen AT, Flockhart DA. Interethnic differences in genetic polymorphisms of CYP2D6 in the U.S. population: clinical implications. Oncologist. 2006;11(2):126–35.
5. Bradford LD. CYP2D6 allele frequency in European Caucasians, Asians, Africans and their decendants. Pharmacogenomics. 2002;3:229–43.
6. Mulder H, Heerdink ER, van Iersel EE, et al. Prevalence of patients using drugs metabolized by cytochrome P450 2D6 in different populations: a cross-sectional study. Ann Pharmacother 2007;41(3):406–13.
7. Seeringer A, Kirchheiner J. Pharmacogenetics-guided dose modifications of antidepressants. Clin Lab Med. 2008;28(4):619–26.
8. Foster A, Mobley E, Wang Z. Complicated pain management in a CYP450 2D6 poor metabolizer. Pain Pract. 2007;7(4):352–6.
9. Fillingim RB, Kaplan L, Staud R, Ness TJ, Glover TL, Campbell CM, et al. The A118G single nucleotide polymorphism of the mu-opioid receptor gene (OPRM1) is associated with pressure pain sensitivity in humans. J Pain. 2005;6(3):159–67.
10. Smith HS. Variations in opioid responsiveness. Pain Physician. 2008;11:237–48.
11. Cohen M, Sadhasivam S, Vinks AA. Pharmacogenetics in perioperative medicine. Curr Opin Anaesthesiol. 2012;25(4):419–27.
12. Klepstad P, Kaasa S, Skauge M, Borchgrevink PC. Pain intensity and side effects during titration of morphine to cancer patients using a fixed schedule dose escalation. Acta Anaesthesiol Scand. 2000;44(6):656–64.
13. Bertilsson L, Dahl ML, Ekqvist B, Jerling M, Lierena A. Genetic regulation of the disposition of psychotropic drugs. In: Meltzer HY, Nerozzi D, editors. Current practices and future developments in the pharmacotherapy of mental disorders. Amsterdam: Elsevier; 1991. pp. 73–80.
14. Armstrong SC, Cozza KL. Pharmacokinetic drug interactions of morphine, codeine, and their derivatives: theory and clinical reality part II. Psychosomatics. 2003;44(6):515–20.
15. Kirchheiner J, Schmidt H, Tzvetkov M, Keulen JT, Lotsch J, Roots I, et al. Pharmacokinetics of codeine and its metabolite morphine in ultra-rapid metabolizers due to CYP2D6 duplication. Pharmacogenomics J. 2007;7(4):257–65.
16. Grond S, Sablotzki A. Clinical pharmacology of tramadol. Clin Pharmacokinet. 2004;43(13):879–923.
17. Otton SV, Schadel M, Cheung SW, Kaplan HL, Busto UE, Sellers EM. CYP2D6 phenotype determines the metabolic conversion of hydrocodone to hydromorphone. Clin Pharmacol Ther. 1993;54(5):463–72.
18. Poyhia R, Seppala T, Olkkola KT, Kalso E. The pharmacokinetics and metabolism of oxycodone after intramuscular and oral administration to healthy subjects. Br J Clin Pharmacol. 1992;33(6):617–21.
19. Steimer W, Zopf K, von Amelunxen S, Pfeiffer H, Bachofer J, Popp J, et al. Amitriptyline or not, that is the question: pharmacogenetic testing of CYP2D6 and CYP2C19 identifies patients with low or high risk for side effects in amitriptyline therapy. Clin Chem. 2005;51(2):376–85.
20. Jannetto PJ, Bratanow NC. Utilization of pharmacogenomics and therapeutic drug monitoring for opioid pain management. Pharmacogenomics. 2009;10(7):1157–67.
21. David SP, Strong DR, Munafo MR, Brown RA, Lloyd-Richardson EE, Wileyto PE, et al. Bupropion efficacy for smoking cessation is influenced by the DRD2 Taq1A polymorphism: analysis of pooled data from two clinical trials. Nicotine Tob Res Official J Soc Res Nicotine Tob. 2007;9(12):1251–7.
22. Savitz J, Hodgkinson CA, Martin-Soelch C, Shen PH, Szczepanik J, Nugent AC, et al. DRD2/ANKK1 Taq1A polymorphism (rs1800497) has opposing effects on D2/3 receptor binding in healthy controls and patients with major depressive disorder. Int J Neuropsychopharmacol/Official Sci J Collegium Int Neuropsychopharmacologicum (CINP). 2013;16(9):2095–101.

23. Pearson-Fuhrhop KM, Dunn EC, Mortero S, Devan WJ, Falcone GJ, Lee P, et al. Dopamine genetic risk score predicts depressive symptoms in healthy adults and adults with depression. PLoS ONE. 2014;9(5):e93772.
24. Bu ZB, Ye M, Cheng Y, Wu WZ. Four polymorphisms in the cytochrome P450 1A2 (CYP1A2) gene and lung cancer risk: a meta-analysis. Asian Pac J Cancer Prev APJCP. 2014;15(14):5673–9.
25. Hu J, Liu C, Yin Q, Ying M, Li J, Li L, et al. Association between the CYP1A2-164 A/C polymorphism and colorectal cancer susceptibility: a meta-analysis. Mol Genet Genomics MGG. 2014;289(3):271–7.
26. Ghoshal U, Tripathi S, Kumar S, Mittal B, Chourasia D, Kumari N, et al. Genetic polymorphism of cytochrome P450 (CYP) 1A1, CYP1A2, and CYP2E1 genes modulate susceptibility to gastric cancer in patients with Helicobacter pylori infection. Gastric Cancer Official J Int Gastric Cancer Assoc Jpn Gastric Cancer Assoc. 2014;17(2):226–34.
27. Totah RA, Allen KE, Sheffels P, Whittington D, Kharasch ED. Enantiomeric metabolic interactions and stereoselective human methadone metabolism. J Pharmacol Exp Ther. 2007;321(1):389–99.
28. Lee HY, Li JH, Wu LT, Wu JS, Yen CF, Tang HP. Survey of methadone-drug interactions among patients of methadone maintenance treatment program in Taiwan. Subst Abuse Treat Prev Policy. 2012;7:11.
29. Llerena A, Berecz R, Penas-Lledo E, Suveges A, Farinas H. Pharmacogenetics of clinical response to risperidone. Pharmacogenomics. 2013;14(2):177–94.
30. Foster A, Wang Z, Usman M, Stirewalt E, Buckley P. Pharmacogenetics of antipsychotic adverse effects: case studies and a literature review for clinicians. Neuropsychiatric Dis Treat. 2007;3(6):965–73.

Chapter 6
Benzodiazepines, Alcohol, and Stimulant Use in Combination with Opioid Use

J. Gregory Hobelmann and Michael R. Clark

Background and Epidemiology

The exponential increase in opioid sales in the USA between 1997 and 2008 has resulted in greater availability of opioids for both legitimate and illicit use of these medications [1]. Over 1 million practitioners prescribe opioids to patients now. Unfortunately, a greater-than-4-fold rise in the deaths from prescription opioids has occurred from 1999 to 2010, and 82 % of those were classified as unintentional. In 2007, the estimated cost of opioid abuse was estimated to be $72.5 billion with no signs of decreasing. These alarming trends have led to the Department of Health and Human Services to deem overdose deaths from prescription opioids an epidemic [2].

The use of benzodiazepines, alcohol, and/or stimulants in combination with opioids can pose great challenges for practitioners and adds another layer of risk in caring for patients with chronic pain. Although it is often underappreciated, the combination of opioids with sedatives and alcohol has led to an increase in opioid-related morbidity and mortality and the risks are not limited to those with aberrant drug-related behavior [3]. Even when patients take medications as prescribed, adverse reactions including death occur. In 2010, there were over 2 million drug-related ED visits resulting from adverse reactions to medications taken as prescribed [4]. Patients tend to underestimate the amount of alcohol they consume, and patients on opioid therapy for chronic pain often do not understand the dangers of combining these substances [3, 5].

J. Gregory Hobelmann (✉)
Department of Psychiatry and Behavioral Sciences, Johns Hopkins University,
600 North Wolfe Street, 205 Midhurst Rd., Baltimore, MD 21287, USA
e-mail: Jhobler1@jhmi.edu

M.R. Clark
Department of Psychiatry and Behavioral Sciences, Johns Hopkins Medicine,
Baltimore, MD, USA

© Springer International Publishing Switzerland 2016
P.S. Staats and S.M. Silverman (eds.), *Controlled Substance
Management in Chronic Pain*, DOI 10.1007/978-3-319-30964-4_6

Furthermore, patients taking benzodiazepines are more likely to be prescribed opioids [6, 7]. Few practice guidelines exist for the use of opioids in combination with benzodiazepines, alcohol, or stimulants.

The use of benzodiazepines in combination with opioids and alcohol can have severe, and sometimes fatal, consequences. The rates of benzodiazepine abuse are increasing, and related hospital admissions have nearly tripled since 1998. Most of these admissions are for concomitant opioid use, followed closely by concomitant alcohol use (The TEDS report: Substance). From 2000 to 2010, hospital admission rates related to coabuse of opioids and benzodiazepines increased by a staggering 570 %, while those related to all other substances declined by approximately 10 % (The TEDS report: Admissions). Emergency department visits secondary to the use of all prescription drugs increased by 76 % between 2005 and 2010 [4].

Accidental fatalities from opioids increased 4-fold from 1999 to 2009, and prescription opioid-related deaths commonly involved sedatives and/or alcohol [8]. According to the data from the Centers of Disease Control and Prevention, 75.2 % of deaths from pharmaceutical agents involved opioids and 29.4 % involved benzodiazepines. Of these deaths, 74.3 % were unintentional and the rest were due to suicide or undetermined causes [9]. The Utah Medical Examiner's office found that in 278 opioid-related overdose deaths, 83 % of the decedents experienced chronic pain suggesting that the drugs were at some point prescribed with the intention of treatment [8]. The most common cause of polysubstance overdose was found to be the combination of opioids and benzodiazepines, and the studies indicate that benzodiazepines play a role in up to 80 % of deaths involving opioids [10, 11].

Patients with chronic pain who are taking both opioids and benzodiazepines had more pain-related and behavioral management problems and were at higher risk of overdose [12]. Concomitant use was also associated with longer periods of being prescribed opioids, taking higher mean doses, greater risk of receiving a psychogenic pain diagnosis, and higher rates of being diagnosed with alcohol-use disorders [13]. Despite these consequences, many patients continue to use opioids concurrently with benzodiazepines and/or alcohol.

Physiology of Respiratory Depression

The majority of deaths resulting from concomitant use of opioids and benzodiazepines or alcohol are caused by respiratory depression. Risk factors for respiratory depression include age >55 years, chronic obstructive pulmonary disease, sleep-disordered breathing problems, airway abnormalities, and other comorbidities such as renal or hepatic impairment [14]. Central medullary respiratory centers with input from peripheral chemoreceptors control respiration. Glutamate is the major excitatory neurotransmitter, and gamma-aminobutyric acid (GABA) is the major inhibitory neurotransmitter involved in the control of respiration. Opioids produce significant inhibition in both the medulla and peripheral chemoreceptors.

Benzodiazepines and alcohol facilitate the effects of GABA (at $GABA_A$ receptor), and alcohol also decreases the excitatory effect of glutamate at N-methyl-D-aspartate (NMDA) receptors. Alone, benzodiazepines and alcohol produce little respiratory depression, but in combination with opioids, the effect can be fatal. The combination tends to prolong and increase the respiratory effects of opioids. Also, the tolerance to respiratory depression is incomplete and may be slower to evolve than the tolerance to euphoria and other side effects, which could explain the high rates of overdose deaths among experienced opioid users [15].

Combination Opioid and Benzodiazepine Use

There are many reasons to combine opioids and benzodiazepines, but it is likely that the motivation of physicians is different from patients in many cases. Clinicians treating pain may utilize benzodiazepines as adjuncts to opioids for their muscle relaxant or sedative effects and to treat comorbid psychiatric disorders. It has been shown that approximately 60 % of patients with depression report pain at the time of diagnosis [16]. In addition, almost 50 % of patients with chronic pain report anxiety symptoms and 30 % of chronic pain patients have a diagnosed anxiety disorder, such as generalized anxiety disorder or panic disorder [17, 18]. These patients report pain of greater intensity and persistence and exhibit more pain behaviors [19]. They also report increased rates of suicidal ideation, suicide attempts, and suicide completion [20]. For these reasons, we recommend consultation with a psychiatrist for any patient with a comorbid psychiatric disorder. In general, benzodiazepines are less effective for these conditions than other pharmacotherapies such as antidepressants, anticonvulsants, mood stabilizers, and neuroleptics.

Patients, however, may take benzodiazepines for other reasons. Benzodiazepines are reported to enhance the euphoric effects of opioids in an additive or synergistic manner. Patients often notice the enhanced feeling of euphoria when opioids and benzodiazepines are used together, especially if the drugs are misused or abused. Data suggest that the vast majority of benzodiazepine use is recreational, rather than therapeutic [10]. Subjective ratings of pleasant effects like "high" and feeling "good" all increase when the drugs are used in combination [21, 22]. Among patients on long-term opioid therapy, over 25 % report initiation of benzodiazepines out of curiosity to explore drug effects (e.g., relaxation, relieve tensions, feel good, get high) [23].

As noted, the primary mechanism of fatal overdose when opioids and benzodiazepines are combined is respiratory depression and this is supported in several older studies. It has been shown that in healthy patients who received both benzodiazepines and opioids, there is an increased rate of apnea and hypoxemia [24, 25]. Among patients undergoing surgical procedures, over 80 % of deaths occurred when midazolam was combined with opioids [24].

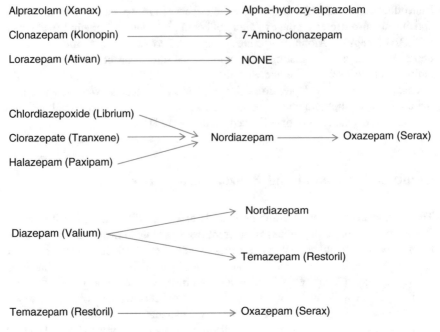

Fig. 6.1 Metabolism of common benzodiazepines

The metabolism of opioids involves the cytochrome P450 enzyme, and some benzodiazepines can interfere with this process [26, 27]. Lorazepam, temazepam, and oxazepam are directly metabolized via glucuronyl transferase and do not affect the metabolism of opioids. Diazepam, clonazepam, and alprazolam, however, are first metabolized by the cytochrome P450 enzyme system and inhibit the clearance of opioids. In addition, diazepam is metabolized to an active metabolite, desmethyldiazepam, which has a prolonged half-life, particularly in the elderly. Also, any additional medication that interferes with cytochrome P450 enzyme can intensify the effects of opioids and/or benzodiazepines leading to increased risk of respiratory depression (Fig. 6.1).

Combination Opioid and Alcohol Use

Alcohol use is pervasive in this country, and alcohol-use disorders are some of the most prevalent substance-use disorders reported. In 2012, 88 % of people 18 years of age or older in the USA reported that they consumed alcohol at some point in their lifetime and 56 % reported that they drank in the last month. Furthermore, 7.2 % of respondents were classified as having an alcohol-use disorder and 27 % of people reported that they binge drank in the past month [28].

Similar to benzodiazepines, the majority of the fatal consequences related to combining opioid and alcohol use are due to respiratory depression [29, 30]. This is due to both peripheral and central nervous system inhibition. When used in combination, ventilator response to hypercapnia is significantly reduced [31]. There is no therapeutic benefit from combining opioids with alcohol, so clinicians should NEVER recommend alcohol consumption to a person on opioid therapy. It is likely, however, that many opioid prescribers do no emphasize the importance of abstinence from alcohol. Patients have been shown to report increases in positive effects such as "drug liking" and "pleasant body sensations" when administered opioids and alcohol compared to either drug alone [32]. These pleasant effects potentially predispose opioid users to continued alcohol use and abuse while increasing the related dangers.

Another important phenomenon to note is referred to as "dose dumping." This refers to the unintended, rapid release of a large proportion of opioid contained in long-acting opioid (LAO) formulations [3]. Alcohol has been linked to dose dumping when combined with several LAO formulations. There is now a black box warning on several LOAs warning patients that consuming alcohol in any form, including medications containing alcohol, may result in rapid release and absorption of the opioid, which can be fatal [33]. In the case of one previously available opioid, Palladone^{TM} (hydromorphone hydrochloride extended-release capsules), dose dumping caused up to a 16-fold increase in plasma concentrations of the drug. This resulted in the drug being withdrawn from the market in 2005 [3]. In addition, alcohol can increase the maximum plasma concentration (Cmax) and decrease the time to maximum concentration (Tmax) of certain opioids with no evidence of dose dumping [34, 35]. The abuse quotient (AQ) of an opioid (or benzodiazepine) is defined as $AQ = Cmax/Tmax$ and the pharmacologic parameter that may be altered via dose dumping with alcohol. Opioids with a high AQ may be sought by abusers and thus be abused or combined with alcohol.

Combination Opioid and Stimulant Use

The prescription of stimulants including amphetamines (Adderall and Dexedrine), methylphenidate (Ritalin), phentermine, and modafinil (Provigil and Nuvigil) have been on the rise over the past two decades. Production of methylphenidate has increased over 8-fold, and amphetamine production has increased over 20-fold during that time (http://www.dea.gov/pubs/cngrtest/ct051600.htm). The vast majority of stimulants are used in the treatment of attention deficit/hyperactivity disorder (ADHD). However, they have also been used to counteract the sedative effects of opioids or as adjuvant treatment in patients with chronic pain.

Stimulants not only have synergistic analgesic effects when used in combination with opioids, but they also have analgesic effects when used alone [36–38]. Despite this finding, little evidence exists that the combination of opioids and stimulants diminishes pain scores or improves function over time. Additionally, there are no readily available guidelines for their combined use in patients with chronic pain. As a result, prescribing both opioids and stimulants to manage pain is not recommended.

Increases in morbidity and mortality from the coadministration of stimulants and opioids have not been well described. However, stimulants, such as opioids, are controlled substances in which tolerance and dependence are known to occur. They possess significant abuse potential alone, and this may be amplified when combined with opioids. The potential for abuse and dependence is reason enough for clinicians to be wary and resist prescribing opioids and stimulants together.

Clinical Considerations

Although there are well-established consequences, many patients continue to combine opioids with benzodiazepines and/or alcohol. Approximately 40 % of patients who are prescribed opioids are also prescribed benzodiazepines [13, 39]. Patients taking opioids and benzodiazepines in combination consume higher doses of opioids for longer periods of time, are more likely to abuse additional substances, are more likely to suffer comorbid psychiatric illness, and utilize more health services compared to those taking opioids alone [40, 41]. Furthermore, patients taking opioids and benzodiazepines have about a 25 % risk of overdose compared to 10 % in the general population [40]. The problem is not limited to benzodiazepines. 12 % of chronic opioid users also drink alcohol, and 3 % of patients report using all three substances. These rates are likely gross underestimations considering that patients frequently underreport their consumption [39].

Given these findings and associated risks, clinicians treating pain should conduct thorough assessments of their patients' pain, medical, psychiatric comorbidities, and current medications. Predictors for concurrent opioid and sedative use include female gender, younger age, using opioids for more than one problem, taking opioids at greater than 120 mg morphine equivalents per day, psychiatric comorbidities, and substance-use disorders. Predictors for concurrent opioid and alcohol use include male gender, taking opioids at greater than 120 mg morphine equivalents per day, lower average pain intensity rating, alcohol-use disorders, and risky drinking behaviors [39]. There are no readily available screening instruments to assess the risks related to benzodiazepine abuse, and the screening tools used to assess alcohol abuse risk, such as the Cut Down, Annoyed, Guilty, Eye-Opener (CAGE) and Alcohol Use Disorder Identification Test-Consumption (AUDIT-C), are of limited utility because they rely on patient self-reports [42, 43].

Treatment adherence monitoring has been shown to increase compliance rates and reduce rates of substance abuse among patients with chronic pain [44]. Available tools for monitoring treatment adherence include baseline and random toxicology screening, prescription monitoring programs, standard risk stratification, and behavioral assessments [45]. Opioid treatment agreements or contracts are also recommended. These may facilitate provider–patient communication, improve adherence rates, and reduce opioid misuse [46]. Also, education about the dangers of combined opioid and benzodiazepine, stimulant, or alcohol use in the treatment agreement is a useful method for encouraging abstinence from these substances.

The accurate prediction of misuse of prescription medications is impossible. Patient demographics and opioid dose are poor predictors of aberrant drug-taking behaviors. Urine toxicology screening has been advocated by many state, policy, and society guidelines to monitor patients in chronic opioid therapy [47–49]. Urine drug testing provides a more objective way to monitor treatment compliance and detect polysubstance abuse [50]. Studies suggest that the majority of patients who are prescribed opioids have invalid urine toxicology screens (positive for non-prescribed substances or negative for prescribed medications) at some point in their treatment. Sources of collateral information address the risks of relying solely on self-reports [45].

Urine toxicology screening should be performed on all patients who are pre-scribed chronic opioids, regardless of risk or known substance abuse histories. A universal drug screening policy for all patients destigmatizes drug testing and helps maintain a therapeutic relationship with patients. However, individualized risk assessments should be performed as well. Practice guidelines recommend stratifying patients into one of the three risk categories (low, moderate, and high) for aberrant drug-taking behavior to guide the frequency of screening [49]. In addition, urine drug screening should be performed at any visit when the patient is suspected of aberrant use or has a change in mental status.

In general, it is preferable to use laboratory testing (gas or liquid chromatog-raphy followed by mass spectrometry) rather than point-of-care (POC) testing. Point-of-care testing often does not screen for synthetic opioids, alcohol, certain benzodiazepines or stimulants, recently ingested drugs, and low levels of drugs (Gudin JA). The practitioner should be familiar with the chosen laboratory and take care of ordering the appropriate screens. The interpretation of test results should carefully consider which medications should be present (e.g., metabolites of pre-scribed parent medications). When a patient is prescribed oxycodone, its active metabolite, oxymorphone, and its end metabolite, noroxycodone, may be present in the urine [51]. When assessing benzodiazepine use, metabolites are usually reported as being detected. Also, reporting cutoff concentrations and presence of cross-reacting substances should be considered when interpreting results that might be the result of false-negative and false-positive results, respectively. Variability in metabolism, age, body composition, nutritional status, duration of drug use, dosage of drug use, and many other parameters may affect screening results [52]. Tables for cross-reacting substances are readily available, but confirmatory testing should be performed when questions arise. Patients should also be educated and encouraged to avoid substances that can interfere with test results.

Alcohol screening poses a unique problem because alcohol use is legal and pervasive. There are no firm guidelines for concomitant opioid and alcohol use, but it is clear that opioids should be used with caution in patients who are at high risk for alcohol abuse [3]. Furthermore, alcohol should be avoided completely in patients utilizing opioids for chronic pain. Because alcohol can increase the risk for adverse reactions, patients should be assessed for risk of abuse and be closely monitored. A breathalyzer or urine screen for ethanol limits the detection of alcohol use to the past several hours and cannot assess chronic consumption. Assaying the alcohol metabolites ethyl glucuronide (EtG) and ethyl sulfate (EtS) has the advantage of an extended window of detection. This allows better identification of recent alcohol use and relapse. These metabolites can be detected reliably for up to 4 days and are often present for considerably longer periods [53]. False-positive results for either metabolite alone are relatively frequent, but if both EtG and EtS are positive, alcohol consumption can be reliably confirmed [54].

Prescription monitoring programs provide data on patterns of prescription medication use and identify patients who are seeking prescriptions from more than one provider, using multiple pharmacies, and paying cash for their medications [55, 56]. Most states have monitoring programs that monitor for controlled substances that are classified as Schedule II–V, and practitioners who prescribe opioids are encouraged to utilize them to monitor compliance. These programs do not provide data on alcohol or other illicit substances, and they do not yet allow for monitoring across states. Furthermore, there is little evidence of their efficacy in reducing harm caused by concomitant use of opioids and other substances, but their potential for reaching this goal appears to be significantly high [48].

Addressing Substance Abuse in Patients

When substance abuse is detected in patients who are treated with opioids, an open dialogue to reinforce abstinence should be pursued. Brief interventions consisting of screening, education, and counseling during office visits have been shown to improve outcomes in patients with aberrant alcohol or drug use [57, 58]. Increasing frequency of office visits along with contingency prescription writing is also a useful technique to help cease aberrant substance abuse. Contingency prescription writing may include requiring the patient to produce a negative urine screen prior to receiving a prescription. Also, limiting the number of pills prescribed to periods of shorter than a month may improve treatment adherence and assist the patient in regaining control of their use of the medication. Communication with the patient's other healthcare providers is always encouraged to help assure that the patient is not receiving prescriptions from multiple sources. As always, practitioners should document thoroughly and include test results, interventions, and any changes in the patient's clinical condition [3]. If aberrant drug-taking behavior persists, referral to a specialist consultation will be needed to provide the patient with expert care for addiction.

Management of Patients with Comorbid Psychiatric Disorders

Chronic pain patients with comorbid psychiatric disorders such as anxiety disorders and attention deficit hyperactivity disorder (ADHD) may be prescribed benzodiazepines or stimulants. However, even when taken as prescribed, combining opioids with these medications increases in the likelihood of significant morbidity and mortality. Therapy for patients taking benzodiazepines or stimulants should be restructured. Alternative medications to treat anxiety such as antidepressants, atypical antipsychotics, or buspirone should be considered [59]. Also, referral for non-pharmacological therapy such as cognitive behavioral therapy can be beneficial in reducing symptoms of anxiety, depression, and/or ADHD [60]. Other psychotherapeutic approaches include visual imagery, distraction, relaxation, meditation, and desensitization [61]. If combining opioids with benzodiazepines and/or stimulants cannot be avoided, the lowest possible effective doses of each should be utilized. Treatment in conjunction with a psychiatrist familiar with chronic pain and its treatments is also recommended for patients with persistent or severe comorbid psychiatric illnesses, including substance-use disorders.

References

1. Okie S. A flood of opioids, a rising tide of deaths. N Engl J Med. 2010; 363(21):1981–1985
2. Volkow ND, Frieen TR, Hyde PS, Cha SS. Medication-assisted therapies—tackling the opioid-overdose epidemic. N Engl J Med. 2014;370(22):2063–7.
3. Gudin JA, Modali S, Jones JD, Comer SD. Risks, management, and monitoring of combination opioid, benzodiazepine, and/or alcohol use. Postgrad Med. 2013;125(4):115–30.
4. Highlights of the 2010 Drug Abuse Warning Network (DAWN) Findings on Drug-Related Emergency Department Visits. Rockville, MD: Center for Behavioral Health Statistics and Quality; 2012. Substance abuse and Mental Health Services Administration (SAMSHA).
5. UK Department of Health. Drinkers can underestimate alcohol habits. 7 Feb 2013. https://www.gov.uk/government/news/drinkers-can-underestimate-alcohol-habits.
6. Skurveit S, Furu K, Bramness J, Selmer R, Tverdal A. Benzodiazepines predict use of opioids—a follow-up study of 17,074 men and women. Pain Med. 2010;11(6):805–14.
7. Webster LR. Considering the risks of benzodiazepines and opioids together. Pain Med. 2010;11(6):801–2.
8. Calcaterra S, Glanz J, Binswagner IA. National trends in pharmaceutical opioid related overdose deaths compared to other substance related overdose deaths: 1999–2009. Drug Alcohol Depend. 2013;131(3):263–70.
9. Jones CM, Mack KA, Paulozzi LJ. Pharmaceutical overdose deaths, United States, 2010. JAMA. 2013; 309(7):657–659
10. Jones JD, Mogali S, Comer SD. Polydrug abuse: a review of opioid and benzodiazepine combination use. Drug Alcohol Depend. 2012;125(1–2):8–18.
11. Pirnay S, Borron SW, Giudicelli CP, Tourneau J, Baud FJ, Ricordel I. A critical review of the causes of heath among post-mortem tozicoogical investigations: analysis of 34 buprenorphine-associated and 35 methadone-associated deaths. Addiction. 2004;99 (8):978–88.

12. Dunn KM, Saunders KW, Rutter CM, Banta-Green CJ, Merrill JO, Sullivan MD, Weisner CM, Silverberg MJ, Campbell CI, Psaty BM, Von Korff M. Opioid prescriptions for chronic pain and overdose: a cohort study. Ann Intern Med. 2010;152(2):85–92.
13. Hermos JA, Young MM, Gagnon DR, Fiore LD. Characterizations of long term oxycodone/acetaminophen prescriptions in veteran patients. Arch Intern Med. 2004;164 (21):2361–6.
14. Jarzyna D, Jungquist CR, Pasero C, et al. American society for pain manaement nursing guidelines on monitoring for opioid-induced sedation and respiratory depression. Pain Manag Murs. 2011;12(13):118–45.
15. White JM, Irvine RJ. Mechanisms of fatal opioid oversose. Addiction. 1999;94(7):961–72.
16. Simon GE, VonKorff M, Piccinelli M, Fullerton C, Ormel J. An international study of the relationship between somatic symptoms and depression. N Engl J Med. 1999; 341:1329–1335
17. Dersh J, Polatin PB, Gatchel RJ. Chronic pain and psychopathology: research findings and theoretical considerations. Psychosom Med. 2002;64:773–86.
18. McWilliams LA, Cox BJ, Enns MW. Mood and anxiety disorders associated with chronic pain: an examination in a nationally representative sample. Pain. 2003;106:127–33.
19. Hassenbring M, Marienfeld G, Kuhlendahl D, et al. Risk factors of chronicity in lumbar disc patients: a prospective investigation of biologic, psychologic, and social predictors of therapy outcome. Spine. 1994;19:2759–65.
20. Magni G, Rigatti-Luchini S, Fracca F, et al. Suicidality in chronic abdominal pain: an analysis of the hispanic health and nutrition examination survey (HHANES). Pain. 1998;76:137–44.
21. Linzteris N, Mitchell TB, Bond AJ, Nestor L, Strang J. Pharmacodynamics of diazepam co-administration with methadone or buprenorphine under high dose conditions in opioid dependent patients. Drug Alcohol Depend. 2007;91(2–3):187–94.
22. Spiga R, Huang DB, Meisch RA, Grabowski J. Human methadone self-administration: effects of diazepam pretreatment. Exp Clin Psychopharmacol. 2001;9(1):40–6.
23. Chen KW, Berger CC, Forde DP, D'Adamo C, Weintraub E, Gandhi D. Benzodiazepine use and misuse among patients in a methadone program. BMC Psychiatry. 2011;11:90.
24. Bailey PL, Pace NL, Ashburn MA, Moll JW, East KA, Stanley TH. Frequent hypozemia and apnea after sedation with midazolam and fentanyl. Anesthesiology. 1990;73(5):826–30.
25. Faroqui MH, Cole M, Curran J. Buprenorphine, benzodiazepines and respiratory depression. Anesthesia. 1983;38(10):1002–3.
26. Altamura AC, Moliterno D, Paletta S, Maffini M, Mauri MC, Bareggi S. Understanding the pharmacokinetics of anxiolytic drugs. Expert Opin Drug Metab, Toxicol. 2013;9(4):423–40.
27. Smith HS. Opioid metabolism. Mayo Clin Proc. 2009;84(7):613–24.
28. SAMSHA. 2012 National Survey on Drug Use and Health (NSDUH) Table 2.7B—alcohol use in lifetime, past year, and past month among persons aged 18 and older, by Geographic Characteristics: Percentages, 2011 and 2012. http://www.samsha.gov/data/sites/default/files/NSDUH-DetTabs2012/HTML/NSDUH-DetTabsSect2peTanbs43to84htm#Tab2.71B.
29. Hakkinen M, Launiainen T, Vouri E, Ojanpera I. Comparison of fatal poisonings by prescription opioids. Forensic Sci Int. 2012;222(1–3):327–31.
30. Webster LR, Cochella S, Dasgupta N, Fakate KL, Fine PG, Fishman SM, Grey T, Johnson EM, Lee LK, Passik SD, Peppin J, Porusznik CA, Ray A, Schnoll SH, Stieg RL, Wakeland W. An analysis of the root causes for opioid-related overdoses in the United States. Pain Med. 2011;12(supp2):S26–35.
31. Ali NA, Marshall RW, Allen EM, Graham DF. Richens A. Comparison of effects of therapeutic doses of meptazinol and dextropropoxyphene/paracetamol mixture alone and in combination with ethanol on ventilatory function and saccadic eye movements. Br J Clin Pharmaol. 1985; 20(6):631–637.
32. Zancy JP, Guitierrez S. Subjective, psychomotor, and physiologic effects of oxycodone alone and in combination with ethanol in healthy volunteers. Psychopharmacology. 2011;218 (3):471–81.
33. Carson S, Thakurta S, Low A, Smith B, Chou R. Drug class review: long acting opioid analgesics final update 6 report, OR. Portland: Oregon Health and Science University; 2011.

34. Fiske WD, Jobes J, Xiang Q, Chang SC, Benedek IH. The effects of ethanol on the bioavailability of oxymorphone extended release tablets and oxymorphone crush-resistant extended release tablets. J Pain. 2012;13(1):90–9.
35. Johnson FK, Ciric S, Boudriau S, Kisicki J, Stauffer J. Effects of alcohol on the pharmacokinetics of morphine sulfate and naltrexone hydrochloride extended release capsules. J Clin Pharmacol. 2012;52(5):747–56.
36. Dalal S, Melzak R. Potentiation of opioid analgesia by psychostimulant drugs: a review. J Pain Symptom Manage. 1998;16(4):245–53.
37. Melzak R, Mount BM, Gordon JM. The Brompton mixture versus morphine solution given orally: effects on pain. Ajemian I, Mount BM, editors. The RVH manual on palliative/hospice care: a resource book. Montreal, Quebec, Canada: Palliative Care Services: Royal Victoria Hospital; 1980.
38. Sasson S, Unterwald EM, Kornetsky C. Potentiation of morphine analgesia by d-amphetamine. Psychopha (Berl). 1986; 90(2):163–165
39. Saunders KW, Von Korff, Cammpbell CI, Banta-Green CJ, Sullivan MD, Merrill JO, Weisner C. Concurrent use of alcohol and sedatives among persons prescribed chronic opioid therapy: prevalence and risk factors. J Pain. 2012; 13(3):266–275.
40. Nielsen S, Lintzeris N, et al. Benzodiazepine use among chronic pain patients prescribed opioids: associations with pain, physical and mental health, and health utilization services. Pain Medicine. 2015;16(2):356–66.
41. Rooney S, Kelly G, Bamford L, Sloan D, O'Connor JJ. Co-abuse of opiates and benzodiazepines. Ir J Med Sci. 1999;168(1):36–41.
42. Bush K, Kivlahan DR, McDowell MB, Fihn SD, Bradley KA. The AUDIT alcohol consumption questions (AUDIT-C): an effective brief screening test for problem drinking. Ambulatory care quality improvement project (ACQUIP). Alcohol ise disorders identification test. Arch Intern Med. 1998;158(16):1789–95.
43. Dhalla S, Kopec JA. The CAGE questionnaire for alcohol misuse: a review of reliability and validity studies. Clin Invest Med. 2007;30(1):33–41.
44. Manchikanti L, Manchukonda R, Pampati V, et al. Does random urine drug testing reduce illicit drug use in chronic pain patients receiving opioids? Pain Phycician. 2006;9(2):123–9.
45. Owen GT, Burton AW, Schade CM, Passik S. Urine drug testing: current recommendations and best practices. Pain Physician. 2012; 15(3):ES119–ES133.
46. Sehgal N, Manchikanti L, Smith HS. Prescription opioid abuse in chronic pain: a review of opioid abuse predictors and strategies to curb opioid abuse. Pain Physician. 2012; 15(3):ES67–ES92.
47. Chou R, Fanciullo GJ, Fine PG, et al. American pain society—american academy of pain medicine opioids guidelines panel. Clinical guidelines for the use of chronic opioid therapy in chronic noncancer pain. J Pain. 2009;10(2):113–30.
48. Manchikanti L, Abdi S, Atluri S et al. American Society of Pain Physicians (ASIPP) guidelines for responsible opioid prescribing in chronic non-cancer pain: Part I-evidence assessment. Pain Physician. 2012; 15(3):S1–S65.
49. Manchikanti L, Abdi S, Atluri S et al. American Society of Pain Physicians (ASIPP) guidelines for responsible opioid prescribing in chronic non-cancer pain: Part II-guidance. Pain Physician. 2012; 15(3):S67–S116.
50. Michna E, Jamison RN, Pham LD, et al. Urine toxicology screening among chronic pain patients on opioid therapy: frequency and predictability of 24 abnormal findings. Clin J Pain. 2007;23(2):173–9.
51. Trescot AM, Helm S, Hansen H, et al. Opioids in the management of chronic non-cancer pain: an update of the American Society of Interventional Pain Physicians' (ASIPP) Guidelines. Pain Physician. 2008;11(2 suppl):S5–62.
52. Katz N, Fanciullo GJ. Role of urine toxicology testing in the management of chronic opioid therapy. Clin J Pain. 2002;18(4 suppl):S76–82.

53. Helander A, Bottcher M, Fehr C, Dahmen N, Beck O. Detection times for urinary ethyl glucuronide and ethyl sulfate in heavy drinkers during alcohol detoxification. Alcohol Alcohol. 2009;44(1):55–61.
54. Kelly AT, Mozayani A. An overview of alcohol testing and interpretation in the 21st century. J Pharm Pract. 2012;25(1):30–6.
55. Fishman SM, Papazian JS, Gonzales S, Riches PS, Gilson A. Regulating opioid prescribing through prescription monitoring programs: balancing drug diversion and treatment of pain. Pain Med. 2004;5(3):309–24.
56. Wang J, Christo PJ. The influence of prescription monitoring programs on chronic pain management. Pain Physician. 2009;12(3):507–15.
57. Harris SK, Louis-Jacques J, Knight JR. Screening and brief intervention for alcohol and other abuse. Adolesc Med State Art Rev. 2014;25(1):126–56.
58. Madras BK, Compton WM, Avula D, Stegbauer T, Stein JB, Clark HW. Screening, brief interventions, referral to treatment (SBIRT) for illicit drug and alcohol use at multiple healthcare sites: comparison at intake an 6 months later. Drug Alcohol Depend. 2009;99 (1–3):280–95.
59. Khong E, Sim MG, Hulse G. Benzodiazepine dependence. Aust Fam Physician. 2004;33 (11):923–6.
60. Otte C. Cognitive behavioral therapy in anxiety disorders: current state of evidence. Dialogues Clin Neurosci. 2011;13(4):413–21.
61. Cottraux J. Nonpharmacologic treatments for anxiety disorders. Dialogues Clin Neurosci. 2002;4(3):305–19.

Chapter 7
Marijuana and Cannabinoids for Pain

Timothy Furnish and Mark Wallace

The History of Marijuana Use in Medicine

Cannabis has been used as medicine and for its mind-altering qualities for centuries. The earliest recorded references are from China around 4000 BC where it was cultivated for fiber [1, 2]. The earliest use of cannabis for medicine is recorded in China in the world's oldest pharmacopoeia, the *pen-ts'ao ching*. Its indications included rheumatic pain, intestinal constipation, disorders of the female reproductive system, and others. The use of cannabis in India was much more widespread than that in China, both for medicinal and for religious and recreational purposes [1, 3]. In Indian medicine, it was claimed to be useful as a sedative, anxiolytic, anticonvulsant, analgesic, and appetite stimulant and for relief of diarrhea [3].

The Irish physician William O'Shaughnessy, who served with the British forces in India, introduced the medicinal use of cannabis to Europe. He documented the medicinal use of cannabis in his 1839 book titled *On The Preparation of the Indian Hemp, or Gunjah*. In this work, he described his own experiments with use of cannabis for rheumatism, convulsions, nausea, and muscle spasms [1, 2]. O'Shaughnessy's publication led to the spread of medicinal cannabis use throughout Europe and America in the mid-nineteenth century. Cannabis was widely used as a sedative, analgesic, and anticonvulsant through the late nineteenth and early twentieth centuries and was mentioned in the United States Dispensatory as early as 1845 [3–5]. The United States Dispensatory remarks that cannabis "is capable of producing most

T. Furnish
Department of Anesthesiology, UC San Diego Medical Center,
9300 Campus Point Drive, Mail Code 7651, San Diego, CA 92037, USA
e-mail: tfurnish@ucsd.edu

M. Wallace (✉)
Department of Anesthesiology, University of California San Diego,
9300 Campus Point Drive, 7651, La Jolla, CA 92037, USA
e-mail: mswallace@ucsd.edu

© Springer International Publishing Switzerland 2016
P.S. Staats and S.M. Silverman (eds.), *Controlled Substance
Management in Chronic Pain*, DOI 10.1007/978-3-319-30964-4_7

of the therapeutical effects of opium, and may be employed as a substitute for that narcotic, when found to disagree with a patient from some peculiarity of constitution" [5]. The analgesic uses of the drug were summarized in *Sajou's Analytic Cyclopedia of Practical Medicine* (1924) and included headaches, migraine, eyestrain, menopause, brain tumors, neuralgia, gastric ulcer, uterine disturbances, dysmenorrhea, chronic inflammation, acute rheumatism, tingling, and relief of dental pain [1, 6]. During this time, tinctures and extracts of cannabis were marketed by a variety of pharmaceutical companies including Merck, Burroughs Wellcome, Bristol-Meyers Squibb, and Eli Lilly [1].

In the early twentieth century, the medicinal use of cannabis began to wane. This is likely due to the fact that the plant-based preparations available were of variable strength and had a short shelf life. Additionally, newer compounds such as opioids, aspirin, chloral hydrate, and barbiturates gained favor and supplanted cannabis extracts for its main indications [1, 3, 6]. After the alcohol prohibition was lifted in the USA, cannabis came under increasing legal scrutiny. In 1937, Congress passed the Marihuana Tax Act, which restricted and taxed the medicinal and non-medicinal use of the drug. Cannabis was ultimately removed from the British Pharmacopoeia in 1932 and the American Pharmacopoeia in 1941 [1–3]. Despite these prohibitions on clinical use, preclinical studies continued. The non-psychoactive compound cannabidiol (CBD) was isolated by two independent investigators in 1940. The psychoactive compound tetrahydro-cannabinol (THC) was isolated in 1964 [3]. Neurobehavioral studies confirmed the analgesic effects of cannabinoids [7–9]. Finally, in the early 1990s, the G-protein-coupled cannabinoid receptors CB1 and CB2 were identified [10]. Resurgent interest in the medicinal use of cannabis in the USA resulted in the passage of medicinal marijuana legalization laws starting with California and Arizona in 1996.

Under direction from the White House Office of Drug Control Policy, the Institute of Medicine issued a report in 1999, which contained several recommendations regarding medicinal marijuana. These recommendations were as follows: (1) Research should continue into the physiologic effects of synthetic and plant-derived cannabinoids, (2) development of new delivery systems should be pursued, (3) the psychological effects of cannabis should be evaluated, (4) studies to define health risks of smoked marijuana should be conducted, and (5) clinical trials should involve short-term use, reasonable expectations of efficacy, and approval by an institutional review board. The report also recommended that use of smoked cannabis must meet the following conditions: (1) failure of approved medications, (2) reasonable expectation of efficacy, (3) administration under medicinal supervision, and (4) inclusion of an oversight strategy [11].

In 1996, the voters of California and Arizona passed the first medicinal marijuana laws to eliminate state penalties for the use of marijuana for medicinal purposes. The ensuing two decades has brought similar laws to a total of 23 states plus the District of Columbia at the time of this writing. Four states have legalized the recreational use, and 15 others have decriminalized possession of small amounts of marijuana. The continued Drug Enforcement Agency (DEA) classification of marijuana as a schedule 1 drug with no medicinal value has resulted in uncertainty for clinicians regarding whether and when to recommend or "prescribe" medicinal marijuana. Additionally, the quasi-legal and unregulated nature of the market for medicinal marijuana has resulted in a lack of uniform drug quality or strength. For those clinicians who are interested in recommending the use of these drugs, it remains difficult to give clear advice on what to buy, how much to use, and by what route to deliver the drug.

There continues to be a broad range of opinions regarding the use of herbal marijuana for clinical purposes. Arguments supporting medicinal use state that (1) the leaf contains numerous active constituents making it more clinically effective than FDA-approved single-constituent cannabinoid medications, (2) marijuana has no lethal dose and in terms of respiratory depression is much safer than the opioid class of medication, and (3) millennia of use support safety and efficacy. Arguments opposing medicinal use state that (1) it will never meet the Food and Drug Administration (FDA) criteria for approval as a medication and (2) approval for medicinal use will lead to more widespread availability for recreational use and lead to public harm. Nonetheless, the momentum for legalizing the medicinal use of marijuana in the USA suggests that it is here to stay. This reality stresses the need for clinicians to prepare for this momentum so that they can provide patients with the best medicinal advice.

Regulatory and Legal Considerations

Regulations for Clinical Use

Neither the FDA nor any other federal regulatory agency in the USA oversees or regulates the production and distribution of herbal marijuana. Growers, processors, and distributors of medicinal marijuana exist in states that have legalized use; however, there is no federal or state oversight holding them accountable for content and purity. Therefore, it is difficult to predict the purity as well as the presence of other additives such as pesticides.

Efforts are emerging to provide better oversight of herbal marijuana processing and distribution. Oregon recently passed a bill (Oregon Measure 19, 2014) that designates the Oregon Liquor Commission to work with the Department of Agriculture and the Department of Health to oversee the growth, processing, and distribution of marijuana into the marketplace. In addition, laboratories that assay the leaf for cannabinoids and contaminants are proliferating across the country. These laboratories, however, are currently not under any regulatory oversight and thus have questionable validity.

Marijuana laws vary widely among those states that have passed some form of legalization, and the clinician must be familiar with the state in which they practice. These states' laws vary on (1) which medicinal conditions marijuana can be used for, (2) the type of marijuana (relative THC:CBD ratio) (3) how physicians are certified, (4) physician responsibilities when recommending marijuana, (5) how

much marijuana patients can possess for medicinal use, (6) possession by designated caregivers, and (7) rules governing the dispensaries. Since marijuana is not
FDA-approved, no state requires a physician to write a prescription and there are no
third-party payors that have provide coverage.

Some states provide guidelines for recommending medicinal marijuana. In the
absence of guidelines, the clinician should manage the patients in accordance with
good medicinal practice. This involves becoming familiar with the safety and
efficacy of medicinal marijuana and counseling patients on their responsibilities and
on the side effects. Patients should then be followed to assess the clinical effects,
side effects, and impact on function and quality of life. Appropriate documentation
of the patient's medicinal record should be made.

Regulations for Clinical Research

As marijuana is subject to control under the Schedule I of the Controlled Substances
Act (CSA) (21 U.S.C. 801 et. Seq), conducting clinical research is quite challenging. Whereas marijuana used for medicinal purposes can be obtained from state
dispensaries, research with marijuana falls under the auspices of multiple agencies
including the Drug Enforcement Agency (DEA), Department of Health and Human
Services (DHHS), Food and Drug Administration (FDA), and the National Institute
of Drug Abuse (NIDA). Obtaining a Schedule I DEA license is required in order to
conduct marijuana research. This license requires a much more intensive application process than that necessary for obtaining a regular Schedule II license. First, the
proposed research must be submitted for review by the Office of Public Health and
Science (an interagency review panel within the DHHS). After approval, an
Investigational New Drug Application must be filed with the FDA. After IND
approval and number assignment, the study is submitted for further review by
NIDA and the Federal DEA. Simultaneous approval must be obtained from the
local DEA office. The local DEA will inspect the location of the proposed study and
practices for storage, safeguarding, and dispensing, which have higher requirements
than for other investigational drugs. Some states have additional review and
approval (i.e., California requires all research with Schedule I or II controlled
substances to undergo review by the Research Advisory Panel of California, a
branch of the Office of the Attorney General in the California State Department of
Justice).

Since 1968, the University of Mississippi has been the sole supplier of marijuana
for research in the USA through a contract with NIDA. The agency has made
marijuana available with different concentrations of THC, with a placebo leaf and
with CBD levels typically being very low (<1 %). CBD oil for use in research is
actively being pursued.

Classification of Cannabinoids

The term "cannabinoid" originally referred to a variety of compounds, which were derived from the cannabis plant. With the discovery of human cannabinoid receptors and the synthesis of non-plant-based compounds with similar effects, the term has come to refer to all compounds which mimic the effects of naturally occurring cannabis or which have an effect at the cannabinoid receptors [12]. The term "phytocannabinoids" is used to identify those cannabinoid compounds derived from the cannabis plant. Endogenous compounds that interact with the cannabinoid receptors are referred to as endocannabinoids [12, 13] (Fig. 7.1).

In the clinical use of cannabinoids, there are three main product types. The first is non-pharmaceutically derived phytocannabinoids from the cannabis plant. These take the form of marijuana, hashish, or their derivatives, which are prepared outside of a pharmaceutical manufacturing facility. The second type of product is pharmaceutically derived plant-based extracts. Lastly, there are synthetic cannabinoids that have been formulated as pharmacologic agents [2, 13, 14].

Herbal Marijuana

Cannabis is a genus of flowering plants, which includes three species: *Cannabis sativa* (the largest variety), *Cannabis indica,* and *Cannabis ruderalis.* The term "marijuana" is a Mexican word, which refers to the dried leaves and flowers of the plant, which is most commonly smoked [2]. Hashish is the Arabic term for hemp and refers to the resin of the plant [2]. Cannabis contains 537 known compounds, of which 107 are cannabinoids [15]. The main psychoactive compound in cannabis is delta-9-tetrahydrocannabinol (Δ9-THC) [2, 12, 16, 17]. Clinically, THC has been shown to have analgesic properties as well as appetite stimulant and antinausea

Fig. 7.1 Sources of cannabinoids

Phytocannabinoids
• Commercial plant -based cannabis extracts
• Nabiximols
• Cannador
• Medical Marijuanna

Endocannabinoids
• Anandamide
• 2-arachidonyl glycerol (2 -AG)

Synthetic Cannabinoids
• Synthetic THC - Dronabinol
• Synthetic analogue of THC - Ajulemic Acid
• Synthetic analogue of THC - Nabilone

effects [2, 16]. Other major cannabinoids found in the cannabis plant are delta-8-tetrahydrocannabinol (Δ8-THC), CBD, and cannabinol (CBN) [2]. The concentration of the various cannabinoids in *cannabis sativa* varies tremendously by variety and growing conditions [16]. The concentration of THC in marijuana has increased from an average of 3 % in the 1980s to 13 % in 2009. The highest concentration of THC found in 2009 was 37 % for cannabis, 66 % for hashish, and 81 % for hash oil [18]. In general, CBD is the second most abundant compound in cannabis plants next to THC [2, 16]. Unlike THC concentration trends, CBD content in marijuana has remained relatively low and stable from the early 1980s to 2008, averaging 0.3–0.4 % [18]. However, the recent promotion of high CBD marijuana for various conditions has resulted in the availability of strains with higher CBD content in some dispensaries [19, 20]. CBD is generally considered to have no psychoactive effects, but clinically may reduce seizure activity, improve muscle spasm, and have anti-inflammatory properties [17, 21, 22]. CBD has a very low affinity for the CB1 and CB2 receptors and may act as an inverse agonist [16, 21]. The complex interactions of CBD with the cannabinoid receptors modulate the clinical and pharmacologic effects of THC. This may include the attenuation of the psychotropic effects of THC [21–23]. Cannabinol (CBN), a metabolite of THC, is minimally psychoactive and found in only trace amounts in the plant [24]. Delta-8-tetrahydrocannabinol is also minimally psychoactive and present at low concentrations [2].

Cannabis-Based Medicine Extracts

Cannabis-based medicine extracts (CBME) are derived by extracting compounds directly from the marijuana plant [25]. There are currently three CBMEs that have undergone clinical trials: Cannador, nabiximols (Sativex, GW Pharmaceuticals, UK), and purified CBD (Epidiolex, GW Pharmaceuticals, UK) [14, 23, 25]. Cannador (Weleda, Arlesheim, Switzerland) is a CBME delivered in oral capsules with a 2:1 ratio of THC to CBD [13, 23]. It has been studied for acute and chronic pain but is not currently clinically available. Nabiximols (Sativex) is a sublingual spray containing a 1:1 ratio of THC to CBD which is currently approved for the treatment of multiple sclerosis-related spasticity in Canada and parts of Europe. It has also been studied for cancer pain [14, 23, 25]. A cannabidiol-based extract (Epidiolex) is being used clinically under an investigational new drug approval to treat certain epilepsies in children.

Synthetic Cannabinoids

Currently, there are two FDA-approved cannabinoids: nabilone (Cesamet—a synthetic molecule similar to THC) and dronabinol (Marinol—a THC molecule).

Nabilone and dronabinol, as well as another cannabinoid, ajulemic acid (CT3), have undergone clinical trials. Dronabinol is Schedule III synthetic delta-9-THC, which is marketed in the USA for the treatment of nausea associated with chemotherapy and as an appetite stimulant for HIV-related wasting syndrome [2, 21, 26]. Nabilone is a Schedule II synthetic analogue of delta-9-THC which is FDA-approved to treat chemotherapy-induced nausea. Both dronabinol and nabilone have been studied for the treatment of chronic pain and spasticity [14, 17]. Ajulemic acid is a synthetic analogue of the terminal metabolite of delta-8-THC. It has potent anti-inflammatory effects and is non-psychoactive. It is currently being investigated as an anti-inflammatory and analgesic agent [2, 27].

The Endocannabinoid System

It was long believed that the clinical effects of lipophilic cannabis-based compounds were due to non-specific disruption of phospholipid biologic membranes. The understanding of the cannabinoid's biologic effects began to change with the discovery of the structure of delta-9-THC in 1964 by Raphael Mechoulam and his subsequent discovery in 1992 of anandamide, an endogenous cannabinoid. This ultimately led to the cloning of human cannabinoid receptors in the early 1990 [12, 28]. The endocannabinoid system consists of the endogenous ligands anandamide and 2-AG, and the cannabinoid receptors CB1 and CB2 [28, 29].

Cannabinoids produce their effects by the activation of G-protein-coupled cannabinoid receptors identified as CB1 and CB2 [28, 29]. Cannabinoid CB1 receptors are located mainly in the central nervous system (CNS) at nerve terminals where they mediate inhibition of transmitter release [12, 29, 30]. CB2 is found mainly on immune cells including microglia, monocytes, macrophages, B, and T lymphocytes where they modulate cytokine release [12, 28, 29]. CB1 and CB2 receptors are coupled through $G_{i/o}$ proteins, negatively to adenylate cyclase (inhibiting the production of cyclic AMP) and positively to mitogen-activated protein kinase (MAPK) [12, 28]. Additionally, CB1 is coupled positively to inwardly rectifying and A-type outward potassium channels and negatively to N-type and P/Q type calcium channels [12, 28]. Within the CNS, there is wide distribution of CB1 receptors including the cerebral cortex, hippocampus, caudate putamen, substantia nigra, pars reticulata, cerebellum, the mesolimbic system, which modulates reward, and the brain stem and spinal cord [12, 29]. Within the spinal cord, CB1 receptors have been localized to multiple areas involved in nociceptive processing including the superficial dorsal horn, dorsolateral funiculus, and lamina X [30]. The activation of CB1 receptors in central nociceptive processing regions and primary afferents inhibits the release of neurotransmitters via decreasing calcium conductance and increasing potassium conductance which forms the anatomic basis for the analgesic action of cannabinoid agonists [28]. Additionally, there are CB1 receptors located in adipocytes of peripheral tissues, liver, lung, reproductive organs, smooth muscle, gastrointestinal tract, immune system, and peripheral sensory nerves [31].

CB2 receptors play a role in mediating analgesia through their effects on inflammation. The CB2 receptors are found in the spleen, tonsils, thymus, and other tissues responsible for immune cell production and regulation. Activation of CB2 receptors down modulates mast cell function, and there is evidence that CB2 receptors can trigger microglial cell migration and regulate cytokine release [12, 30]. The effect of CB2 on mast cells may play a role in modulating nerve growth factor (NGF)-driven sensitization of nerve terminals during inflammation, which has been implicated in the development of inflammatory hyperalgesia [30]. There is also some evidence that CB2 receptors are located on and play a role in nociceptive regulation of primary sensory neurons [31].

The primary endocannabinoids are anandamide and 2-arachidonoyl glycerol (2-AG), both of which are eicosanoids [12]. Both are synthesized in postsynaptic neurons and act as retrograde signaling messengers. They regulate the presynaptic release of a variety of neurotransmitters [12, 31, 32].

There are additional compounds that have been proposed as possible endocannabinoids. These include noladin ether, virodhamine, and N-arachidonoyldopamine (NADA) [12, 29, 30]. Currently, the endocannabinoid-like properties of these compounds remain unclear.

Both anandamide and 2-AG are both produced from cell membrane lipid precursors on demand [12, 29, 31]. The synthesis of 2-AG results from the enzymatic cleavage (using phospholipase C) of membrane precursors to produce diacylglycerol. This is followed by the enzymatic cleavage (using diacylglycerol lipase) of diacylglycerol to produce 2-AG [29, 31]. Anandamide is an amide of ethanolamine and arachidonic acid. It is generated from its membrane precursor, N-arachidonoyl phosphatidylethanolamine (NAPE), through cleavage by phospholipase D. These endocannabinoids are released and then enter presynaptic neurons by some combination of simple diffusion and facilitated, carrier-mediated transport [12, 28]. 2-AG is degraded in the presynaptic terminal by monoacylglycerol lipase (MAG). Anandamide is degraded by fatty acid amino hydrolase (FAAH) [12, 29, 31].

Anandamide is widely distributed and has been shown to evoke analgesia as an agonist at CB1 receptors. It has also been shown to act as a weak agonist at the transient receptor potential vanilloid 1 (TRPV-1) receptors [29, 30]. The TRPV-1 receptors are expressed in nociceptive sensory neurons and respond to noxious mechanical, thermal, and chemical stimuli. Anandamide and capsaicin share the same TRPV-1-binding site, but high concentrations of anandamide are required in order to activate TRPV-1 [29]. At low concentrations, it may antagonize the classic effects of delta-9-THC [30].

2-AG is a full agonist at both CB1 and CB2 receptors but with low binding affinity and is found in the brain at concentrations 170-fold higher than anandamide [29, 30]. It is believed to be the primary natural ligand at CB2 receptors [30]. It has been shown to limit lymphocyte proliferation [30].

Cannabinoid receptors and endocannabinoids are located within spinal, supraspinal, and peripheral nervous system nociceptive pathways and processing centers [28, 29]. Activation of CB1 receptors at supraspinal [33–35], spinal [33, 36, 37], and peripheral [38, 39] sites has been shown to independently produce antinociception.

CB1 receptors in the brain are found in the periaqueductal gray, thalamus, basolateral amygdala, and rostroventral medulla. Activation of CB1 receptors in these regions can have local effects on nociceptive processing and affect bulbospinal pathways, which regulate dorsal horn excitability [29]. Electrical stimulation of the dorsolateral periaqueductal gray has been shown to mobilize anandamide and produce antinociception in mice. This analgesia was blocked by the administration of a specific CB1 receptor antagonist [29, 40].

Cannabinoid receptors have been found on primary afferent neurons both pre- and postsynaptically in the spinal cord. CB1 receptors have been identified on interneurons in the dorsal horn. Both anandamide and 2-AG are increased in the spinal cord in animal models of neuropathic pain and spinal cord injury. The intrathecal administration of cannabinoids has been shown to produce antinociception and modulate nociceptive signal processing by suppressing C-fiber-evoked responses of dorsal horn neurons.

At the peripheral level, cannabinoid receptors are present in dorsal root ganglion (DRG) cells. In animal models of neuropathic pain by spinal nerve ligation, the cannabinoid receptors and endocannabinoids are increased in the DRG ipsilaterally [29, 41]. Additionally, both CB1 and CB2 receptors are found in human cutaneous nerve fibers [29, 42].

Pharmacology of Marijuana and Cannabinoids

Herbal Marijuana

For centuries, the primary means of delivering cannabinoids has been via the inhaled smoke of marijuana or hashish. The concentration of THC and other cannabinoids in marijuana varies greatly depending on growing conditions, plant genetics, and processing after harvest [43]. The lack of controlled production and testing in most medicinal marijuana products and diversity of delivery routes (smoked, vaporized, eaten, topically applied) make prediction of pharmacologic effects difficult [44].

Patients who prefer not to smoke are increasingly using marijuana that has been processed into edibles (foods and drinks). The sale of marijuana-laced edibles (often in the form of baked goods and candies) has come under criticism for fear that children will mistakenly ingest them. The oral administration of marijuana produces slow but relatively high absorption with peak plasma concentrations at 60–120 min. However, first-pass metabolism results in a low bioavailability of 6–20 % with significant variability [46]. The delay in peak blood levels of THC from oral administration makes self-titration more difficult. Psychotropic effects begin within 30–90 min after oral ingestion, reach maximal effect after 2–3 h, and may last 4–12 h [45].

Inhaled marijuana, on the other hand, is easy to titrate with fast and predictable onset. Smoking cannabis results in rapid absorption. Smoking marijuana yields approximately 50 % of its THC content in the inhaled smoke with the rest lost to heat. Another 50 % or more of the inhaled THC is then lost to exhalation or localized metabolism in the lung, leaving a bioavailability for the active drug between 10 and 35 % [45–47]. Bioavailability varies depending on the depth of inhalation, puff duration, and breath holding with regular users being more efficient [45]. Vaporization is another means of inhaled delivery without burning the cannabis and results in higher bioavailability. The volatile cannabinoids are vaporized when heated air is drawn through the cannabis [44, 47]. Alveolar absorption results in maximal plasma concentration within minutes and psychotropic effects starting within a few seconds and reaching maximal effect within 15–30 min. Psychotropic effects with inhalation will last 2–3 h [45].

Metabolism of THC primarily occurs in the liver via the cytochrome P450 systems, CYP2C subfamily of isoenzymes. Some metabolism occurs in the lungs as well as other tissues. Elimination is primarily in the form of acid metabolites both renally and through biliary excretion with only 5 % eliminated unchanged [45]. Extensive tissue storage of metabolites results in prolonged elimination. The detection of metabolites in urine will fluctuate between positive and negative results for days after last use. For infrequent users, the average time to the first negative urine test is 8.5 days with 12.9 days to the last positive test. For frequent users, the average time to first negative test is 19.1 days with 31.5 days to the last positive test [48].

The coadministration of CBD and THC in both animals and humans has been shown to modulate some of the effects of THC. Studies in mice have shown that administration of CBD blocked catatonia from THC but potentiated the analgesia [23]. Human studies have shown that CBD attenuated the anxiety, disturbed time tasks, and tachycardia produced by THC [23, 49].

Pharmaceutical Cannabinoids

Nabiximols (Sativex) is a sublingual spray containing the cannabis-based mrdical extract (CBME) combination of THC and CBD in a roughly 1:1 ratio. It is manufactured by the extraction from cloned cannabis plants with reproducible yields of THC and CBD [23]. It is approved in Canada and Europe to treat spasticity related to multiple sclerosis and is in phase III trials in the USA to treat cancer-related pain. Each spray delivers 2.7 mg of THC and 2.5 mg of CBD [23]. The bioavailability and pharmacokinetics of both sublingual spray and oral delivery are similar [50].

Dronabinol (Marinol) is a synthetic preparation of the (-)-trans isomer of delta-9-THC dissolved in sesame oil. It is available as capsules in 2.5, 5, and 10 mg strengths [45]. It is FDA-approved for the treatment of nausea associated with chemotherapy and as an appetite stimulant for HIV-related wasting syndrome [2, 21, 26]. Nabilone is a synthetic analogue of delta-9-THC that is significantly more potent with a longer clinical duration [2, 21, 26]. In the USA, it is FDA-approved to treat chemotherapy-induced nausea [13].

Side Effects of Cannabinoids: Acute and Chronic

Acutely, THC induces a psychoactive, mildly euphoric intoxication or "high" which leads to changes in psychomotor and cognitive function. This intoxication will vary depending on the strain and dose and may include sedation, relaxation, hunger, and heightened sensory input. Physiologic changes include decreased body temperature, muscle relaxation, conjunctival injection, hyposalivation and dry mouth, tachycardia, vasodilation, orthostatic hypotension, and bronchodilation. Acutely, there is also impairment in attention, balance, cognition, memory, judgment, and sense of time [17, 45, 51]. Less commonly, cannabis can induce unpleasant effects including anxiety, panic, and paranoia [17, 51]. In rare cases, cannabis use may lead to acute psychosis involving delusions and hallucinations. There is an association between heavy cannabis use in adolescence and the development of schizophrenia as well as an association between cannabis use and worsening symptoms in schizophrenia [17, 45, 52]. Strains of cannabis with higher CBD content may be associated with a lower risk of adverse psychiatric effects, presumably due to modulating (depressant) effect of CBD on the excitatory effects of THC [17]. CBD alone is not psychoactive but has significant anticonvulsant, sedative, and other pharmacologic activities [17].

The median lethal dose (LD50) of oral THC in rats was found to be 800–1900 mg/kg. There have been no deaths in animal studies in dogs (up to 3000 mg/kg THC) and monkeys (up to 9000 mg/kg THC). There are no substantiated human cases of death from THC overdose [45]. In a systemic review of studies of oral and oral mucosal cannabis for various medicinal conditions, the majority of adverse events' reports were considered non-serious (96.6 %) [53]. The non-serious averse events were significantly more common in the cannabinoid groups compared to placebo with the most common events being nervous system disorders such as dizziness. The number of serious adverse events was not significantly different than in control groups and involved relapse of multiple sclerosis, vomiting, urinary tract infections, and respiratory infections [53].

The chronic effects of regular marijuana use have been the subject of significant investigation and controversy. A review of 40 articles on the use of cannabis found no consistent evidence for persisting neuropsychological deficits in cannabis users. However, half of the studies reported at least some subtle impairment. Another review of 11 articles covering 623 cannabis users and 409 non- or minimal users concluded that there may be decrements in the ability to learn and remember new information, whereas other cognitive abilities are unaffected [54, 55]. However, there are several studies that show early age use leads to persistent cognitive deficits and reduced educational achievement. Adolescent-onset users diagnosed before age 18 tended to become more persistent users. After comparing adolescent- and adult-onset users on total number of cannabis-dependent diagnoses, adolescent-onset users showed greater IQ decline [56–58].

Adult-onset cannabis users did not appear to experience IQ decline as a function of persistent cannabis use. However, this was challenged in a subsequent analysis of data stating that when socioeconomic status was factored, the true effect was closer to zero [59].

These effects appear to be mild and present only in frequent heavy users of cannabis [51].

- In chronic heavy smokers of marijuana, there is some evidence of an increased risk of bronchitis and other respiratory disorders [56, 60]. There is conflicting evidence on long-term pulmonary function. A longitudinal study of 972 tobacco and marijuana smokers found increased FVC, TLC, and FRC independent of the effects of tobacco use [61]. Other studies have failed to find similar associations. A review of 34 articles on cannabis smoking and pulmonary function found no association between long-term use and airflow obstruction but did find increased chronic cough, sputum production, and wheezing [62]. In a study of cannabis-only smokers compared to tobacco-only smokers, the effect on FEV-1 of one cannabis cigarette was found to be 2.5–5 times as pronounced as one tobacco cigarette [63]. This may be in part because each inhalation of a cannabis cigarette is typically 2/3 larger, inhaled 1/3 deeper, and is held 4 times longer. Additionally, cannabis cigarettes were found to be 50 % higher in tar [64]. Per cigarette, cannabis smoke contains many of the same chemicals and carcinogens as tobacco smoke, including benzene (76 mcg vs. 67 mcg), acetone (443 mcg vs. 578 mcg), and ammonia (228 mcg vs. 199 mcg) [65]. Epidemiologic studies have not consistently found an increased risk of lung cancer in chronic marijuana smokers when controlled for the concurrent use of tobacco [56, 60]. However, some studies have found an increased risk of head and neck cancers in chronic marijuana users [56, 60].

Cannabis withdrawal syndrome has been demonstrated in frequent, heavy users. The syndrome is characterized by increased anxiety, restlessness, anger and aggression, and irritability with decreased appetite, weight loss, sleeplessness, depressed mood, and stomach pains [51, 66]. These symptoms may emerge two days after cessation of use and remit in one to two weeks [51]. Unlike the withdrawal syndromes associated with opioids, alcohol, and benzodiazepines, cannabis withdrawal lacks significant physiologic symptoms or deleterious effects [66].

Cannabinoids as Analgesics

Human clinical studies of cannabinoids for pain have thus far been relatively small. Careful interpretation of these studies is necessary as there are several variables that can affect outcomes. These include the route of administration (oral or inhaled) and the drugs studied and their constituents such as synthetic Δ9-THC, other synthetic single-compound cannabinoids, mixed synthetic or natural cannabinoids, and whole plant inhaled or ingested cannabis. Additionally, the dosages of study drug will play a role in study outcome. Other factors include the study design and experimental pain models versus clinical pain studies [67].

Studies in Healthy Volunteers

Experimental pain model studies using healthy volunteers have produced mixed results. Several studies have shown that cannabis increases the pain threshold suggesting an analgesic effect. Other studies have found either no effect on pain thresholds or a lowering of the pain threshold [68–73]. In one trial of smoked cannabis on capsaicin-induced pain and hyperalgesia, cannabis cigarettes with 2 % THC produced no effect on pain, 4 % THC significantly decreased pain, and 8 % THC significantly increased pain compared to placebo [74]. Another study found that 4 % THC had a significant effect on both neuropathic pain and experimental capsaicin-induced pain in HIV patients [75]. These studies suggest that there may be a therapeutic window for analgesia from cannabis. Another study of cannabis extracts found a hyperalgesic effect in human experimental models of acute pain [76].

Studies in Clinical Pain

Large, well-designed clinical studies for cannabinoids are limited. The largest number of studies has been conducted for various neuropathic pain states with smaller numbers for other acute, cancer, and chronic pain states. A summary of the evidence for various pain indications shows relatively solid evidence for multiple sclerosis pain and spasticity. Modest efficacy has been reported for certain cannabinoid drugs in other neuropathic pain states and for cancer-related pain. Mixed or limited evidence exists for acute pain and inflammatory and nociceptive pain states.

Neuropathic Pain

The majority of studies of cannabinoids for neuropathic pain states have been for multiple sclerosis (MS) pain as well as MS-related spasticity. However, there are several studies in other types of neuropathic pain. A meta-analysis of cannabinoid medications including nabiximols, dronabinol, and CBD studied for MS-related and neuropathic pain found significant evidence of analgesic efficacy [77].

Nabiximols (Sativex) has been evaluated in studies with various types of neuropathic pain. In patients with pain from brachial plexus avulsion, nabiximols and delta-9-THC were compared with placebo. Both nabiximols and delta-9-THC produced significant improvements in pain as well as quality of sleep [78]. In unilateral neuropathy patients, nabiximols reduced pain, improved mechanical and punctate allodynia, and improved sleep disturbances [79].

Two studies have evaluated the effects of inhaled cannabis for HIV-associated peripheral neuropathy [80, 81]. Both found a significant effect in pain reduction compared to placebo. In studies of mixed etiology neuropathic pain, higher doses of smoked cannabis (7–9.4 %) resulted in analgesia when compared to placebo or low doses of smoked cannabis [82, 83].

Patients with multiple sclerosis (MS) have both neuropathic pain and painful spasticity. Both of these symptoms have been targets of cannabinoid therapy studies. A study of patients with MS-related neuropathic pain found a significant improvement in pain and pain-related sleep disturbance with nabiximols [84]. A three-arm trial with 630 MS patients comparing either oral delta-9-THC or a cannabis extract (Cannador) containing both THC and CBD versus placebo found subjective improvement in spasticity and pain for both cannabinoid compounds compared to placebo, but no objective improvement in spasticity on the Ashworth Spasticity Scale. A one-year continuation study found both THC and THC + CBD improved objective spasticity on the Ashworth Spasticity Scale at 1 year compared to baseline [85]. A multicenter trial of 160 patients with MS compared nabiximols to placebo and found a decrease in pain intensity but not spasticity [13, 86]. Smoked marijuana studies in MS-related pain and spasticity have been small and produced mixed results [13, 87].

The Canadian Pain Society's consensus statement regarding the treatment of neuropathic pain lists cannabinoids as a recommended third-line analgesic ahead of SSRIs, methadone, and topical lidocaine [88]. Additionally, a systematic review by the American Academy of Neurology's Guidelines Subcommittee found that oral cannabis extract and smoked marijuana were effective for reducing patient-reported symptoms of spasticity and that nabiximols was effective at both patient-reported spasticity and objective measures of spasticity [87]. For the treatment of MS-related pain, the same review found oral cannabis extracts effective and both nabiximols and dronabinol probably effective [87].

Cancer Pain

Several early studies of oral dronabinol showed it to be effective for cancer pain at higher doses (15–20 mg) with efficacy similar to codeine 60–120 mg but with more significant adverse effects than codeine [89]. There have been two published studies showing efficacy of nabiximols as add-on therapy with opioids for intractable cancer pain when compared to placebo [90, 91]. At the time of this writing, there are an additional three studies of nabiximols underway for cancer pain. One of these three trials was recently reported to have been negative although official results have not yet been published [92].

Acute Pain

Only a few studies have evaluated the effects of cannabinoids on acute pain. Cannador was evaluated in a multicenter dose escalation study in 30 patients with postoperative pain and showed a dose-dependent reduction in pain [93]. However, two studies with the synthetic cannabinoids, dronabinol (abdominal hysterectomy) and nabilone, failed to show any effect on postoperative pain [94, 95].

Chronic Non-neuropathic Pain

Compared to neuropathic pain, few studies have evaluated cannabinoids for nociceptive or inflammatory pain states. One study of dronabinol in mixed etiology chronic non-cancer pain found that single daily doses of 10 and 20 mg resulted in a dose-dependent decrease in pain [96]. Nabiximols has been compared to placebo in patients with chronic pain due to rheumatoid arthritis. The nabiximols group experienced significant reduction in pain with movement and at rest, and improved quality of sleep compared to placebo. However, nabiximols did not decrease morning stiffness [97].

Medicinal Marijuana Use in the Pain Clinic

Given the quasi-legal status of medicinal marijuana in the 23 states where it has been allowed, there are a number of questions regarding how to address the use of marijuana in the pain clinic setting. These include such areas as appropriate evaluation and patient selection, where to send patients to obtain the drug and in what form they should administer it, monitoring and coadministration of other controlled substances, and what disclosures are necessary regarding the potential risks of medicinal marijuana.

Physicians Recommending Medical Marijuana Should:

1. Take a history and conduct a good faith examination of the patient
2. Develop a treatment plan with objectives
3. Provide informed consent including discussion of adverse effects
4. Periodically review the treatment's efficacy
5. Obtain consultations as necessary
6. Keep proper records supporting the decision to recommend the use of medical marijuana

---

Fig. 7.2 California medical board guidelines for recommending medicinal marijuana. *Source* http://www.mbc.ca.gov/Licensees/Prescribing/medical_marijuana_cma-recommend.pdf

Patient Selection

There are no published guidelines for risk stratification or patient selection for medicinal marijuana use. Nabilone (DEA Schedule II) and dronabinol (DEA Schedule III) have some abuse potential, as does marijuana itself. Evaluation of a patient's risk for substance abuse should be a part of any patient selection process although the widely used tools for opioid risk evaluation such as the Opioid Risk Tool (ORT) or the Screener and Opioid Assessment for Patients with Pain—Revised (SOAPP-R) have not been studied specifically for marijuana abuse risk. Those patients who have failed first- and second-line therapies, especially for cancer-related or neuropathic pain, may be the most likely candidates. The Medical Board of California has published some basic guidelines for the evaluation of patients prior to recommending medicinal marijuana (Fig. 7.2) [98, 99]. Additionally, those patients with a history of serious mental illness such as schizophrenia or bipolar disorder likely are not acceptable candidates [100]. The tachycardia and blood pressure fluctuations may limit the acceptability of cannabis therapy for those with substantial coronary artery disease.

The drugs dronabinol and nabiximols have been evaluated for abuse potential in various studies. Clinical use of dronabinol has not been shown to be associated with significant diversion, drug seeking, or street value. In studies with recreational marijuana users, both dronabinol and nabiximols were found to have some abuse potential although nabiximols was significantly lower than dronabinol. While dronabinol is known to have significant psychoactive effects, it has been found less desirable than marijuana by regular users due to higher incidence of dysphoria, slower onset, and less flexible titration of effect. Nabiximols has been found to have significantly lower euphoria or psychoactive effects compared to dronabinol [101].

Dispensaries and Routes of Administration

In California, as with most states, any physician can recommend the use of marijuana to a patient for the treatment of a medicinal condition. Provision of a letter verifying this recommendation provides the patient with some protections against state and local prosecution for possession and use of marijuana up to the statutorily prescribed limits. Such a letter provides no protection against prosecution by federal authorities. Additionally, patients may take their letter to a state agency and obtain a medicinal marijuana ID card. Obtaining a state-issued ID card is optional in several states but required in some other states. The registration of an ID card places the patient's name in a state database accessible by marijuana dispensaries and law enforcement to aid in identifying those with the required physician recommendations. medicinal marijuana dispensaries sell the drug in various forms. These may include the dried buds of the plant for smoking or vaporizing, oils and tinctures that can be ingested, creams or solutions for topical application, and prepared cookies and other edible products made with marijuana-infused oils and fats. Some of the pulmonary adverse effects may be attenuated with the use of a vaporizer device instead of smoking [100]. The potency of marijuana products available in dispensaries will vary considerably. In most locations, there will not be any independent testing or labeling of THC or CBD content. A reputable and knowledgeable dispensary may provide some assistance in educating patients and directing them to lower THC- and higher CBD-content products than those cultivated primarily for recreational purposes. In 15 of the 23 states with medicinal marijuana laws, patients or their caregivers may cultivate their own marijuana at home with some limits on the number of plants per patient. The quantity of marijuana an individual patient may possess varies among the 23 states from 1 up to 24 oz [102].

Combining Medicinal Marijuana with Opioids

Studies in healthy adults have shown an additive or synergistic effect with cannabinoids and opioids in combination [47]. In cancer-related pain, nabiximols was studied as add-on therapy along with opioids. However, the combination of different controlled substances with addictive and psychomimetic effects should be considered with caution. No clear guidelines yet exist regarding the coadministration of opioids and cannabinoids. Cannabis use in patients on chronic opioids has been associated with future aberrant opioid-related behaviors [100]. At minimum, clinicians should exercise careful evaluation of patients' substance abuse risk. There should also be ongoing monitoring for aberrant drug-seeking behaviors, positive analgesic and functional effects, and appropriate use of only the prescribed or recommended drugs via urine drug screening. Some have advocated the use of a medicinal cannabis agreement, analogous to opioid agreements, which outline the various risks and expected responsibilities and behaviors of patients on this therapy [100].

Medicinal Marijuana Risk Disclosures

There are several risks associated with the possession and use of medicinal marijuana, which should be part of any patient disclosure prior to recommending the drug. First is the legal risk for possessing and using a controlled substance that is still categorized as Schedule I by the DEA. Accidental pediatric exposures have increased along with the spread of medicinal marijuana laws [17]. Foods and drinks containing cannabis are a particular risk for pediatric exposures, and patients should be warned to keep cannabis-containing products out of reach of children. While likely lowering the risk for addiction than opioids or alcohol, there remains a dependence, addiction, and withdrawal risk, which should be discussed with patients [98]. The pulmonary and cancer risks of smoking cannabis remain unclear; however, some discussion of potential pulmonary complications is worth considering [13]. Cannabis use impairs the ability to operate a vehicle, and this impairment is exacerbated when combined with alcohol. Patients should be cautioned not to drive while using cannabis or cannabinoid medications, especially those containing THC [98].

Conclusion

Therapeutic use of cannabis use has a very long history in medicine. Similar to opioids, its use has undergone fluctuations in acceptability and availability over the past 150 years. The current momentum of public opinion is clearly shifting toward more widespread acceptance despite the continuing regulatory limbo in which the drug resides. Pain physicians will increasingly be encountering the use of cannabinoids in their practice whether or not they choose to recommend medicinal cannabis or prescribe cannabis-derived pharmaceuticals. It has been suggested by many that cannabinoids are a potentially safer alternative to the use of opioids for chronic non-terminal pain. However, the data thus far suggest they are unlikely to be a panacea or completely replace opioids in the majority of cases. A careful consideration of the pros and cons of this therapy along with proper patient selection and monitoring may help in avoiding the simple replacement of one controlled substance problem for another.

References

1. Zuardi AW. History of cannabis as a medicine: a review. Rev Bras Psiquiatr. 2006;28:153–7.
2. Amar MB. Cannabinoids in medicine: a review of their therapeutic potential. J Ethnopharmacol. 2006;105:1–25.
3. Kalant H. Medicinal use of cannabis: history and current status. Pain Res Manage. 2001;6:80–91.
4. Mikuriya TH. Marijuana in medicine: past, present and future. Calif Med. 1969;110:34–40.
5. Wood GB, Bache F. The dispensatory of the United States of America. 6th ed. Philadelphia: Grigg and Elliot; 1845. p. 1238.
6. Aldrich M. History of therapeutic cannabis. In: Mathre ML, editor. Cannabis in medical practice. Jefferson, NC: Mc Farland; 1997. p. 35–55.
7. Sofia RD, et al. Antiedema and analgesic properties of D9 tetrahydrocannabinol. J Pharmacol Exp Ther. 1973;186:646–54.
8. Kosersky DS, Dewey WL, Harris L. Anitpyretic analgesic and antiinflammatory effects of delt 9-tetrahyodrocannabinol in the rat. Eur J Pharmacol. 1973;24:1–7.
9. Bloom AS, et al. 9-Nor-9B-hydroxyhexahydrocannabinol a cannabiniod with potent antinociceptive activity: comparisons with morphine. J Phamacol Exp Therap. 1977;200:263–70.
10. Cravatt BF, Lichtman AH. The endogenous cannabinoid system and its role in nociceptive behavior. J Neurobiol. 2004;61:149–60.
11. Joy JE, Watson SJ, Benson JA. Marijuana and medicine: assessing the science base. Institute of Medicine National Academy Press; 1999.
12. Pertwee RG. Pharmacological actions of cannabinoids. HEP. 2005;168:1–51.
13. Elikottil J, Gupta P, Gupta K. The analgesic potential of cannabinoids. J Opioid Manag. 2009;5:341–57.
14. Robson PJ. Therapeutic potential of cannabinoid medicines. Drug Text Anal. 2014;6:24–30.
15. Mechmedic Z, Chandra S, Slade D, Denham H, Foster S, Patel AS, Ross SA, Khan IA, ElSohly MA. Potency trends of delta9-THC and other cannabinoids in confiscated cannabis preparations from 1993–2008. J Forensic Sci. 2010;55:1209–17.
16. Appendino G, Chianese G, Taglialatela-Scafati O. Cannabinoids: occurrence and medicinal chemistry. Curr Med Chem. 2011;18:1085–99.
17. Borgelt LM, Franson KL, Nussbaum AM, Wang GS. The pharmacologic and clinical effects of medical cannabis. Pharmacother. 2013;33:192–209.
18. ElSohly MA. Quarterly report potency monitoring project. Report 104. In: NIDA Marijuana Project, National center for natural products research division of the resean institute of pharmaceutical sciences. The School of Pharmacy, University of Mississippi; 2009.
19. El Sohly MA, Ross SA, Mehmedic Z, Arafat R, Yi B, Banahan BF. Potency trends of delta 9-THC and other cannabinoids in confiscated marijuana from 1980–1997. J Forensic Sci. 2000;45:24–30.
20. Maa E, Figi P. The case for medical marijuana in epilepsy.y. Epilepsia. 2014;55:783–6.
21. Pertwee RG. The diverse CB1 and CB2 receptor pharmacology of three plant cannabinoids: delta-9-tetrahydrocanabidiol, cannabidiol and delta-9-tetrahydrocannabivarin. Br J Pharmacol. 2008;153:199–215.
22. Hayakawa K, Mishima K, Hazekawa M, Sano K, Irie K, Orito K, Egawa T, Kitamura Y, Uchida N, Nishimura R, Egashira N, Iwasaki K, Fujiwara M. Cannabidiol potentiates pharmacological effects of delta-9-tetrahydrocannabinol via CB1 receptor-dependent mechanism. J Brain Res. 2008;1188:157–64.
23. Russo EB, Guy GW. A tale of two cabanninoids: the therapeutic rationale for combining tetrahydrocannibinol and cannabidiol. Med Hypotheses. 2006;66:234–46.
24. Mahadevan A, Siegel C, Martin BR, Abood ME, Beletskaya I, Razdan RK. Novel cannabinol probes for CB1 and CB2 cannabinoid receptors. J Med Chem. 2000;43:3778–85.
25. Robson P. Human studies of cannabinoids and medicinal cannabis. HEP. 2005;168:719–56.

26. Di Marzo V, De Petrocellis L. Plant, synthetic, and endogenous cannabinoids in medicine. Annu Rev Med. 2006;57:553–74.
27. Burstein SH, Tepper MA. In vitro metabolism and metabolic effects of ajulemic acid, a synthetic cannabinoid agonist. Pharma Res Per. 2013;1:1–9.
28. Pacher P, Batkai S, Kunos G. The endocannabinoid system as an emerging target of pharmacotherapy. Pharmacol Rev. 2006;53:389–462.
29. Guindon J, Hohmann AG. The endocannabinoid system and pain. CNS Neurol Disord: Drug Targets. 2009;8:403–21.
30. Rice ASC, Farquhar-Smith WP, Nagy I. Endocannabinoids and pain: spinal and peripheral analgesia in inflammation and neuropathy. Prostaglandins Leukot Essent Fatty Acids. 2002;66:243–56.
31. La Porta C, Bura SA, Negrete R, Maldonado R. Involvement of the endocannabinoid system in osteoarthritis pain. Eur J Neuroscience. 2014;39:485–500.
32. Davis MP. Cannabinoids in pain management: CB1, CB2 and non-classic receptor ligands. Expert Opin Invest Drugs. 2014;23:1123–40.
33. Lichtman AH, Martin BR. Spinal and supraspinal mechanisms of cannabinoid-induced antinociception. J Pharmacol Exp Ther. 1991;258:517–23.
34. Lichtman AH, Cook SA, Martin BR. Investigation of brain sites mediating cannabinoid-induced antinociception in rats: evidence supporting periaqueductal gray involvement. J Pharmacol Exp Ther. 1996;276:585–93.
35. Monhemius R, Azami J, Green DL, Roberts MH. CB1 receptor mediated analgesia from the nucleus reticularis gigantocellularis pars alpha is activated in an animal model of neuropathic pain. Brain Res. 2001;908:67–74.
36. Yaksh TL. The antinociceptive effects of intrathecally administered levoantradol and deacetyllevonatradol in the rat. J Clin Pharmacol. 1981;21:334S–40S.
37. Smith FL, Fujimori K, Lowe J, Welch SP. Characterization of delta-9-tetrahydrocannabinol and anadamide antinociception in nonarthritic and arthritic rats. Parmacol Biochem Behav. 1998;60:183–91.
38. Richardson JD, Kilo S, Hargreaves KM. Cannabinoids reduce hyperalgesia and inflammation via interaction with peripheral CB1 receptors. Pain. 1998;75:111–9.
39. Calignano A, La Rana G, Giuffrida A, Piomelli D. Control of pain initiation by endogenous cannabinoids. Nature. 1998;394:277–81.
40. Walker JM, Huang SM, Strangman NM, Tsou K, Sanudo-Pena MC. Pain modulation by release of the endogenous cannabinoid anandamide. Proc Natl Acad Sci. 1999;96:12198–203.
41. Mitrirattanakul S, Ramakul N, Guerrero AV, Matsuka Y, Ono T, Iwase H, Mackie K, Faull KF, Spigelman I. Site-specific increases in peripheral cannabinoid receptors and their endogenous ligands in a model of neuropathic pain. Pain. 2006;126:102–14.
42. Stander S, Schmelz M, Metze D, Luger T, Rukwied R. Distribution of cannabinoid receptor 1 (CB1) and 2 (CB2) on sensory nerve fibers and adnexal structures in human skin. J Dermatol Sci. 2005;38:177–88.
43. de Meijer E. The breeding of cannabis cultivars for pharmaceutical end uses. In: Guy GW, Whittle BA, Robson P, editors. Medicinal uses of cannabis and cannabinoids. London: Pharmaceutical Press; 2004. p. 55–70.
44. Borgelt LM, Franson KL, Nussbaoum AM, Wang GS. The pharmacologic and clinical effects of medical cannabis. Pharmacother. 2013;33:195–209.
45. Grotenhermen F. Pharmacokinetics and pharmacodynamics of cannabinoids. Clin Pharmacokinet. 2003;42:327–60.
46. Agurell S, Halldin M, Lindgren JE. Pharmacokinetics and metabolism of delta-1-tetrahydrocannabinol and other cannabinoids with emphasis on man. Pharmacol Rev. 1986;38:21–43.
47. Elikottil J, Gupta P, Gupta K. The analgesic potential of cannabinoids. J Opioid Manag. 2009;5:341–57.

48. Ellis GM, Mann MA, Judson BA, Schramm NT, Tashchian A. Excretion patterns of cannabinoid metabolites after last use in a group of chronic users. Clin Pharmacol Ther. 1985;38:572–8.
49. Zuardi AW, Shirakawa I, Finkelfarb E, Karniol IG. Action of cannabidiol on the anxiety and other effects produced by delta 9-THC in normal subjects. Psychopharmacology. 1982;76:245–50.
50. Karschner EL, Darwin WD, Goodwin RS, Wright S, Huestis MA. Plasma cannabinoid pharmacokinetics following controlled oral delta9-tetrahydrocannabinol and oromucosal cannabis extract administration. Clin Chem. 2011;57:66–75.
51. Gonzalez R. Acute and non-acute effects of cannabis on brain functioning and neuropsychological performance. Neuropsychol Rev. 2007;17:347–61.
52. Hall W, Degenhardt L. Cannabis use and psychosis: a review of clinical evidence and epidemiological evidence. Aust NZ J Psychiatry. 2000;34:26–34.
53. Wang T, Collet JP, Shapiro S, Ware M. Adverse effects of medical cannabinoids: a systematic review. CMAJ. 2008;178:1669–78.
54. Gonzalez R, Carey C, Grant I. Nonacute (residual) neuropsychological effects of cannabis use: a qualitative analysis and systematic review. J Clin Pharm. 2002;42:48S–57S.
55. Grant I, Gonzalez R, Carey CL, Natarajan L, Wolfson T. Non-acute (residual) neurocognitive effects of cannabis use: a meta-analytic study. J Int Neuropsychol Soc. 2003;9:679–89.
56. Hall W, Degenhardt L. The adverse health effects of chronic cannabis use. Drug Test Anal. 2014;6:39–45.
57. Meier MH, Caspi A, Ambler A, Harrington H, Houts R, Keefe RS, McDonlad K, Ward A, Poulton R, Moffitt TE. Persistent cannabis users show neuropsychological decline from childhood to midlife. Proc Natl Acad Sci USA. 2012;109:E2657–64.
58. Horwood L, Fergusson D, Hayatbakhsh M, Najman J, Coffey C, Patton G, Silins E, Hutchinson DM. Cannabis use and educational achievement: findings from three Australian cohort studies. Drug Alcohol Depend. 2010;110:247–53.
59. Rogeberg O. Correlations between cannabis use and IQ change in the Dunedin cohort are consistent with confounding from socioeconomic status. Proc Natl Acad Sci. 2013;110:4251–4.
60. Gordon AJ, Conley JW, Gordon JM. Medical consequences of marijuana use: a review of current literature. Curr Psychiatry Rep. 2013;15:419.
61. Hancoz RJ, Poulton R, Ely M, Welch D, Taylor DR, McLachian CR, Greene JM, Moffitt TE, Caspi A, Sears MR. Effects of cannabis on lung function: a population-based cohort study. Eur Respir J. 2010;35:42–7.
62. Tetrault JM, Crothers K, Moore BA, Mehra R, Concato J, Fiellin DA. Effects of marijuana smoking on pulmonary function and respiratory compliance: a systematic review. Arch Intern Med. 2007;167:221–8.
63. Aldington S, Williams M, Nowitz M, Weatherall M, Prichard A, McNaughton A, Robinson G, Beasley R. Effects of cannabis on pulmonary structure, function and symptoms. Thorax. 2007;62:1058–63.
64. Wu TC, Tashkin DP, Djahed B, Rose JE. Pulmonary hazards of smoking marijuana as compared with tobacco. NEJM. 1988;318:347–51.
65. Relman AS. Committee to study the health-related effects of cannabis and its derivatives. Marijuana and health. Washington, DC: Institute of Medicine, National Academy Press; 1982. p. 16–8.
66. Bundy AJ, Hughes JR. The cannabis withdrawal syndrome. Curr Opin Psychiatry. 2006;19:233–8.
67. Walker JM, Huang SM. Cannabinoid analgesia. Pharmacol Ther. 2002;95:127–35.
68. Greenwald MK, Stitzer ML. Antinociceptive, subjective and behavioral effects of smoked marijuana in humans. Drug Alcohol Depend. 2000;59:261–75.
69. Milstein SL, MacCannell K, Karr G, Clark S. Marijuana-produced impairments in coordination. Experienced and nonexperienced subjects. J Nerv Ment Dis. 1975;161:26–31.

70. Naef M, Curatolo M, Petersen-Felix S, Arendt-Nielsen L, Zbinden A, Brenneisen R. The analgesic effect of oral delta-9-tetrahydrocannabinol (THC), morphine, and a THC-morphine combination in healthy subjects under experimental pain conditions. Pain. 2003;105:79–88.

71. Zeidenberg P, Clark WC, Jaffe J, Anderson SW, Chin S, Malitz S. Effect of oral administration of delta-9-tetrahydrocannabinol on memory, speech, and perception of thermal stimulation: results with four normal human volunteer subjects. Compr Psychiatry. 1973;14:549–56.

72. Hill SY, Schwin R, Goodwin DW, Powell BJ. Marihuana and pain. J Phamacol Exp Ther. 1974;188:415–8.

73. Clark WC, Janal MN, Zeidenberg P, Nahas GG. Effects of moderate and high doses of marihuana on thermal pain: a sensory decision theory analysis. J Clin Pharmacol. 1981;21:299S–310S.

74. Wallace M, Schulteis G, Atkinson JH, Wolfson T, Lazzaretto D, Bentley H, Gouaux B, Abramson I. Dose-dependent effects of smoked cannabis on capsaicin-induced pain and hyperalgesia in healthy volunteers. Anesthesiology. 2007;107:785–96.

75. Abrams DI, Jay CA, Shade SB, Vizoso H, Reda H, Press S, Kelly ME, Rowbotham MC, Petersen KL. Cannabis in painful HIV-associated sensory neuropathy: a randomized placebo-controlled trial. Neurology. 2007;68:515–21.

76. Kraft B, Frickey NA, Kaufmann RM, Reif M, Frey R, Gustorff B, Kress HG. Lack of analgesia by oral standardized cannabis extract on acute inflammatory pain and hyperalgesia in volunteers. Anesthesiology. 2008;109:101–10.

77. Iskedjian M, Bereza B, Gordon A, Piwko C, Einarson T. Meta-anlysis of cannabis based treatements for neuropathic and multiple sclerosis-related pain. Curr Med Res Opin. 2007;23:17–24.

78. Berman JS, Symonds C, Birch R. Efficacy of two cannabis based medicinal extracts for relief of central neuropathic pain from brachial plexus avulsion: results of a randomized controlled trial. Pain. 2004;112:299–306.

79. Nurmikko TJ, Serpell MG, Hoggart B, Toomey PJ, Morlion BJ, Haines D. Sativex successfully treats neuropathic pain characterized by allodynia: a randomized, double-blind, placebo-controlled clinical trial. Pain. 2007;133:210–20.

80. Abrams DI, Jay CA, Shade SB, Vizoso H, Reda H, Press S, Kelly ME, Rowbotham MC, Petersen KL. Cannabis in painful HIV-associated sensory neuropathy: a randomized placebo-controlled trial. Neurology. 2007;68:515–21.

81. Ellis RJ, Toperoff W, Vaida F, van den Brande G, Gonzales J, Gouaux B, Bentley H, Atkinson JH. Smoked medicinal cannabis for neuropathic pain in HIV: a randomized, crossover clinical trial. Neuropsychopharmacology. 2009;34:672–80.

82. Ware MA, Wang T, Shapiro S, Robinson A, Ducret T, Huynh T, Gamsa A, Bennett GJ, Collet JP. Smoked cannabis for chronic neuropathic pain: a randomized controlled trial. CMAJ. 2010;182:E694–701.

83. Wilsey B, Marcotte T, Tsodikov A, Millman J, Bentley H, Gouaux B, Fishman S. A randomized, placebo controlled, crossover trial of cannabis cigarettes in neuropathic pain. J Pain. 2008;9:506–21.

84. Rog DJ, Nurmikko TJ, Friede T, Young CA. Randomized, controlled trial of cannabis-based medicine in central pain in multiple sclerosis. Neurology. 2005;65:812–9.

85. Zajicek JP, Fox P, Sanders H, Wright D, Vickery J, Nunn A, Thompson A. Cannabinoids for treatment of spasticiy and other symptoms related to multiple sclerosis (CAMS study): multicenter randomized placebo-controlled trial. Lancet. 2003;362:1517–26.

86. Wade DT, Makela P, Robson P, House H, Bateman C. Do cannabis-based medicinal extracts have general or specific effects on symptoms in multiple sclerosis? A double-blind, randomized, placebo-controlled study on 160 patients. Mult Scler. 2004;10:434–41.

87. Koppel BS, Brust JCM, Fife T, Bronstein J, Youssof S, Gronseth G, Gloss D. Systematic review: Efficacy and safety of medical marijuana in selected neurological disorders. Report of the guideline development subcommittee of the American Academy of Neurology. Neurology. 2014;82:1556–63.

88. Moulin DE, Boulanger A, Clark AJ, Clarke H, Dao T, Finley GA, Furlan A, Gilron I, Gordon A, Morley-Forster PK, Sessle BJ, Squire P, Stinson J, Taenzer P, Velly A, Ware MA, Weinberg EL, Williamson OD. Pharmacological management of chornic neuropathic pain: revised consensus statement from the canadian pain society. Pain Res Manag. 2014;19:328–35.

89. Noyes R, Brunk SF, Baram DA, Canter A. Analgesic effect of delta-9-tetrahydrocannabinol. J Clin Pharmacol. 1975;15:139–43.

90. Johnson JR, Burnell-Nugent M, Lossignol D, Ganae-Motan ED, Potts R, Fallon MT. Multicenter, double-blind, randomized, placebo-controlled, parallel-group study of the efficacy, safety, and tolerability of THC: CBD extract and THC extract in patients with intractable cancer-related pain. J Pain Symptom Manage. 2010;39(2):167–79.

91. Portenoy RK, Ganae-Motan ED, Allende S, Yanagihara R, Shaiova L, Weinstein S, Fallon MT. Nabiximols for opioid-treated cancer patients with poorly-controlled chronic pain: a randomized, placebo-controlled, graded-dose trial. J Pain. 2012;13(5):438–49.

92. Hirschler B. GW Pharma's cannabis drug fails in cancer pain study, shares fall. Reuters.com. 8 Jan 2015. http://www.reuters.com/article/2015/01/08/us-gw-pharma-epilepsy-idUSKBN0KH13U20150108

93. Holdcroft A, Maze M, Dore C, Tebbs S, Thompson S. A multicenter dose-escalation study of the analgesic and adverse effects of an oral cannabis extract (Cannador) for postoperative pain management. Anesthesiology. 2006;104:1040–6.

94. Buggy DJ, Toogood L, Maric S, Sharpe P, Lambert DG, Rowbotham DJ. Lack of analgesic efficacy of oral delta-9-tetrahydrocannabinol in postoperative pain. Pain. 2003;106:169–72.

95. Beaulieu P. Effects of nabilone, a synthetic cannabinoid, on postoperative pain. Can J Anaesth. 2006;53:769–75.

96. Narang S, Gibson D, Wasan AD, Ross EL, Michna E, Nedeljkovic SS, Jamison RN. Efficacy of dronabinol as an adjuvant treatment for chronic pain patients on opioid therapy. J Pain. 2008;9:254–64.

97. Blake DR, Robson P, Ho M, Jubb RW, McCabe CS. Preliminary assessment of the efficacy, tolerability and safety of a cannabis-based medicine (Sativex) in the treatment of pain caused by rheumatoid arthritis. Rheumatology. 2006;45:50–2.

98. Grant I, Atkinson H, Gouaux B, Wilsey B. Medical marijuana: clearing away the smoke. Open Neurology Journal. 2012;6:18–25.

99. Physician recommendation of medical cannabis: guidelines of the council on scientific affairs subcommittee on medical marijuana practice advisory. Rev Aug 2011. California Medical Association. http://www.mbc.ca.gov/Licensees/Prescribing/medical_marijuana_cma-recommend.pdf

100. Wilsey B, Atkinson JH, Marcotte TD, Grant I. The medicinal cannabis treatment agreement: providing information to chronic pain patients through a written document. Clin J Pain. 2015;31(12):1087–96.

101. Robson P. Abuse potential and psychoactive effects of Delta-9-tetrahydrocannabinol and cannabidiol oromucosal spray (Sativex), a new cannabinoid medicine. Expert Opin Drug Saf. 2011;10:675–85.

102. 23 Legal marijuana states and DC. @ Pro-Con.org http://medicalmarijuana.procon.org/view.resource.php?resourceID=000881

Chapter 8
Adjuvant Agents in Chronic Pain Therapy

Joseph V. Pergolizzi

Introduction

With our increasing understanding of the multimechanistic nature of chronic pain, the role of adjuvant agents, also called coanalgesics, in multimodal pain control therapy is expanding. Americans, who spend about $17.8 billion on prescription drugs for chronic pain annually, spend more on adjuvant agents ($12.3 billion) than opioids ($3.6 billion) and non-opioid analgesics ($1.9 billion) combined [1]. If one considers biologics as an adjuvant therapy in rheumatologic disorders, adjuvant therapy accounts for 69 % of total pain medication costs [1]. Yet despite the costs to the healthcare system and patients, there is not a wealth of evidence-based literature about adjuvant agents for chronic pain to guide prescribing choices.

Adjuvant agents may be defined as medications whose primary effects are not analgesic but who have secondary analgesic effects that can be useful in treating pain syndromes [2]. Adjuvant agents may be considered when the patient's analgesic therapy is ineffective or does not address a specific type of pain (such as a neuropathic component of chronic pain) [3]. In chronic pain, the most commonly prescribed adjuvant agents fall into the categories of antidepressants, anticonvulsants, and muscle relaxants. Typically, these adjuvant agents are combined with opioid pharmacotherapy and may offer additive or synergistic analgesic benefits, broaden the therapeutic spectrum, and possibly reduce cumulative opioid consumption. In this way, they may help to prevent opioid-associated adverse events or postpone the development of opioid tolerance [4]. A short summary of some leading adjuvant agents and their indications and clinical considerations appears in Table 8.1.

J.V. Pergolizzi (✉)
Department of Medicine, Johns Hopkins University School of Medicine,
3384 Woods Edge Circle, Suite 102, Bonita Springs, FL 34134, USA
e-mail: jpjmd@jhu.edu

© Springer International Publishing Switzerland 2016
P.S. Staats and S.M. Silverman (eds.), *Controlled Substance
Management in Chronic Pain*, DOI 10.1007/978-3-319-30964-4_8

Table 8.1 A brief overview of adjuvant agents and how they might be used in combination with analgesic therapy

Agents	Indications	Concerns	Duration of treatment
TCAs	Neuropathic pain; depression	Side effects include constipation, dizziness, and dry mouth; may be associated	May be appropriate for long-term use under clinical supervision
Antiepileptics	Neuropathic pain	Unsteadiness, blurry vision, weight gain, suicidal ideation (rare)	May be appropriate for long-term use under clinical supervision
Nonsteroidal anti-inflammatory drugs	Inflammatory pain	GI adverse events; cardiovascular risk	Use at the lowest possible dose for the shortest amount of time
Muscle relaxants	Pain associated with muscle spasms	Drowsiness, dizziness, dry mouth; abuse potential	<3 months
Steroids	Inflammatory pain	Hypertension, glaucoma, weight gain	Use at the lowest possible dose for the shortest amount of time; do not discontinue abruptly
Alpha-2 agonists	Complex regional pain syndrome; opioid withdrawal; attention deficit/hyperactivity disorder	Hypertension, vasoconstriction, sedation; abuse potential	These are relatively new agents but appear to be suitable for long-term use under clinical supervision

Multimechanistic Chronic Pain and Multimodal Therapy

Appropriate multimodal pain control requires that clinicians first identify the type(s) of pain they are treating as well as any comorbid conditions. A detailed patient history and interview should be conducted, with the patient describing each pain site. Patients should be asked about when the pain at each site began, if anything alleviates or exacerbates that pain, whether the pain is continuous or intermittent, pain intensity (a numeric rating scale or visual analog scale should be used rather than descriptions), and pain characteristics [5]. Patients may struggle to describe their pain, so clinicians may prompt them, suggesting terms such as deep, throbbing, stabbing, electrical, jabbing, jolting, sudden, dull, and aching. It is common for patients with chronic pain to have difficulty localizing the pain, to describe migrating pains, and to have multiple types of pain. Analgesic therapy should be based on the patient's pain mechanisms; this may necessitate multimodal pain therapy with adjuvant agents (see Table 8.2) [6].

Table 8.2 Clinicians should first determine the type of pain syndrome(s) in their patients before considering primary and adjuvant pain control treatments

Syndrome	Nerve fibers	Description	Examples	Of note	Primary pharmacotherapy	Adjuvants to consider
Somatic (nociceptive)	Nociceptor activation in peripheral region, mediated mainly by A (delta) and C fibers [12]	Pain is typically localized and easy to pinpoint and may include tenderness and swelling at site	Acute traumatic injury; metastatic bone disease; musculoskeletal pain such as low back pain	If pain becomes chronic, it becomes more diffuse and more difficult to localize	Mild to moderate pain can be treated with acetaminophen or NSAIDs; opioids are appropriate for moderate to severe pain. Combination therapy (non-opioid + opioid) may be effective	Antidepressants may be helpful. Somatic pain associated with inflammation may be treated with steroids. For low back pain or other muscular pain, short-term use of muscle relaxants can be helpful
Visceral	Activated by a distortion, stretching, ischemia, or invasion of an organ; by A (delta) and C fibers [12]	Deep, squeezing, cramping pain, often diffuse, poorly localized, sometimes accompanied by nausea and vomiting	Tumor-related pain in organs; irritable bowel syndrome; pancreatitis	Complicated by the extensive nerve structures of some internal organs	Opioid therapy is a first-line approach; opioid-induced constipation ("narcotic bowel syndrome") must be considered [126]	Antidepressants may be helpful; for inflammation, corticosteroids may be used. If bacterial infection is present, antibiotics are required. Antispasmodics (hyoscyamine) may help patients with functional abdominal pain [126]
Neuropathic	Mediated by A (delta) and A (beta) fibers and C fibers [12]	Sharp, electrical, "shocking" pain (likely associated with A fibers) and chronic burning sensation (C fibers)	Related to diabetes; induced by chemotherapy	May be accompanied by paradoxical sensations of numbness or lack of feeling	Anticonvulsants may be used as monotherapy in purely neuropathic pain; in multimechanistic pain, opioids may be combined with anticonvulsants	Anticonvulsants should be considered first; antidepressants may also be useful [127]

The use of adjuvant agents must be undertaken with clinical prudence. Many adjuvant agents are associated with potentially treatment-limiting side effects, and the long-term use of certain agents may result in organ toxicity [3]. Adjuvant agents often have a much more narrow therapeutic window than opioids and offer less flexibility in terms of routes of administration. Adjuvants are not useful in managing breakthrough pain, a challenging condition that occurs in both cancer and non-cancer pain syndromes [7]. On the other hand, tolerance—frequently observed with chronic opioid therapy—does not typically occur with the adjuvants discussed in this chapter.

Antidepressants

Mechanisms of Action

While there are clear associations between mental health disorders, chronic pain, and the fact that a patient's affective state can influence pain perception, it is important to preface this section with the fact that the analgesic properties of antidepressants are different and distinct from the antidepressant effects of those same agents [8]. The analgesic benefits of antidepressants typically occur more rapidly and at lower doses than their antidepressant effects [8, 9]. On the other hand, an elevated mood might contribute to overall functional improvement which, in turn, might then contribute to pain relief [10]. Mood and pain may indeed be more closely linked in ways that remain to be elucidated. Evidence has suggested that there may be certain common neurobiological mechanisms involved in mood and pain processing [11].

In simple terms, the primary mechanism of action of tricyclic antidepressants (TCAs) is the blockade of norepinephrine (NE) and serotonin (5-HT) at the spinal dorsal synapses [12]. TCAs may be considered NE and 5-HT reuptake inhibitors, resulting in increased bioavailability of NE and 5-HT in the intersynaptic space. Both NE and 5-HT modulate the dual descending pain pathways in the body that inhibit pain signals [13]. One pain pathway originates at midbrain level in the periaqueductal gray and nucleus raphe magnus (5-HT), while the other pain pathway starts at the locus coeruleus in the medulla (NA) [8]. Our understanding of these pain pathways is not complete. At times these pathways inhibit but at other times may facilitate pain transmission and they likely interact with each other in ways that have not yet been thoroughly described [8]. TCAs may act on or via the endogenous opioid system, and it is known that selective opioid antagonists such as naloxone can negate the analgesic benefits of TCAs [8]. Further, chronic TCA therapy increases endogenous opioid levels and may affect the opioid receptor density in the patient [14].

The mechanisms of analgesic effects of TCAs are extensive and may include the following: monoamine reuptake inhibition, endogenous opioid interactions, NMDA receptor antagonism, immune factor expression modulation, enhancement of gamma-aminobutyric acid beta (GABA$_B$) receptor activity, histamine inhibition [9, 15, 16], and adenosine system involvement [17, 18]. The discovery of peripheral effects of TCAs has given rise to work on topical formulations for analgesia [19]. TCAs are also known to block ion channels and antagonize N-methyl-d-aspartate (NMDA) receptors [8]. The role of glutamate, a key neurotransmitter in centralized pain sensation, is to allow calcium to enter the cell via the NMDA receptor. In this way, glutamate acts to prolong cellular depolarization and may activate other neurotransmitters. In other words, NMDA allows for a higher level of intracellular calcium, which has been associated with chronic pain. One function of TCAs is to antagonize the NMDA receptor and, in that way, lower intercellular calcium levels [8]. TCAs may affect sodium and potassium ion channels as well. Indeed, the effect of TCAs on sodium channels has long been evident from electrocardiograms, showing that TCAs can prolong the cardiac QRS interval [20].

TCAs are considered a first-line approach to neuropathic pain [21–23], mainly on account of their strong NA and 5-HT reuptake inhibition plus their sodium and calcium channel blockade [9, 16]. Thus, TCAs may be considered for patients with pure neuropathic pain, such as fibromyalgia, or for patients with multimechanistic chronic pain with a neuropathic component. Furthermore, TCAs may be considered as adjuvant agents for patients with nociceptive and/or inflammatory pain. In this context, it is important for the clinician and patient to recognize that the analgesic contributions of TCAs are typically modest and may involve side effects [24]. Despite our growing knowledge about neuropathy and numerous recent break-throughs in pharmacology, clinicians should recognize that about 30 % of neuro-pathic pain patients will not respond well to even optimized pharmacotherapy and a substantial subset of these poor responders may be refractory to all forms of medical analgesia [25].

As a rule of thumb, TCAs are more effective for pain control than selective sero-tonin reuptake inhibitors (SSRIs) because TCAs are less selective. The number needed to treat (NNT) for 50 % relief of neuropathic pain is 6.7 for SSRI therapy compared to 2.4 for TCAs [8]. Many TCAs and SSRIs are commercially available; the most commonly prescribed agents include amitriptyline (tertiary amine) and nortriptyline (secondary amine which is actually the demethylated metabolite of amitriptyline). There is a paucity of high-quality evidence in terms of head-to-head clinical trials.

Clinical Efficacy

In an open-label study of 228 peripheral neuropathy patients which found amitriptyline and nortriptyline to be similarly effective and tolerated, the use of TCAs reduced pain on a visual analog scale by 23–26 % [26]. This reduction in pain intensity occurred whether the agents were used as monotherapy or adjuvants to another pharmacological regimen. In a double-blind study of diabetic and non-diabetic painful polyneuropathy patients, amitriptyline and maprofiline pro-vided significantly better pain relief than placebo at week 4 of the study ($p < 0.001$

and $p < 0.01$, respectively) with no significant difference between amitriptyline and maprofiline [27]. A systematic review of the use of amitriptyline in neuropathic pain and fibromyalgia patients (21 studies, $n = 1437$) recommended that amitriptyline be used as part of the treatment for neuropathic pain or fibromyalgia, although evidence in support of the drug was limited [28]. A similar review (5 studies, $n = 177$) found little evidence to support for desipramine for neuropathic pain [29]. However, a systematic review of various two-drug combination pharmacotherapy for neuropathic pain (including various regimens such as an opioid plus a TCA, an anticonvulsant plus a TCA, and fluphenazine plus TCA, among others) found all of these two-drug combinations to be effective (21 studies, $n = 578$) [30]. Gabapentin plus a TCA (nortriptyline) was shown to be more effective in treating neuropathic pain than either drug alone in a double-blind study of 45 patients with diabetic polyneuropathy or postherpetic neuralgia [31].

Amitriptyline combined with chronic behavioral therapy was effective in reducing the number of total headache days for pediatric patients suffering from chronic migraines (from a mean of 21/28 days to 6.8/28 days) [32]. Amitriptyline plus stress management programs have been effective for reducing tension headaches in adults [33]. Moreover, these studies suggest the important role non-pharmacological treatments can play in chronic pain control.

A meta-analysis of studies of duloxetine (a serotonin–norepinephrine reuptake inhibitor) monotherapy found that duloxetine was effective in treating painful diabetic peripheral neuropathy at doses of 60–120 mg/day, but lower doses were not effective (18 trials, $n = 6407$) [34]. Duloxetine was part of an effective multimodal regimen for controlling pain associated with chronic prostatitis or chronic pelvic pain ($n = 38$, drug regimen consisted of duloxetine, alpha blockade, and saw palmetto extract) [35].

In order to achieve greater than 50 % relief with venlafaxine in patients with painful diabetic neuropathy, the NNT was 4.5 [36]. Venlafaxine was shown to reduce postoperative analgesic requirements [37], effectively treat painful neuropathy [38], and relieve headache pain [39, 40].

Clinical experience with these drugs plus the literature support their use for certain chronic pain patients, providing prescribers and patients do not overestimate their contribution to total pain control.

Adverse Events

The rate of adverse events with TCA can be considerable. In the study of 228 neuropathy patients, about one-third of the patients (26–37 %) discontinued TCA therapy because of adverse events [26]. Among the most commonly reported adverse events associated with TCAs are drowsiness, sexual dysfunction, weight gain, dry mouth, constipation, and blurred vision [8]. Since TCAs may prolong the QRS interval and could in that way trigger arrhythmias [20], they may be contraindicated in patients with heart disease, prior myocardial infarction, or history of

Table 8.3 A list of selected TCAs and SSRIs that may be considered as adjuvant agents for chronic pain patients

Drug	Mechanism of action	Considerations
Amitriptyline	One of the best known and most prescribed TCAs, potent sodium channel blocker	May have a peripherally mediated analgesic effect [128]
Clomipramine	A highly selective serotonin reuptake inhibitor used as primary treatment for obsessive–compulsive disorder	A retrospective analysis ($n = 1997$) found that diabetes was significantly higher in patients treated with clomipramine than those not treated (26 % vs. 8 %, $p < 0.00001$) [129]
Desipramine	A selective norepinephrine reuptake inhibitor with minor effect on serotonin. It is the active metabolite of imipramine	May have a peripherally mediated analgesic effect [130]
Duloxetine	A serotonin–norepinephrine reuptake inhibitor (SNRI) with a short half-life and elevated risk for withdrawal symptoms if discontinued suddenly [24]	May be effective in reducing chronic pain associated with osteoarthritis [131] May be an effective adjuvant agent for diabetic peripheral neuropathy, fibromyalgia, chronic musculoskeletal pain, and low back pain [132]
Fluoxetine	A frequently prescribed SSRI and also a selective brain steroidogenic stimulator; it has no appreciable effect on norepinephrine reuptake	May have a peripherally mediated analgesic effect [130]
Imipramine	A tertiary amine that inhibits both serotonin and norepinephrine reuptake	The first TCA approved to treat depression in the USA in 1958 [8] and whose analgesic effects were already discussed in the literature by 1960 [133]
Milnacipran	An SNRI which is conjugated to the inactive glucuronide and excreted renally. Strong selective noradrenaline reuptake inhibitor [134]	Recently approved in the USA for the treatment of fibromyalgia
Mirtazapine	A noradrenergic and specific serotonergic antidepressant (NaSSA) with side effects similar to venlafaxine; appears to activate opioid-mediated analgesia [8]	Has a unique side effect profile and is associated with increased appetite and weight gain but is less likely to cause nausea, vomiting, or sexual dysfunction [135]
Nortriptyline	The active metabolite of amitriptyline	
Venlafaxine	Blocks reuptake of noradrenaline and 5-HT and is relatively free of muscarinic cholinergic, histaminic, and alpha-adrenergic receptor activity [8]. Analgesic action appears to involve endogenous opioid system [136]	May be most promising TCA for analgesia [8], but caution is advised with respect to serotonin syndrome

arrhythmias [8]. However, a recent study from Japan ($n = 87$) found that median daily doses of 25 mg/day of amitriptyline or 10 mg/day of nortriptyline resulted in a QRS prolongation of ≤60 ms and did not provoke any hazardous rhythm disorders [41].

Prescribing Considerations

TCAs are metabolized via the cytochrome P450 (CYP450) enzyme and the isoenzyme CYP2D6 [12]. About 10 % of Caucasians have a mutated CYP2D6 gene which can affect their ability to metabolize this drug, making them poor metabolizers [12]. Thus, some patients will not respond well to TCA therapy and others discontinue otherwise effective therapy because of adverse events. When prescribing TCAs, it is important to consider if the patient is taking other drugs that affect 5-HT because of the possibility of serotonin syndrome (discussed later in this chapter) [42].

While TCAs are not associated with tolerance, as are opioids, they can cause dependence with the result that their abrupt discontinuation may provoke withdrawal symptoms that include headache, nausea, vomiting, and extreme malaise [43]. To discontinue long-term TCA therapy, taper the drug gradually under close clinical supervision [43].

There are several different types of TCAs and SSRIs available and multiple commercial products (see Table 8.3). Patients who suffer side effects or do not find a particular drug effective may benefit from another type of TCA.

Anticonvulsants

Mechanism of Action

Anticonvulsants decrease ectopic neuronal activity and stabilize neuronal cell membranes through modulation of the voltage-gated sodium or calcium ion channels. These drugs may inhibit sodium channels (phenytoin, lamotrigine, and others) or inhibit calcium channels (gabapentinoids, that is, gabapentin and pregabalin) and are widely used in the treatment of seizure disorders [12, 44]. A particularly well-known anticonvulsant, gabapentin, is an analog of the gamma-aminobutyric acid (GABA), a substance which, among other things, regulates conduction across calcium ion channels. The analgesic effects of anticonvulsants may be explained by the fact that demyelinated or injured nerves display a redistribution of ion channels which appear to contribute to ectopic hyperexcitability. While all anticonvulsants have different mechanisms of action, they all decrease this ectopic hyperexcitability [45, 46].

Neuropathic pain has been associated with excessive ectopic activity near the areas of damaged nerve cells and/or near the dorsal root ganglion [47]. Chronic pain exhibits a characteristic activation of spinal glia, and recent preclinical work has found that gabapentin can decrease the activation of spinal glia [48]. Further, gabapentin may act on the supraspinal regions to stimulate NE-mediated descending inhibition, a contributor to neuropathic pain [49].

Gabapentinoids and antidepressants are recommended as frontline treatments for chronic neuropathic pain or chronic pain with a neuropathic component [50–52]. Gabapentinoids include gabapentin and the newer agent, pregabalin. Pregabalin is a lipophilic analog of GABA which is inactive at the GABA receptors [53]. Pregabalin may be titrated more rapidly than gabapentin [12]. But both agents are associated with potentially treatment-limiting adverse events. The therapeutic window of gabapentinoids can be relatively narrow. Preclinical studies suggest that low-dose pregabalin can improve analgesia when combined with morphine in a dose-dependent fashion, but only at low doses and not at high doses (defined as ≥17 mg/kg) [54].

A meta-analysis of anticonvulsants used for painful diabetic neuropathy, postherpetic neuralgia, central neuropathic pain, or fibromyalgia found evidence to support only gabapentin and pregabalin; for the many other anticonvulsants, the evidence to support their use is less clear [55]. It should be noted that for some chronic pain patients, anticonvulsants may improve quality of life or function rather than relieve pain, and these improvements may contribute to a holistic improvement that is not specifically a pain reduction.

Carbamazepine, another anticonvulsant, appears to inhibit voltage-gated sodium channels and, in that way, reduce inflammatory pain [56]. It may be used to treat trigeminal neuralgia and other chronic myofascial pain syndromes. Levetiracetam is a novel anticonvulsant agent which appears to exert a synergistic antihyperalgesic effect against inflammatory pain when combined with a nonsteroidal anti-inflammatory drug (NSAID) plus caffeine [57]. Topiramate and valproate are anticonvulsants that have been effective in the treatment of episodic migraine [58] and neuropathic pain [59].

Clinical Efficacy

In a study of 120 cancer patients with neuropathic pain, patients were randomized to receive either oral pregabalin monotherapy or transdermal fentanyl monotherapy for 28 days. At the end of the study, significantly more pregabalin-only patients reported ≥30 % reduction of pain measured on a visual analog scale compared to the fentanyl-only patients ($p < 0.001$). Moreover, the pregabalin group had fewer adverse events and a higher degree of patient-reported satisfaction with their treatment [60].

In a systematic review (16 randomized clinical trials), gabapentin for postoperative pain control significantly decreased opioid consumption and at doses

<1200 mg significantly reduced pain intensity. The use of gabapentin in this study was associated with a significantly higher risk of sedation, but a lower rate of vomiting and pruritus [61]. However, the use of gabapentin for acute burn pain management did not reduce pain score or reduce opioid consumption ($n = 50$) [62].

In a study of 101 total knee arthroplasty patients, patients were randomized to receive oral gabapentin 600 mg preoperatively followed by oral gabapentin 200 mg every 8 h for two days or placebo. All patients received oral acetaminophen 1 g and oral ketorolac 15 mg preoperatively and then patient-controlled anesthesia (PCA) with morphine following surgery along with oral acetaminophen 1 g plus oral ketorolac 15 mg every six hours. At 72 h, cumulative morphine consumption was 66.3 mg in the gabapentin group compared to 72.5 mg in the placebo group ($p = 0.59$) and pain scores at rest or with movement, patient satisfaction scores, and hospital lengths of stay were similar between groups [63]. In another study of 262 total knee arthroplasty patients, patients who were administered pregabalin plus opioid analgesia had significantly lower rates of postsurgical respiratory, renal, or hemodynamic complications compared to those who received opioid therapy alone [64].

In a randomized, double-blind study of 64 patients undergoing internal fixation of the tibia under spinal anesthesia, patients received either a single dose of oral gabapentin 300 mg or placebo following surgery. This study found no significant differences in pain intensity scores at 2, 12, and 24 h after surgery [65]. On the other hand, in a study of 80 craniotomy patients randomized to receive oral gabapentin (3 doses of 400 mg) or oral phenytoin (3 doses of 100 mg) for a seven-day period that spanned the preoperative to postoperative phases, gabapentin patients had significantly lower postoperative pain intensity scores and less morphine consumption [66]. Patients with persistent pain following spinal surgery reported significantly better pain control with gabapentin at a maximum daily dose of 1800 mg compared to naproxen at a maximum daily dose of 1500 mg [67].

Chronic pancreatitis may be associated with moderate to very severe visceral pain. In a study of 64 chronic pancreatitis patients, patients were randomized to receive pregabalin or placebo. At three weeks, more patients in the pregabalin group had more effective pain relief than placebo patients (36 % vs. 24 %, respectively, mean difference 12 %, $p = 0.02$) [68]. Functional status, quality of life, and adverse events were similar in both groups.

Adverse Events

Adverse events associated with anticonvulsant agents are common and may be treatment-limiting. Some of the most frequently reported adverse events include drowsiness, headache, and increased appetite [69]. Intriguing work is ongoing to develop an aqueous pregabalin solution for possible transdermal drug delivery, thus minimizing or even preventing this agent's potential central nervous system (CNS) side effects [70]. Effective July 28, 2005, the Deputy Administrator of the

Drug Enforcement Administration (DEA) issued a final rule to place pregabalin [(S)-3-(aminomethyl)-5-methylhexanoic acid] including its salts and all products containing pregabalin into Schedule V of the Controlled Substances Act (CSA). It is estimated that approximately 10 % of patients studied exhibited "likability" of the drug, hence prompting the scheduling of the drug. As a result of this rule, the regulatory controls and criminal sanctions of Schedule V will be applicable to the manufacture, distribution, dispensing, importation, and exportation of pregabalin and products containing pregabalin [71]. A rare but troubling side effect associated with pregabalin is self-harm [69, 72], while carbamazepine, oxcarbamazepine, valproate, and lamotrigine appear to possess antisuicidal properties [73]. Topiramate, tiagabine, vigabatrin, levetiracetam, and zonisamide are anticonvulsants which may exert negative effects on mood and cognition, but whose association with suicide has not been well established [73].

Many drugs, including anticonvulsants and SSRIs, may negatively impact bone metabolism and have been associated with osteoporosis [74, 75].

Side effects of anticonvulsants can vary by agent. Carbamazepine has been associated with side effects such as drowsiness, dizziness, constipation, ataxia, and hepatotoxicity and in rare cases aplastic anemia [12]. Oxcarbamazepine has no known hepatic adverse events, but has been associated with potentially life-threatening hyponatremia [12]. Phenytoin has been associated with gait abnormalities, nausea and vomiting, and sedation [12].

Myorelaxants

Mechanism of Action

Myorelaxants can be grouped into two broad categories with different mechanisms of action, tolerability profiles, and indications: the antispastics and the antispasmodics [76]. Antispastics, such as baclofen and dantrolene, work on the spinal cord or skeletal muscles to improve muscle hypertonicity and relieve involuntary spasms. Antispasmodics also reduce muscle spasms, but they accomplish this by . altering conduction through the CNS. Antispasmodics can be further divided into benzodiazepines (which inhibit transmission of the postsynaptic gamma-aminobutyric acid or GABA neurons) and non-benzodiazepines, which act on the brain stem and spinal cord [77]. Benzodiazepines can be further subdivided into sedative agents, anxiolytics, and anticonvulsants. Non-benzodiazepine antispasmodics are the most frequently prescribed agents for chronic painful conditions such as low back pain and include agents such as carisoprodol, cyclobenzaprine, metaxalone, and methocarbamol [76].

Carisoprodol is an oral, centrally acting, skeletal muscle relaxant indicated for the treatment of acute musculoskeletal pain. Its mechanism of action involves altered neuronal communication at the reticular formation and spinal cord, which, in turn, reduces pain perception [78]. Carisoprodol is indicated for short-term treatment of two to three weeks. Its association with side effects has placed it on the Beers list (risks of side effects outweigh potential benefits of treatment) [79]. Carisoprodol is metabolized via the CYP2C19 enzyme with meprobamate as the active metabolite; meprobamate is a Schedule IV controlled substance with anxiolytic effects [76]. The accumulation of metabolites may exacerbate CNS side effects with long-term use. Patients who have taken carisoprodol long term should not discontinue the drug abruptly as they may experience withdrawal symptoms, including anxiety, irritability, tremors, muscle twitches, and ataxia [80, 81].

With a structure similar to TCAs, cyclobenzaprine is a muscle relaxant thought to act on the supraspinal area of the brain stem as an agonist at the descending noradrenergic neurons [82]. Cyclobenzaprine offers serotonergic antagonism, but its mechanism of action as an antispasmodic is not entirely clear [82]. Indicated for acute musculoskeletal pain unrelated to a CNS condition, it is sometimes prescribed off-label for fibromyalgia pain [83]. Cyclobenzaprine has a half-life of 36 h and, for that reason, should be prescribed only with clinical caution in the elderly [84]. Cyclobenzaprine is intended for short-term use.

Although frequently considered as a muscle relaxant, metaxalone is actually a CNS depressant whose mechanism of action is sedative rather than antispasmodic [76]. Metaxalone is metabolized via CY-450 isoenzymes 1A2, 2D6, 2E1, and 3A4 [85]. When compared to other muscle relaxants such as cyclobenzaprine and carisoprodol, metaxalone has the fewest reports of side effects and the least safety issues [86].

Clinical Efficacy

Myorelaxants are typically prescribed to help treat myalgia and musculoskeletal conditions, including chronic low back pain (cLBP) [87, 88]. Antispastics, such as baclofen, are often prescribed for patients with cerebral palsy, multiple sclerosis, or spinal cord injury [89]. Guidelines for cLBP recommend acetaminophen or NSAIDs as first-line treatment with muscle relaxants recommended if those first-line agents fail [77]. There is no strong evidence in the literature supporting the use of muscle relaxants in patients with inflammatory arthritis or rheumatoid arthritis [90, 91]. However, muscle relaxants may be helpful in the short-term setting for relieving a flare of muscle spasms. About a third of patients (35 %) with non-specific back pain will be prescribed some form of muscle relaxant [87, 88, 92, 93], but their use may be controversial because of potential side effects, added costs, and limited effectiveness [76]. Muscle relaxants may be more widely prescribed than stated above; in a prospective cohort study, a secondary analysis of data from 1633 patients who sought medical attention for acute back pain found that 64 % were prescribed a muscle relaxant [94]. Muscle relaxants are appropriate for short-term use, even in the setting of chronic pain, although data suggest that a substantial number of patients are on long-term muscle relaxant therapy [95].

In placebo-controlled clinical studies, skeletal muscle relaxants have been shown to offer short-term relief of acute low back pain [93, 96]. There are few direct comparative studies of muscle relaxants in cLBP patients, with the result that there is little guidance for the clinician in selecting one particular agent over others. An older study found carisoprodol more effective than diazepam [97]. A more recent meta-analysis (8 studies, $n = 2030$) of carisoprodol, cyclobenzaprine, and metaxalone found carisoprodol and metaxalone effective in treating low back pain [98].

Eperisone (a centrally acting muscle relaxant) combined with tramadol was compared to tizanidine plus tramadol in 60 cLBP patients [99]. Both drug combinations resulted in significant pain reduction versus baseline; the two groups did not differ statistically from each other, except that significantly fewer eperisone patients experienced somnolence (16.6 % vs. 43.3 %, respectively) [99]. Eperisone was found to be an effective pain reliever in a study of 240 low back pain patients with acute muscle spasms randomized to eperisone 150 mg/day or placebo [100]. In a double-blind study of patients with acute lower back spasms ($n = 285$), carisoprodol (250 mg three times a day) was significantly more effective than placebo in patient-rated global impression of change ($p < 0.0001$) [101]. Cyclobenzaprine extended-release formulation was effective in treating muscle spasm associated with painful back and neck conditions after four days of treatment in two identically designed studies with a total of 834 patients [102]. A pooled analysis ($n = 504$) likewise reported cyclobenzaprine extended-release was effective in relieving acute muscle spasm [103].

Adverse Events

While skeletal muscle relaxants can provide short-term relief for acute low back pain, they increase the risk of adverse events by 50 % [93, 96]. Among the most commonly reported side effects are sedation, headaches, and visual disturbances [76]. Other adverse events reported with the use of myorelaxants include drowsiness, fatigue, and dizziness [98]. The safety of these drugs may involve more than the traditional adverse event report. A recent retrospective study in Norway found that patients with a carisoprodol prescription were at elevated risk for traffic accidents involving personal injury (incidence ratio 3.7, 95 % confidence interval, 2.9–4.8) [104], suggesting that the drug may be associated with psychomotor impairment. Patients taking these drugs should be appropriately counseled about driving.

Cyclobenzaprine has anticholinergic effects (dry mouth, burry vision, constipation, urinary retention) as well as dizziness, drowsiness, and possible prolongation of the QT interval [84]. Common side effects of metaxalone include dizziness, drowsiness, nausea, and vomiting; it should not be taken by patients with severe hepatic and/or renal dysfunction [85]. The antispasmodic agent dantrolene carries a black box warning for hepatotoxicity [89].

Because muscle relaxants are associated with CNS adverse events, they should be used with great clinical caution (if at all) in geriatric patients who are at particular risk of anticholinergic adverse events, sedative effects, and potential falls [79]. In a case-control study of Medicare patients, the use of skeletal muscle relaxants had been associated with a 40 % increased risk of fracture (adjusted odds ratio 1.40, 95 % confidence interval 1.15–1.72, $p < 0.001$) [105].

Although the literature reports comparatively little about muscle relaxant abuse, over 50,000 emergency department (ED) visits were caused by muscle relaxant misuse or abuse in 2011 [106]. The most frequently misused muscle relaxants were carisoprodol and cyclobenzaprine [106]. Carisoprodol may be abused in order to enhance the effects of other drugs, particularly the sedating effects; it may mitigate the jitteriness accompanying cocaine use and smooth out the "bumps" between ingestions in steady cocaine abusers. Carisoprodol may also have a synergistic effect on relaxation and euphoria produced by more familiar drugs of abuse, such as opioids [107]. In 2012, carisoprodol was added to Schedule IV of the CSA [76]. The abuse potential of carisoprodol is not trivial. In a survey of patients taking carisoprodol for three months or longer ($n = 40$), half had a history of substance abuse. Of those individuals ($n = 20$), 40 % said they took more carisoprodol than prescribed, 10 % said they took it for reasons other than why it was prescribed, and 5 % said they used it to counteract the effects of other drugs [108].

Muscle relaxants also pose a danger for patients with suicidal ideation. Nearly 5 % of attempted suicides involve the use of a muscle relaxant as the primary agent, about half of which involved cyclobenzaprine [106].

Prescribing Considerations

Muscle relaxants may offer relief to patients dealing with muscle spasms in the setting of chronic musculoskeletal pain. Muscle relaxants are intended for short-term use, and indeed, clinical prudence dictates short-term use owing to their potential side effects and tolerability issues. There are numerous muscle relaxants available; clinicians should consider tolerability and adverse events when making a selection as these can vary among drugs.

Serotonin Syndrome

Serotonin syndrome may occur when a patient takes agent(s) which increase serotonergic agonism in the central and peripheral nervous system serotonergic receptors [109]. Symptoms include neuromuscular hyperactivity (such as tremor, clonus), autonomic hyperactivity (including diaphoresis, fever, tachycardia), and altered mental state (including agitation and excitement). The increasing use of drugs with some degree of serotonergic activity makes this condition increasingly prevalent. It may be potentially life-threatening, but can be managed effectively when diagnosed early [110].

The Hunter Serotonin Toxicity Criteria is a useful diagnostic tool; cyproheptadine may be used as an antidote, and moderate to severe cases may require hospitalization [111]. The sudden onset of new or worsening headache together with the use of serotonergic drugs may be a presenting feature of serotonin syndrome [112]. Potentially dangerous drugs with respect to serotonin syndrome may include combinations of TCAs, SSRIs, monoamine oxidase inhibitors (MAOIs), and the opioid agent tramadol [113]. Note that tramadol is not necessarily contraindicated for use with all of these agents, although it is contraindicated in patients taking MAOIs [114]. Other factors that can contribute to serotonin syndrome include advanced age, higher doses, and the use of other agents which inhibit the CYP450-2D6 substrate [114].

Present and Future Challenges in the Use of Adjuvant Agents for Chronic Pain

Patients with chronic pain often take multiple medications, and multimodal therapy is often advocated for such patients to address multimechanistic painful conditions. In a survey of 224 pain patients (average pain duration 10.3 years), the Medication Quantification Scale III (MQS-III) test was used to measure potential harm exposure [115]. In this survey, medications were grouped into four analgesic categories: simple analgesics, adjuvants, opioids, and benzodiazepines. Ten percent of respondents took medications from all four categories, 35 % took medicine from three of the four categories, and 37 % took medicine from two categories. Eighty percent of respondents took opioids. Patients taking multiple medications had higher harm exposure, and the greatest risk for harm came from medicines other than opioids [115]. This is not to minimize the potential harms of opioid therapy but rather to emphasize to clinicians that all drugs, especially adjuvant therapy, be carefully considered for use in individual patients.

Polypharmacy carries with it the risk of potential pharmacokinetic drug–drug interactions. When adding new agents to the patient's pharmacological regimen, clinicians should be mindful of potential interactions, which can be dangerous to the patients and burdensome to the healthcare system [116–119].

Prescribers often face challenges in selecting agents for multimodal pharmacotherapy, and there are few direct head-to-head comparisons of specific categories of agents. This may be due to the fact that the Food and Drug Administration (FDA) relies primarily on placebo-controlled studies for drug approvals and not comparative trials. Regardless of the reasons, there is a paucity of high-quality evidence in the literature to advocate for certain specific agents over others, and this situation is unlikely to change. For that reason, prescribers should familiarize themselves with the agents and select drugs most appropriate for individual patients. Adjuvant agents that are not well tolerated by the patient may be discontinued (usually by tapering) and other agents selected.

Finally, it is important that clinicians neither overestimate nor undervalue the effect of adjuvant agents in a multimodal regimen for chronic pain control. In many cases, the contribution of an adjuvant agent to the patient's overall pain control may be modest. Some adjuvants improve the patient's holistic status (e.g., functional improvement or better sleep) rather than offer substantial pain control. For chronic pain patients struggling with daily life, these can be important benefits.

Prescribing Choices

The literature offers some important studies that compare drug categories (for instance, antidepressants versus anticonvulsants) in pain patients. For example, in a study of 257 patients with diabetic peripheral neuropathy, patients were randomized to receive carbamazepine, venlafaxine, or pregabalin for pain control as assessed with a visual analog scale. Pregabalin was more effective than carbamazepine and venlafaxine; the latter two drugs were similar in efficacy [120]. All of the patients in this study showed improvements in sleep, mood, and productivity. It should be noted that in this study, drugs were administered as monotherapy, not as adjuncts.

In a study of 88 adult cancer patients with neuropathic pain, patients were administered oral tramadol for pain control and one group received gabapentin as an adjuvant agent, while the other group received amitriptyline. At six months, both groups derived similar analgesic relief; there was no significant difference in terms of efficacy, safety, or rate of adverse events [121]. A comparative study of gabapentin monotherapy versus amitriptyline monotherapy for peripheral neuropathic pain found similar pain relief for both groups, although gabapentin was more effective for treating paroxysmal shooting pain [122].

Adjuvant agents may be combined together. In a study of 52 cancer patients with neuropathic pain, low-dose gabapentin (200 mg every 12 h) combined with imipramine (10 mg every 12 h) was more effective in reducing pain than either gabapentin or imipramine monotherapy [123]. In a study of 37 cancer patients with painful bone metastases prescribed opioid therapy, patients were randomized to three groups: Group one took oral pregabalin 60 mg every 8 h, group two took oral pregabalin 25 mg every 8 h plus oral imipramine 5 mg every 12 h, and the third group took oral pregabalin 25 mg every 8 h and 7.5 mg of oral mirtazapine every 12 h. All three regimens provided effective pain control, and the combination adjuvant groups (pregabalin and imipramine or pregabalin or mirtazapine) had significantly greater pain relief than the patient group receiving pregabalin alone [124].

In a randomized clinical trial of 75 cancer patients with painful neuropathy, patients were assigned to group A with fixed doses of oxycodone and escalating doses of pregabalin or group B with fixed doses of pregabalin and escalating doses of oxycodone [125]. Patients were evaluated at 3, 7, 10, and 14 days by a numerical rating scale, a neuropathic pain scale, and a scale for their well-being. Both groups reported effective control of their neuropathic pain, but more patients in group A achieved ≥1/3 overall pain reduction than group B (76 % vs. 64 %, respectively) and side effects were lower in group A (constipation 52.8 % vs. 66.7 %; nausea 27.8 % vs. 44.4 %; drowsiness 44.4 % vs. 55.6 %; confusion 16.7 % vs. 27.8 %; pruritus 8.3 % vs. 19.4 % for groups A and B, respectively) [125]. In this study, both treatment options were effective, but group A could be considered clinically preferable to group B.

Conclusion

Chronic pain can be a devastating condition for patients and a challenge for clinicians to treat. Growing understanding of the multimechanistic nature of chronic pain has given rise to multimodal pharmacotherapy, including the use of chronic opioid therapy plus one or more adjuvant agents. Although there are many drugs that can be considered adjuvants in this context, antidepressants, anticonvulsants, and myorelaxants are likely the most familiar and are widely prescribed. Antidepressants and anticonvulsants have analgesic properties apart from their main actions. Muscle relaxants can help provide relief to patients suffering muscle spasms in the setting of musculoskeletal pain, but their use often improves overall well-being rather than providing pain relief. Antidepressants, anticonvulsants, and muscle relaxants may offer greater relief to chronic pain patients, but they present clinical challenges in terms of managing tolerability, toxicity, and drug–drug interactions associated with polypharmacy. Adjuvant agents should be prescribed with clinical caution, usually for short-term rather than long-term use, and monitored closely. Patients should be advised of potential side effects and encouraged to report adverse events. Clinicians should be mindful of the potential for serotonin syndrome, a potentially life-threatening adverse event that can be readily and safely managed when diagnosed early. Adjuvant agents offer great hope for chronic pain patients but must be used prudently.

References

1. Rasu RS, Vouthy K, Crowl AN, Stegeman AE, Fikru B, Bawa WA, et al. Cost of pain medication to treat adult patients with nonmalignant chronic pain in the United States. J Managed Care Pharm JMCP. 2014;20(9):921–8 Epub 2014/08/29.
2. Lussier D, Portenoy R. Adjuvant analgesics in pain management. In: Doyle D, Hanks G, Christakis N, editors. Oxford textbook of palliative medicine. 3rd ed. Oxford, England: Oxford University Press; 2003. pp. 349–77.
3. Khan MI, Walsh D, Brito-Dellan N. Opioid and adjuvant analgesics: compared and contrasted. Am J Hospice Palliat Care. 2011;28(5):378–83 Epub 2011/05/31.
4. Gilron I, Max M. Combination pharmacotherapy for neuropathic pain: current evidence and future directions. Expert Rev Neurother. 2005;5(6):823–30.
5. Pergolizzi JV, Gharibo C, Ho KY. Treatment considerations for cancer pain: a global perspective. Pain Pract Official J World Inst Pain. 2014 Epub 2014/12/04.

6. Muller-Schwefe G, Ahlbeck K, Aldington D, Alon E, Coaccioli S, Coluzzi F, et al. Pain in the cancer patient: different pain characteristics CHANGE pharmacological treatment requirements. Curr Med Res Opin. 2014;30(9):1895–908 Epub 2014/05/21.
7. Smith H. A comprehensive review of rapid-onset opioids for breakthrough pain. CNS Drugs. 2012;26(6):509–35 Epub 2012/06/07.
8. Coluzzi F, Mattia C. Mechanism-based treatment in chronic neuropathic pain: the role of antidepressants. Curr Pharm Des. 2005;11(23):2945–60 Epub 2005/09/24.
9. Sawynok J. Antidepressants as analgesics: an introduction. J Psychiatry Neurosci JPN. 2001;26(1):20 Epub 2001/02/24.
10. Robinson MJ, Sheehan D, Gaynor PJ, Marangell LB, Tanaka Y, Lipsius S, et al. Relationship between major depressive disorder and associated painful physical symptoms: analysis of data from two pooled placebo-controlled, randomized studies of duloxetine. Int Clin Psychopharmacol. 2013;28(6):330–8 Epub 2013/07/23.
11. Jaracz J, Gattner K, Moczko J, Hauser J. Comparison of the effects of escitalopram and nortriptyline on painful symptoms in patients with major depression. General Hospital Psychiatry. 2014 Epub 2014/12/07.
12. Mitra R, Jones S. Adjuvant analgesics in cancer pain: a review. Am J Hospice Palliat Care. 2012;29(1):70–9 Epub 2011/06/30.
13. Basbaum A, Fields H. Endogenous pain control mechanisms: review and hypothesis. Ann Neurol. 1978;4:451–62.
14. De Felipe M, De Ceballos M, Gil CF. Chronic antidepressant treatment increases enkephalin levels in nucleus accumbens and striatum of the rat. Eur J Pharmacol. 1985;112:119.
15. Mico J, Ardid D, Berrocoso E, Eschalier A. Antidepressants and pain. Trends Pharmacol Sci. 2006;27:348–54.
16. Sawynok J, Esser MJ, Reid AR. Antidepressants as analgesics: an overview of central and peripheral mechanisms of action. J Psychiatry Neurosci: JPN. 2001;26(1):21–9 Epub 2001/02/24.
17. Liu J, Reid AR, Sawynok J. Spinal serotonin 5-HT7 and adenosine A1 receptors, as well as peripheral adenosine A1 receptors, are involved in antinociception by systemically administered amitriptyline. Eur J Pharmacol. 2013;698(1–3):213–9 Epub 2012/11/13.
18. Sawynok J, Reid AR, Fredholm BB. Caffeine reverses antinociception by amitriptyline in wild type mice but not in those lacking adenosine A1 receptors. Neurosci Lett. 2008;440(2):181–4 Epub 2008/06/20.
19. Sawynok J. Topical and peripherally acting analgesics. Pharmacol Rev. 2003;55(1):1–20 Epub 2003/03/05.
20. Giardina E, Bigger J, Glassman A, Perel J, Kantor S. The electrocardiographic and antiarrhythmic effects of imipramine hydrocloride at therapeutic plasma concentrations. Circulation. 1979;60:1045–52.
21. Moulin DE, Clark AJ, Gilron I, Ware MA, Watson CP, Sessle BJ, et al. Pharmacological management of chronic neuropathic pain—consensus statement and guidelines from the Canadian Pain Society. Pain Res Manage J Can Pain Soc (Journal de la societe canadienne pour le traitement de la douleur). 2007;12(1):13–21 Epub 2007/03/21.
22. Bril V, England J, Franklin GM, Backonja M, Cohen J, Del Toro D, et al. Evidence-based guideline: treatment of painful diabetic neuropathy: report of the American Academy of Neurology, the American Association of Neuromuscular and Electrodiagnostic Medicine, and the American Academy of Physical Medicine and Rehabilitation. Neurology. 2011;76(20):1758–65 Epub 2011/04/13.
23. Finnerup N, Otto M, McQuay H, Jensen T, Sindrup S. Algorithm for neuropathic pain treatment: an evidence based proposal. Pain Manage Nurs Official J Am Soc Pain Manage Nurs. 2005;118:289–305.
24. Watson CP, Gilron I, Sawynok J, Lynch ME. Nontricyclic antidepressant analgesics and pain: are serotonin norepinephrine reuptake inhibitors (SNRIs) any better? Pain. 2011;152(10):2206–10 Epub 2011/07/05.

25. Vranken J. Mechanisms and treatment of neuropathic pain. Cent Nerv Syst Agents Med Chem. 2009;9(1):71–8.
26. Liu WQ, Kanungo A, Toth C. Equivalency of tricyclic antidepressants in open-label neuropathic pain study. Acta Neurol Scand. 2014;129(2):132–41 Epub 2013/08/14.
27. Vrethem M, Boivie J, Arnqvist H, Holmgren H, Lindstrom T, Thorell LH. A comparison a amitriptyline and maprotiline in the treatment of painful polyneuropathy in diabetics and nondiabetics. Clin J Pain. 1997;13(4):313–23 Epub 1998/02/12.
28. Moore RA, Derry S, Aldington D, Cole P, Wiffen PJ. Amitriptyline for neuropathic pain and fibromyalgia in adults. Cochrane Database Syst Rev (Online). 2012;12:CD008242 Epub 2012/12/14.
29. Hearn L, Moore RA, Derry S, Wiffen PJ, Phillips T. Desipramine for neuropathic pain in adults. Cochrane Database Syst Rev (Online). 2014;9:CD011003 Epub 2014/09/24.
30. Chaparro LE, Wiffen PJ, Moore RA, Gilron I. Combination pharmacotherapy for the treatment of neuropathic pain in adults. Cochrane Database Syst Rev (Online). 2012;7: CD008943 Epub 2012/07/13.
31. Gilron I, Bailey JM, Tu D, Holden RR, Jackson AC, Houlden RL. Nortriptyline and gabapentin, alone and in combination for neuropathic pain: a double-blind, randomised controlled crossover trial. Lancet. 2009;374(9697):1252–61 Epub 2009/10/03.
32. Powers SW, Kashikar-Zuck SM, Allen JR, LeCates SL, Slater SK, Zafar M, et al. Cognitive behavioral therapy plus amitriptyline for chronic migraine in children and adolescents: a randomized clinical trial. JAMA, J Am Med Assoc. 2013;310(24):2622–30 Epub 2013/12/26.
33. Holroyd KA, O'Donnell FJ, Stensland M, Lipchik GL, Cordingley GE, Carlson BW. Management of chronic tension-type headache with tricyclic antidepressant medication, stress management therapy, and their combination: a randomized controlled trial. JAMA, J Am Med Assoc. 2001;285(17):2208–15 Epub 2001/05/18.
34. Lunn MP, Hughes RA, Wiffen PJ. Duloxetine for treating painful neuropathy, chronic pain or fibromyalgia. Cochrane Database Syst Rev (Online). 2014;1:CD007115 Epub 2014/01/05.
35. Giannantoni A, Porena M, Gubbiotti M, Maddonni S, Di Stasi SM. The efficacy and safety of duloxetine in a multidrug regimen for chronic prostatitis/chronic pelvic pain syndrome. Urology. 2014;83(2):400–5 Epub 2013/11/16.
36. Rowbotham M, Goli V, Kunz N, Lei D. Venlafaxine extended release in the treatment of painful diabetic neuropathy: a double blind, placebo controlled study. Pain Manage Nurs Official J Am Soc Pain Manage Nurs. 2004;110:697–706.
37. Amr Y, Yousef A. Evaluation of efficacy of the perioperative administration of venlafaxine or gabapentin on acute and chronic post-mastectomy pain. Clin J Pain. 2010;26:381–5.
38. Sindrup S, Bach F, Madsen C, Gram L, Jensen T. Venlafaxine versus imipramine in painful polyneuropathy: a randomized controlled trial. Neurology. 2003;60:1284–9.
39. Ozyalcin S, Talu G, Kizitlan E, Yucel B, Ertas M, Disci R. The efficacy and safety of venlafaxine in the propylaxis of migraine. Headache. 2005;45:144–52.
40. Zissis N, Harmoussi S, Vlaikidis N, Mitsikostas D, Thomaidis T, Georgiadis GS, et al. A randomized, double-blind, placebo-controlled study of venlafaxine XR in out-patients with tension-type headache. Cephalalgia Int J Headache. 2007;27:315–24.
41. Funai Y, Funao T, Ikenaga K, Takahashi R, Hase I, Nishikawa K. Use of tricyclic antidepressants as analgesic adjuvants results in nonhazardous prolongation of the QTc interval. Osaka City Med J. 2014;60(1):11–9 Epub 2014/10/03.
42. Martin T. Serotonin syndrome. Ann Emerg Med. 1996;28(5):520–6.
43. Zajecka J, Fawcett J, Amsterdam J, Quitkin F, Reimherr F, Rosenbaum J, et al. Safety of abrupt discontinuation of fluoxetine: a randomized, placebo-controlled study. J Clin Psychopharmacol. 1998;18(3):193–7.
44. Burchiel K. Carbamezepine inhibits spontaneous activity in experimental neuromaas. Exp Neurol. 1988;102(2):249–53.
45. Devour M. Pathophysiology of injured nerve. In: Wall P, Melzack E, editors. Textbook of pain. 3rd ed. London, England: Churchill Livingstone; 1994. p. 79–100.

46. England JD, Happel LT, Kline DG, Gamboni F, Thouron CL, Liu ZP, et al. Sodium channel accumulation in humans with painful neuromas. Neurology. 1996;47(1):272–6 Epub 1996/07/01.

47. Wall P, Devor M. Sensory afferent impulses originate from dorsal root ganglia as well as from the periphery in normal and nerve injured rats. Pain Manage Nurs Official J Am Soc Pain Manag Nurs. 1983;17(4):321–39.

48. Yang JL, Xu B, Li SS, Zhang WS, Xu H, Deng XM, et al. Gabapentin reduces CX3CL1 signaling and blocks spinal microglial activation in monoarthritic rats. Mol Brain. 2012;5:18 Epub 2012/06/01.

49. Kukkar A, Bali A, Singh N, Jaggi AS. Implications and mechanism of action of gabapentin in neuropathic pain. Arch Pharmacal Res. 2013;36(3):237–51 Epub 2013/02/26.

50. Moulin D, Boulanger A, Clark AJ, Clarke H, Dao T, Finley GA, et al. Pharmacological management of chronic neuropathic pain: revised consensus statement from the Canadian Pain Society. Pain Res Manage J Can Pain Soc (journal de la societe canadienne pour le traitement de la douleur). 2014;19(6):328–35 Epub 2014/12/06.

51. Dworkin RH, O'Connor AB, Backonja M, Farrar JT, Finnerup NB, Jensen TS, et al. Pharmacologic management of neuropathic pain: evidence-based recommendations. Pain. 2007;132(3):237–51 Epub 2007/10/09.

52. O'Connor AB, Dworkin RH. Treatment of neuropathic pain: an overview of recent guidelines. Am J Med. 2009;122(10 Suppl):S22–32 Epub 2009/10/07.

53. Miljevic C, Crnobaric C, Nikolic S, Lecic-Tosevski D. A case of pregabalin intoxication. Psychiatrike = Psychiatriki. 2012;23(2):162–5 Epub 2012/07/17.

54. Shamsi Meymandi M, Keyhanfar F. Assessment of the antinociceptive effects of pregabalin alone or in combination with morphine during acetic acid-induced writhing in mice. Pharmacol Biochem Behav. 2013;110:249–54 Epub 2013/08/08.

55. Wiffen PJ, Derry S, Moore RA, Aldington D, Cole P, Rice AS, et al. Antiepileptic drugs for neuropathic pain and fibromyalgia—an overview of Cochrane reviews. Cochrane Database Syst Rev (Online). 2013;11:CD010567 Epub 2013/11/13.

56. Iwamoto T, Takasugi Y, Higashino H, Ito H, Koga Y, Nakao S. Antinociceptive action of carbamazepine on thermal hypersensitive pain at spinal level in a rat model of adjuvant-induced chronic inflammation. J Anesthesia. 2011;25(1):78–86 Epub 2010/11/30.

57. Tomic MA, Micov AM, Stepanovic-Petrovic RM. Levetiracetam interacts synergistically with nonsteroidal analgesics and caffeine to produce antihyperalgesia in rats. J Pain Official J Am Pain Soc. 2013;14(11):1371–82 Epub 2013/08/21.

58. Miller S. The acute and preventative treatment of episodic migraine. Ann Indian Academy Neurol. 2012;15(Suppl 1):S33–9 Epub 2012/10/02.

59. Smith HS, Argoff CE. Pharmacological treatment of diabetic neuropathic pain. Drugs. 2011;71(5):557–89 Epub 2011/03/30.

60. Raptis E, Vadalouca A, Stavropoulou E, Argyra E, Melemeni A, Siafaka I. Pregabalin vs. opioids for the treatment of neuropathic cancer pain: a prospective, head-to-head, randomized, open-label study. Pain Pract Official J World Inst Pain. 2014;14(1):32–42. Epub 2013/03/08.

61. Ho KY, Gan TJ, Habib AS. Gabapentin and postoperative pain—a systematic review of randomized controlled trials. Pain. 2006;126(1–3):91–101 Epub 2006/07/19.

62. Wibbenmeyer L, Eid A, Liao J, Heard J, Horsfield A, Kral L, et al. Gabapentin is ineffective as an analgesic adjunct in the immediate postburn period. J Burn Care Res Official Publ Am Burn Assoc. 2014;35(2):136–42 Epub 2013/03/21.

63. Paul JE, Nantha-Aree M, Buckley N, Cheng J, Thabane L, Tidy A, et al. Gabapentin does not improve multimodal analgesia outcomes for total knee arthroplasty: a randomized controlled trial. Can J Anaesth (Journal canadien d'anesthesie). 2013;60(5):423–31 Epub 2013/03/13.

64. Sawan H, Chen AF, Viscusi ER, Parvizi J, Hozack WJ. Pregabalin reduces opioid consumption and improves outcome in chronic pain patients undergoing total knee arthroplasty. Physician Sportsmedicine. 2014;42(2):10–8 Epub 2014/05/31.

65. Panah Khahi M, Marashi S, Khajavi MR, Najafi A, Yaghooti A, Imani F. Postoperative gabapentin to prevent postoperative pain: a randomized clinical trial. Anesthesiol Pain Med. 2012;2(2):77–80. Epub 2013/11/14.
66. Ture H, Sayin M, Karlikaya G, Bingol CA, Aykac B, Ture U. The analgesic effect of gabapentin as a prophylactic anticonvulsant drug on postcraniotomy pain: a prospective randomized study. Anesth Analg. 2009;109(5):1625–31 Epub 2009/08/29.
67. Khosravi MB, Azemati S, Sahmeddini MA. Gabapentin versus naproxen in the management of failed back surgery syndrome; a randomized controlled trial. Acta Anaesthesiol Belg. 2014;65(1):31–7 Epub 2014/07/06.
68. Olesen SS, Bouwense SA, Wilder-Smith OH, van Goor H, Drewes AM. Pregabalin reduces pain in patients with chronic pancreatitis in a randomized, controlled trial. Gastroenterology. 2011;141(2):536–43 Epub 2011/06/21.
69. Kustermann A, Mobius C, Oberstein T, Muller HH, Kornhuber J. Depression and attempted suicide under pregabalin therapy. Ann Gen Psychiatry. 2014;13(1):37 Epub 2014/12/10.
70. Fukasawa H, Muratake H, Nagae M, Sugiyama K, Shudo K. Transdermal administration of aqueous pregabalin solution as a potential treatment option for patients with neuropathic pain to avoid central nervous system-mediated side effects. Bio Pharm Bull. 2014;37(11):1816–9 Epub 2014/09/13.
71. Office of diversion control. schedules of controlled substances: placement of Pregabalin into Schedule V. Washington, D.C.: U.S. Department of Justice 2005 [cited 2015 27 February]; Available from: http://www.deadiversion.usdoj.gov/fed_regs/rules/2005/fr0728.htm.
72. Andersohn F, Schade R, Willich SN, Garbe E. Use of antiepileptic drugs in epilepsy and the risk of self-harm or suicidal behavior. Neurology. 2010;75(4):335–40 Epub 2010/07/28.
73. Kalinin VV. Suicidality and antiepileptic drugs: is there a link? Drug Safety Int J Med Toxicol Drug Experience. 2007;30(2):123–42 Epub 2007/01/27.
74. Panday K, Gona A, Humphrey MB. Medication-induced osteoporosis: screening and treatment strategies. Ther Adv Musculoskeletal Dis. 2014;6(5):185–202 Epub 2014/10/25.
75. Wu FJ, Sheu SY, Lin HC. Osteoporosis is associated with antiepileptic drugs: a population-based study. Epileptic Dis Int Epilepsy J Videotape. 2014;16(3):333–42 Epub 2014/08/29.
76. Witenko C, Moorman-Li R, Motycka C, Duane K, Hincapie-Castillo J, Leonard P, et al. Considerations for the appropriate use of skeletal muscle relaxants for the management of acute low back pain. P & T: Peer-Reviewed J Formulary Manage. 2014;39(6):427–35 Epub 2014/07/23.
77. Chou R, Qaseem A, Snow V, Casey D, Cross JT Jr, Shekelle P, et al. Diagnosis and treatment of low back pain: a joint clinical practice guideline from the American College of Physicians and the American Pain Society. Ann Intern Med. 2007;147(7):478–91.
78. DailyMed.com. Carisoprodol. Bethesda, MD: US National Library of Medicine; 2012 [updated January 2012; cited 2014 29 December]; Available from: http://dailymed.nlm.nih.gov/dailymed/drugInfo.cfm?setid=1fa79b11-6491-4543-8548-8aaa624f7ff8#section-1.
79. The American Geriatrics Society 2012 Beers Criteria Expert Panel. American Geriatrics Society updated Beers Criteria for potentially inappropriate medication use in the elderly. J Am Geriatric Soc. 2012;60(4):616–31.
80. Reeves RR, Beddingfield JJ, Mack JE. Carisoprodol withdrawal syndrome. Pharmacotherapy. 2004;24(12):1804–6 Epub 2004/12/09.
81. Gatch MB, Nguyen JD, Carbonaro T, Forster MJ. Carisoprodol tolerance and precipitated withdrawal. Drug Alcohol Depend. 2012;123(1–3):29–34 Epub 2011/11/08.
82. DailyMed.com. AMRIX-cyclobenzaprine hydrochloride capsule, extended release. Bethesda, MD: U.S. National Library of Medicine; 2011 [updated February 2011; cited 2014 29 December]; Available from: http://dailymed.nlm.nih.gov/dailymed/drugInfo.cfm?setid=b8ca1d80-6ea9-4a3f-ab06-beedf845de8f.
83. Carette S, Bell MJ, Reynolds WJ, Haraoui B, McCain GA, Bykerk VP, et al. Comparison of amitriptyline, cyclobenzaprine, and placebo in the treatment of fibromyalgia. A randomized, double-blind clinical trial. Arthritis Rheum. 1994;37(1):32–40 Epub 1994/01/01.

84. Douglass MA, Levine DP. Hallucinations in an elderly patient taking recommended doses of cyclobenzaprine. Arch Intern Med. 2000;160(9):1373.
85. DailyMed.com. Skelaxin-metaxalone tablet. Bethesda, MD: U.S. National Library of Medicine; 2014 [updated April 2014; cited 2014 29 December]; Available from: http://dailymed.nlm.nih.gov/dailymed/drugInfo.cfm?setid=7a4163f2-c553-4d14-7e98-d14c5c7f772a.
86. Harden RN, Argoff C. A review of three commonly prescribed skeletal muscle relaxants. J Back Musculoskelet Rehabil. 2000;15(2):63–6 Epub 2000/01/01.
87. See S, Ginzburg R. Skeletal muscle relaxants. Pharmacotherapy. 2008;28(2):207–13.
88. See S, Ginzburg R. Choosing a skeletal muscle relaxant. Am Fam Physician. 2008;78 (3):365–70.
89. Chou R. Pharmacological management of low back pain. Drugs. 2010;70(4):387–402.
90. Richards BL, Whittle SL, Buchbinder R. Muscle relaxants for pain management in rheumatoid arthritis. Cochrane Database Syst Rev (Online). 2012;1:CD008922 Epub 2012/01/20.
91. Richards BL, Whittle SL, van der Heijde DM, Buchbinder R. The efficacy and safety of muscle relaxants in inflammatory arthritis: a Cochrane systematic review. J Rheumatol Suppl. 2012;90:34–9 Epub 2012/09/04.
92. Luo X, Pietrobon R, Curtis LH, Hey LA. Prescription of non-steroidal anti-inflammatory drugs and muscle relaxants for back pain in the United States. Spine. 2004;29(23):E531–7.
93. van Tulder MW, Touray T, Furlan AD, Solway S, Bouter LM. Muscle relaxants for non-specific low back pain. Cochrane Database Syst Rev (Online). 2003;(2):CD004252 Epub 2003/06/14.
94. Bernstein E, Carey TS, Garrett JM. The use of muscle relaxant medications in acute low back pain. Spine. 2004;29(12):1346–51 Epub 2004/06/10.
95. Dillon C, Paulose-Ram R, Hirsch R, Gu Q. Skeletal muscle relaxant use in the United States: data from the Third National Health and Nutrition Examination Survey (NHANES III). Spine. 2004;29(8):892–6 Epub 2004/04/15.
96. van Tulder MW, Touray T, Furlan AD, Solway S, Bouter LM, Cochrane Back Review G. Muscle relaxants for nonspecific low back pain: a systematic review within the framework of the Cochrane collaboration. Spine. 2003;28(17):1978–92 Epub 2003/09/16.
97. Boyles W, Glassman J, Soyka J. Management of acute musculoskeletal conditions: thoracolumbar strain or sprain. A double-blind evaluation comparing the efficacy and safety of carisoprodol with diazepam. Today's Ther Trends. 1983;1(1–16).
98. Toth PP, Urtis J. Commonly used muscle relaxant therapies for acute low back pain: a review of carisoprodol, cyclobenzaprine hydrochloride, and metaxalone. Clin Ther. 2004;26(9):1355–67 Epub 2004/11/09.
99. Rossi M, Ianigro G, Liberatoscioli G, Di Castelnuovo A, Grimani V, Garofano A, et al. Eperisone versus tizanidine for treatment of chronic low back pain. Minerva Med. 2012;103 (3):143–9 Epub 2012/06/02.
100. Chandanwale AS, Chopra A, Goregaonkar A, Medhi B, Shah V, Gaikwad S, et al. Evaluation of eperisone hydrochloride in the treatment of acute musculoskeletal spasm associated with low back pain: a randomized, double-blind, placebo-controlled trial. J Postgrad Med. 2011;57(4):278–85 Epub 2011/11/29.
101. Ralph L, Look M, Wheeler W, Sacks H. Double-blind, placebo-controlled trial of carisoprodol 250-mg tablets in the treatment of acute lower-back spasm. Curr Med Res Opin. 2008;24(2):551–8 Epub 2008/01/16.
102. Malanga GA, Ruoff GE, Weil AJ, Altman CA, Xie F, Borenstein DG. Cyclobenzaprine ER for muscle spasm associated with low back and neck pain: two randomized, double-blind, placebo-controlled studies of identical design. Curr Med Res Opin. 2009;25(5):1179–96 Epub 2009/03/28.
103. Weil AJ, Ruoff GE, Nalamachu S, Altman CA, Xie F, Taylor DR. Efficacy and tolerability of cyclobenzaprine extended release for acute muscle spasm: a pooled analysis. Postgrad Med. 2010;122(4):158–69 Epub 2010/08/03.

104. Bramness JG, Skurtveit S, Morland J, Engeland A. The risk of traffic accidents after prescriptions of carisoprodol. Accident Anal Prev. 2007;39(5):1050–5 Epub 2007/09/15.
105. Peron EP, Marcum ZA, Boyce R, Hanlon JT, Handler SM. Year in review: medication mishaps in the elderly. Am J Geriatr Pharmacother. 2011;9(1):1–10 Epub 2011/04/05.
106. SAMHSA. Drug abuse warning network, 2011: national estimates of drug-related emergency department visits. Rockville, MD: Health and Human Services; 2013.
107. Reeves RR, Burke RS. Carisoprodol: abuse potential and withdrawal syndrome. Current Drug Abuse Rev. 2010;3(1):33–8.
108. Reeves RR, Carter OS, Pinkofsky HB, Struve FA, Bennett DM. Carisoprodol (soma): abuse potential and physician unawareness. J Addict Dis. 1999;18(2):51–6 Epub 1999/05/20.
109. Boyer EW, Shannon M. The serotonin syndrome. N Engl J Med. 2005;352(11):1112–20 Epub 2005/03/24.
110. Jimenez Andrade JM, Mantyh P. Cancer pain: from the development of mouse models to human clinical trials translational pain research: from mouse to man. Kruger L, Light AR, editors. Boca Raton, FL: Llc.; 2010.
111. Ables AZ, Nagubilli R. Prevention, recognition, and management of serotonin syndrome. Am Fam Physician. 2010;81(9):1139–42 Epub 2010/05/04.
112. Prakash S, Belani P, Trivedi A. Headache as a presenting feature in patients with serotonin syndrome: a case series. Cephalalgia Int J Headache. 2013 Epub 2013/07/06.
113. Breivik H. Pain management discussion forum: serious interaction among frequently used drugs for chronic pain. J Pain Palliat Care Pharmacother. 2014;28(2):170–1 Epub 2014/05/08.
114. Park SH, Wackernah RC, Stimmel GL. Serotonin syndrome: is it a reason to avoid the use of tramadol with antidepressants? J Pharm Pract. 2014;27(1):71–8 Epub 2013/10/25.
115. Giummarra MJ, Gibson SJ, Allen AR, Pichler AS, Arnold CA. Polypharmacy and chronic pain: harm exposure is not all about the opioids. Pain Med (Malden, Mass). 2014 Epub 2014/10/04.
116. Pergolizzi JV. Quantifying the impact of drug-drug interactions associated with opioids. Am J Managed Care. 2011;17(Suppl 11):S288–92 Epub 2011/10/26.
117. Pergolizzi JV, Jr., Labhsetwar SA, Amy Puenpatom R, Ben-Joseph R, Ohsfeldt R, Summers KH. Economic impact of potential CYP450 pharmacokinetic drug-drug interactions among chronic low back pain patients taking opioids. Pain Pract Official J World Inst Pain. 2012;12(1):45–56 Epub 2011/09/20.
118. Pergolizzi JV Jr, Labhsetwar SA, Puenpatom RA, Joo S, Ben-Joseph R, Summers KH. Exposure to potential CYP450 pharmacokinetic drug-drug interactions among osteoarthritis patients: incremental risk of multiple prescriptions. Pain Pract Official J World Inst Pain. 2011;11(4):325–36 Epub 2011/01/05.
119. Pergolizzi JV Jr, Labhsetwar SA, Puenpatom RA, Joo S, Ben-Joseph RH, Summers KH. Prevalence of exposure to potential CYP450 pharmacokinetic drug-drug interactions among patients with chronic low back pain taking opioids. Pain Pract Official J World Inst Pain. 2011;11(3):230–9 Epub 2010/09/03.
120. Razazian N, Baziyar M, Moradian N, Afshari D, Bostani A, Mahmoodi M. Evaluation of the efficacy and safety of pregabalin, venlafaxine, and carbamazepine in patients with painful diabetic peripheral neuropathy. A randomized, double-blind trial. Neurosciences (Riyadh, Saudi Arabia). 2014;19(3):192–8 Epub 2014/07/02.
121. Banerjee M, Pal S, Bhattacharya B, Ghosh B, Mondal S, Basu J. A comparative study of efficacy and safety of gabapentin versus amitriptyline as coanalgesics in patients receiving opioid analgesics for neuropathic pain in malignancy. Indian J Pharmacol. 2013;45(4):334–8 Epub 2013/09/10.
122. Keskinbora K, Pekel AF, Aydinli I. [Comparison of efficacy of gabapentin and amitriptyline in the management of peripheral neuropathic pain]. Agri: Agri (Algoloji) Dernegi'nin Yayin organidir = The journal of the Turkish Society of Algology. 2006;18(2):34–40 Epub 2006/11/08. Periferik noropatik agrinin kontrolunde gabapentin ve amitriptilinin etkinliginin karsilastirilmasi.

123. Arai YC, Matsubara T, Shimo K, Suetomi K, Nishihara M, Ushida T, et al. Low-dose gabapentin as useful adjuvant to opioids for neuropathic cancer pain when combined with low-dose imipramine. J Anesth. 2010;24(3):407–10 Epub 2010/03/11.

124. Nishihara M, Arai YC, Yamamoto Y, Nishida K, Arakawa M, Ushida T, et al. Combinations of low-dose antidepressants and low-dose pregabalin as useful adjuvants to opioids for intractable, painful bone metastases. Pain Physician. 2013;16(5):E547–52 Epub 2013/10/01.

125. Garassino MC, Piva S, La Verde N, Spagnoletti I, Iorno V, Carbone C, et al. Randomised phase II trial (NCT00637975) evaluating activity and toxicity of two different escalating strategies for pregabalin and oxycodone combination therapy for neuropathic pain in cancer patients. PloS One. 2013;8(4):e59981 Epub 2013/04/12.

126. Srinath A, Young E, Szigethy E. Pain management in patients with inflammatory bowel disease: translational approaches from bench to bedside. Inflamm Bowel Dis. 2014;20 (12):2433–49 Epub 2014/09/11.

127. Jongen JL, Huijsman ML, Jessurun J, Ogenio K, Schipper D, Verkouteren DR, et al. The evidence for pharmacologic treatment of neuropathic cancer pain: beneficial and adverse effects. J Pain Symptom Manage. 2013;46(4):581–90 e1 Epub 2013/02/19.

128. Sawynok J, Reid AR, Esser MJ. Peripheral antinociceptive action of amitriptyline in the rat formalin test: involvement of adenosine. Pain. 1999;80(1–2):45–55 Epub 1999/04/16.

129. Mumoli N, Cocciolo M, Vitale J, Mantellassi M, Sabatini S, Gambaccini L, et al. Diabetes mellitus associated with clomipramine treatment: a retrospective analysis. Acta Diabetol. 2014;51(1):167–8 Epub 2013/07/05.

130. Sawynok J, Esser MJ, Reid AR. Peripheral antinociceptive actions of desipramine and fluoxetine in an inflammatory and neuropathic pain test in the rat. Pain. 1999;82(2):149–58 Epub 1999/09/01.

131. Chappel A, Ossanna M, Liu-Seifert H, Ivengar S, Skjarevski V, Li L, et al. Duloxetine, a centrally-acting analgesic in the treatment of patients with osteoarthritis knee pain: a 13 week, randomized, placebo-controlled trial. Pain. 2009;146:253–60.

132. Pergolizzi JV Jr, Raffa RB, Taylor R Jr, Rodriguez G, Nalamachu S, Langley P. A review of duloxetine 60 mg once-daily dosing for the management of diabetic peripheral neuropathic pain, fibromyalgia, and chronic musculoskeletal pain due to chronic osteoarthritis pain and low back pain. Pain Pract Official J World Inst Pain. 2013;13(3):239–52 Epub 2012/06/22.

133. Paoli F. G C, p C. [Prelimary notes on the effect of imipramine in depressed states]. Rev Neurol. 1960;2:503.

134. Mease P. D C. The efficacy and safety of milnacipran for the treatment of fibromyalgia: a randomized, double-blind, placebo-controlled trial. J Rheumatol. 2009;36(2):398–409.

135. Watanabe N, Omori IM, Nakagawa A, Cipriani A, Barbui C, Churchill R, et al. Mirtazapine versus other antidepressive agents for depression. Cochrane Database Syst Rev (Online). 2011(12):CD006528 Epub 2011/12/14.

136. Hall H, Ogren S-O. Effects of antidepressant drugs on different receptors in the brain. Eur J Pharmacol. 1981;70:393–407.

Chapter 9
Complications of Opioid Therapy

Gerald M. Aronoff

Chronic pain is a major public health problem affecting about 30 % of the US population at an estimated $100 billion a year in medical costs, lost workdays, and compensation payments. The frequency and impact of chronic pain is expected to increase over the next decade. It is generally accepted that using accepted principles from the WHO for the management of non-cancer and cancer pain, when patients with moderate to severe pain do not get adequate pain relief from non-opioid analgesics, it often is appropriate to begin treatment with opioid analgesics and to continue to titrate the opioid analgesic medication in combination with non-opioids and adjuvants combined with non-pharmacological management treatments in attempt to control pain and suffering and improve function and quality of life.

Optimal management of chronic pain depends on comprehensive assessment. We still have much to learn about identifying which patients are most appropriate for which treatments, e.g., improving treatment specificity. In their latest joint consensus statement, the AAPM and the APS published in 2009 the *Clinical Guidelines for the Use of Chronic Opioid Therapy in Chronic Noncancer Pain* [1].

There is a subgroup of the non-malignant chronic pain population that can be treated effectively with long-term opioids. With balanced analgesia, often in combination with principles of physical rehabilitation, behavioral medicine, interventional treatments, and cognitive behavioral techniques, these patients can remain active and productive rather than feeling the need to apply for disability because they cannot cope with their pain.

Two important properties of opioids are physical dependence and tolerance. Physical dependence consists of a physiologic property, which occurs after more than several days of continuous opioid use in which either abrupt discontinuation of the drug or administering an opioid antagonist provokes an abstinence syndrome. In

G.M. Aronoff (✉)
Department of Pain Medicine, Carolina Pain Associates,
PA, 1900 Randolph Road, Ste 1016, Charlotte, NC 28207, USA
e-mail: geraldaronoffmd@msn.com

© Springer International Publishing Switzerland 2016
P.S. Staats and S.M. Silverman (eds.), *Controlled Substance
Management in Chronic Pain*, DOI 10.1007/978-3-319-30964-4_9

clinical practice, physical dependence is rarely a problem and should not be viewed as a pathological property of the drug or of the patient. In my experience, when a pain patient has experienced an abstinence syndrome, it has generally been a result of poor communication between the patient and prescribing physician, or an overly aggressive drug taper (initiated by the physician or the patient.) It must be emphasized that drug dependence does not indicate either drug abuse or addiction [2].

General principles in pain management suggest that moderate to severe pain that is not anticipated to last more than a short time period may be more appropriate for immediate-release opioids (if an opioid is clinically indicated), but that sustained-acting, time-released, or long-acting opioid analgesics are often preferred for continuous pain [3]. In addition, based upon studies with cancer patients, when using mu-agonist opioids not in combination with acetaminophen or NSAIDs, there is generally no ceiling dose when using potent opioids for very severe intractable pain, other than the limitations by adverse side effects [4]. Recently, there have been suggestions that opioid dosages for non-cancer pain should be limited because of risks of serious adverse side effects [5] including respiratory depression and death [6, 7].

Human studies in patients with cancer suggested long-term opioid treatment is not generally associated with major organ toxicity (with the exception generally of hypogonadism associated with low testosterone in men and low estrogen in women) [8]. Clinical experience supports this finding and certainly suggests significantly less gastrointestinal, hepatic, and renal pathology related to opioid treatment than to chronic use of acetaminophen, aspirin, or NSAIDs. Hepatic dysfunction has been reported in patients on long-term methadone treatment, in patients with comorbid alcoholism, or in patients with viral hepatitis [9]. Since adverse effects of opioids are related to 1.8–6 % of drug-related hospitalizations in adults, it is imperative for clinicians to familiarize themselves with the most frequent side effects [10]. Before clinicians initiate treatment with opioids, in accordance with the *Model Policy for Controlled Substance for Chronic Pain, Treatment Guidelines*, it is recommended for patients to be cautioned in writing as to the potential adverse effects of opioid therapy [11].

Opioid Adverse Side Effects

- Nausea and vomiting
- Constipation
- Sedation and somnolence
- Pruritus
- Urinary retention
- Myoclonus
- Cardiac effects
- Endocrine effects including Hypogonadism

- Opioid-induced hyperalgesia
- Respiratory depression
- Xerostomia
- Hypersensitivity reactions
- Peripheral edema
- Pulmonary edema
- Reactivation of a substance use disorder that had been in remission

Although adverse side effects are not uncommon with opioid treatment, they are generally transient, easily managed, and are not debilitating. The most common opioid side effects are GI related, and these should all be discussed with the patient prior to treatment as it is the exception rather than the rule that patients on opioid therapy do not have one or more of these adverse side effects.

Nausea and Vomiting

Due to direct stimulation of the chemoreceptor trigger zone (CTZ), reduced GI motility, and vestibular sensitivity, nausea and vomiting occur in 25 % of opioid-treated patient populations [12, 13]. Although nausea and vomiting generally are transient (last for an estimated 7 days after starting opioid treatment), mild, and self-limited, they can be sufficiently bothersome to interfere with treatment compliance.

Clinicians can choose from multiple antiemetics; in addition, they may initially lower the opioid dosage, titrate the opioid more slowly, or switch to a different opioid. Patients must be given appropriate strategies to deal with this problem ranging from dietary to pharmacological.

Antipsychotics have often been used as agents that block dopamine receptors in the CTZ [14, 15]. First-line options in the past have been haloperidol (Haldol) and prochlorperazine (Compazine) to control nausea; however, adverse effects such as alkathesia, dystonic reactions, sedation, and orthostatic hypotension may occur when used. In more recent years, metoclopramide (Reglan) and antidopaminergic drugs are most frequently used for weaker-grade opioid-induced nausea and vomiting [16, 17]. If the nausea is associated with movement or vertigo, consider scopolamine; if nausea is associated with satiety, consider metoclopramide which will block dopamine receptors in the CTZ aiding peristalsis by increasing the release of acetycholine (warning may cause sedation and extrapyramidal effects) [18]. Antiemetic medication such as promethazine (Phenergan) or ondansetron (Zofran) may be useful for short term, and generally, as tolerance develops to the nausea and vomiting, the antiemetic medication may be discontinued [19, 20]. Recent studies have revealed the use of droperidol and ondansetron to be associated with prolonged QTc and cardiac complications, and the FDA has endorsed the use of palonosetron as its use has not been noted [21]. The study by Appel et al. did reveal not only the decreased risks in using palonosetron (Aloxi) but also the increased effectiveness in comparison with ondansetron with reduction of opioid-induced nausea in the subjects by 42 %. Other commonly used treatments are metoclopramide, prochlorperazine, and hydroxyzine (Vistaril). Extrapyramidal effects were often associated with the use of metoclopramide, and this promoted studies in search of more appropriate antiemetics to relieve acute nausea. Recent studies by Moon et al. also suggest palonosetron as a superior choice to ondansetron in both efficacy and safety [22–24]. Since serotonin antagonists restrict the release of serotonin within the GI tract, they have a secondary benefit in controlling nausea; recent medications such as olanzapine/fluoxetine HCL (Symbyax) have been used as antiemetics. The advantage to the use of such medications in opioid-related adverse effects is that there are no related extrapyramidal adverse effects [25]. However, due to cost–effectiveness, this class of antiemetic medication is not considered first line of care.

Opioid-Induced Constipation (OIC)

Opioid-induced constipation occurs in 40–90 % of the chronic pain population [26]. Unlike other opioid-induced adverse effects, the rate of constipation does not decrease with time. It must be treated; when untreated, the consequences could be hemorrhoid formation, possible ruptured bowel, rectal pain, rectal burning, and bowel obstruction. Opioids induce mu receptors in the GI tract which may cause decrease in contractility and motility in the small and large intestine, generally resulting in constipation. They also decrease secretions into the bowel, increase reabsorption of fluids from the bowel, and increase anal and pyloric sphincter tone. This is a predictable adverse side effect and is the only common side effect to which patients do not develop tolerance. Because constipation can be a management problem, it will be discussed in detail below. As a general rule, advise the patient that constipation generally occurs with opioid treatment, and stool softeners/laxatives should be taken prophylactically. They should also be told that at times making dietary changes may prevent the need for significant use of medication. When constipation is inadequately treated, there is a significant risk of impaction, especially in the at-risk elderly debilitated patient or the sedentary patient on multiple medications. Therefore, the problem should be treated aggressively. (I can recall the wisdom imparted to me from a professor during residency who said "The hand that causes the impaction is the hand that should take care of the dis-impaction" Most of us prefer that this is not our hand!) However, at times, constipation can be extremely difficult to manage, and therefore, the physician may underutilize opioids and, in doing so, not provide adequate analgesia.

My clinical experience is consistent with the literature, which suggests that when constipation becomes a significant management problem despite careful evaluation and treatment as described, consideration should be given to using transdermal fentanyl or transdermal buprenorphine as the opioids of choice. The incidence of constipation is significantly less with these transdermal medications than it is with other sustained-acting or long-acting opioids [27, 28].

The following section on opioid-induced constipation is excerpted from gastroenterologist, Thomas Carr, M.D.'s contribution to my text submitted for publication, *Medication Management of Chronic Pain: What you Need to Know* [29].

- Exclude non-opiate causes of constipation.
- All patients should be encouraged to maintain hydration and exercise moderately.
- If aggressive treatment of constipation fails, rule out fecal impaction.

Therapeutic Agents

Bulking Agents (psyllium) They *must* be taken with adequate water for dose, or they become counterproductive. It takes several weeks for each added amount of therapy to become fully effective.

Stool-Modifying Agents or "Stool Softeners" (docusate sodium) They are often not very effective alone in serious constipation, but are a very useful adjunct to fiber.

Osmotic Laxatives (polyethylene glycol and lactulose) They are relatively safe with several that can be titrated for refractory cases.

Stimulant Laxatives (Senna) They are safe chronically if not used more than 3 times a week. Daily use can cause laxative dependence. Dependence can take a while to develop, so it should not be discounted in patients with a short time frame of therapy.

Motility Agents (metoclopramide, misoprostol) These are not well studied for this indication (and for some, off-label) but are worth a try in refractory cases.

Rectally Administered Agents This is generally the route of last resort, but several important agents are administered in this fashion. Most often used in breakthrough treatment. All of these agents generally work in an hour or less.
Note:

Chloride Channel Blockers (lubiprostone) Only one agent in this category exists which block the chloride channels and increase secretions into the bowel. Lubiprostone (Amitiza®) is approved for OIC and constipation caused by irritable bowel syndrome.

Peripherally Acting Mu-Opioid Receptor Antagonists (PAMORAs) (Methylnatrexone, Naloxegol) This class of medications has been recently developed specifically for OIC. PAMORAs utilize an opioid antagonist to reverse the mu-agonist effect on the bowel. These medications do not penetrate the CNS and therefore will not reverse analgesia or cause significant withdrawal. Two agents available subcutaneously are methylnaltrexone (Relistor) and alvimopan (ENTEREG ®); however, the indications for use are restricted. For example, methylnaltrexone is indicated for use in patients with advanced medical illnesses; alvimopan is used for decreasing postoperative ileus.

In 2014, studies resulted in the use of naloxegol (MOVANTIK ™), a pegylated derivative of the μ-opioid receptor in vitro. Naloxegol has the unique properties provided by pegylation processes. Pegylation presents P-glycoprotein transporter–substrate properties limiting the ability of naloxegol to cross the blood–brain barrier. This is a once-daily dose, and it comes in both 25 and 12.5 mg the PI recommends that it be prescribed in the 25 mg dose first, and should adverse effects be noted, the dose can be lessened to 12.5 mg. It is taken on an empty stomach one hour prior to the first meal of the day, it is not to be combined with any other laxative therapies, and thus, physicians must have patience to stop all other therapies before beginning naloxegol. Although naloxegol is a pegylated naloxone derivative, it does not require alteration in analgesic therapy.

Precautions to be taken with use of naloxegol:

- Monitor for severe, persistent abdominal pain; should this occur, discontinuation of naloxegol is warranted.
- Monitor for symptoms of opioid withdrawal as this is an opioid antagonist derivative—sweating, chills, diarrhea, abdominal pain, anxiety irritability, and somnolence (increased yawning).
- PAMORA medications are not indicated for patients with bowel obstruction.

Guanylate Cyclase C activators (linaclotide) One medication in this class (Linzess®) activates guanylate cyclase C which then stimulates production of cGMP, increasing intestinal fluid secretion and motility.

Behavioral Measures Often neglected, this can be a fairly important aspect of the management of chronic constipation.

Clinical Approaches

Mild–Moderate Constipation

Frequently, this responds to daily use of a bulking agent with or without a stool-modifying agent. The patient will need a movement every 48 h, and the use of a stimulant laxative (up to TIW), osmotic agent, or rectally administered agent may be required for rescue. It is best to start with a low level of bulking agent and titrate upward every 3–4 weeks until the use of the rescue agent is infrequent. The patient should be instructed on behavioral measures.

In patients intolerant of fiber, a higher dose of osmotic laxative (milk of magnesia, lactulose, PEG, sorbitol, or molasses would be best) could be used at bedtime in lieu of the fiber and stool-modifying agent. An example would be 40 gm of lactulose (Kristalose®) at bedtime. The 48-h rescue could be accomplished with a stimulant laxative or rectally administered agent.

Regrettably, most OIC is more involved than this, and many practitioners skip to moderate–severe therapy. In particular, bulking agents can be problematic in these individuals; they can exacerbate the problem if not effective and should be used with caution.

Moderate–Severe Constipation

Continue with a base of a bulk-forming agent plus a stool-modifying agent (consider mineral oil or orlistat (Xenical). Add an osmotic laxative that can be titrated upward (sorbitol, lactulose, milk of magnesia, and molasses) and aggressively titrate it upward until the use of the rescue agent is infrequent. A careful trial of a motility agent might be done if control is less than satisfactory [30]. Rescue is often more difficult in these patients and frequently requires a rectally administered agent. Lubiprostone, PAMORAs, and linaclotide may be used for moderate to severe OIC. Again, review behavioral measures and consider biofeedback. If it is becoming difficult, this would be the time to consult gastroenterology.

Severe Constipation

Continue with high-dose fiber, 1–2 stool-modifying agents, and a high dose of osmotic laxative. You will probably require a gastroenterology consult at this point. Frequently, a motility agent will be tried and a regimen of TIW enemas and/or stimulant laxatives.

Sedation

Although sedation and somnolence are not uncommon in the initial phase of opioid treatment and following dose escalation, fortunately, patients generally become tolerant as treatment progresses, especially those patients maintained on chronic opioid therapy with sustained-acting, time-released medications. Opioid-induced sedation is likely related often to opioid anticholinergic activity. The populations most at risk are the elderly and patients taking concurrent CNS active sedating medication. Extended sedation can occur with other comorbidities such as dementia, metabolic encephalopathy, or brain metastases. Generally, the first strategy for treatment is to decrease the opioid dosage, but this may lead to inadequate analgesia. At times, opioid rotation should be considered. Numerous studies over the past ten years have revealed reduction of adverse effects such as sedation, hallucinations, somnolence, and cognitive impairment [31]. Many have found genetic factors play a role in the reaction to specific opioids and the variations of sensitivity to dose conversion during opioid rotation [32].

When sedation is not self-limited or does not respond to other treatments, patients occasionally will benefit from psychostimulants (make the patient aware that this is not an FDA-approved indication). Although these medications have been used in refractory depression, to decrease sedation and to augment analgesia (non-FDA-approved indications), this author generally avoids the traditional psychostimulants because of the appetite suppression, potential for dependency, and anxiety at times associated with tachycardia as well as other dopaminergic-related problems. At times, methylphenidate (Ritalin) may be helpful and the literature supports its use in carefully selected patients. I do not recommend regular use of amphetamines as not uncommonly they may lead to drug dependence and abuse. I have found modafinil (Provigil®) and armodafinil (Nuvigil®) helpful in patients with excessive daytime sleepiness related to opioids (also an off-label use) and have not seen significant concurrent adverse side effects in most patients (it is mediated by the hypothalamus and not the dopamine system). They are also my drugs of choice in medication-related somnolent patients who have a history of substance abuse although I generally avoid all nonessential medications in this population especially psychoactive medications. If sedation persists, consider dose reduction but with medication given more frequently, use of non-sedating adjuvants, or opioid rotation. At times, dietary changes or activity modification may be helpful.

Responses to be monitored:

Somnolence, a state of feeling drowsy, appears much more prevalent in patients taking benzodiazepines and sedating antihistamines than that of those taking stable doses of sustained-acting opioids.

Sedation: The effect of calm, soothing, or tranquil—the absence of anxiety, excitability, or irritability.

Delirium: mental confusion that develops quickly and fluctuates [33]. At times in the at-risk population of the elderly or frail patient, even small increments in opioid doses can bring on a delirium associated with significant mental confusion. Most patients respond to tapering or discontinuing the opioid or opioid rotation

Respiratory Depression

Respiratory depression is the rise in peripheral PCO_2 combined with the decrease in peripheral oxygen [34]. The occurrence is the most feared adverse side effect because of the potential for apnea and death; therefore, opioids must be used cautiously (although studies reveal its prevalence in 0.5 % of cases) [35]. Respiratory depression is most likely to occur in opioid-naïve patients given too large an opioid dose when treatment is initiated and is associated with other signs of CNS depression [36, 37]. Elderly, debilitated patients, head injury patients—especially with increased intracranial pressure—and patients with preexisting severe pulmonary problems are most at risk. In general, all opioid-naïve patients and their significant others (especially with the above at-risk populations) should be told that it is important, especially for the first 24 h after beginning short-acting, immediate-release opioids and the first 72 h for sustained-acting, time-released medications, to monitor the mental status for signs of overmedication or intoxication, especially excessive somnolence, decrease in mental acuity, word slurring, or cardiopulmonary problems [38]. Any difficulty in these areas (even in the absence of respiratory problems) should warrant holding the next dose. If the symptoms are progressive or severe, patients should call the prescriber's office or go to the emergency room as the effects of respiratory depression are potentially fatal. When there is possibility that the patient has had respiratory compromise, if the drug is later restarted, it should be at a lower dosage and titrated more slowly [28]. Respiratory depression generally does not occur with a normal mental status. Respiratory depression is preceded by sedation, and the process from sedation through reduction and cessation of respiration is a time period generally of 5–15 min [39]. The prescriber is advised to carefully monitor the mental status at each office visit. The patient and significant others should also be alerted of the need to monitor alertness, speech, and other mental status parameters when opioid medication is increased. Boom et al reported that with the use of the opioid receptor antagonist naloxone, the effects can be reversed [40]. Therefore, when treating high-risk patients using opioid analgesics, consider writing for naloxone self-injection to be used only in an emergency situation [41]. This should be followed by emergency room evaluation.

Respiratory depression reversal is often achieved with the use of 3 main agents: potassium channel blockers, 5-hydroxytryptamine (serotonin, 5HT) receptor agonists, and ampakines [42]. These agents are known as respiratory stimulants that act on non-opioid receptor systems restoring breathing to acceptable levels, or at times, they are used as prophylactics to prevent OIRD.

Doxapram (Dopram) is one of the oldest known potassium channel blockers, and although effective, it does not come without adverse effects such as panic attacks, sweating, sympathoexcitation, and convulsions [43]. Doxapram also stimulates the cardiovascular system causing hypertension and increased cardiac output and has been known to reduce plasma concentration which, in turn, will reduce the level of opioid analgesia [44]. Studies of 5-hydroxytryptamine (serotonin, 5HT) receptor agonists reveal these agents as not sufficiently effective against OIRD possibly due to the low potency or the lower brain concentrations and may cause adverse effects such as nausea and vomiting with increased doses. Therefore, this line of therapy is not advisable [45, 46]. Ampakine studies have revealed that the most effective agent is CX717, preventing alfentanil-induced respiratory depression without decreasing the effects of analgesia; however, this agent may cause increased sedation. These agents are non-opioid antagonists which in some cases may be preferable over naloxone especially when the opioid analgesia contains a higher affinity for the μ-opioid receptor than that of naloxone, i.e., buprenorphine [47]. Otherwise, all the clinical findings point to naloxone and its safety as the primary agent for reversal of respiratory depression in OIRD [48].

Other less common adverse side effects include urinary retention, especially in the elderly and multifocal myoclonus at high opioid doses and especially with repeated dosing of parenteral meperidine.

Organ Toxicity

Human studies with cancer patients had suggested that long-term opioid treatment is generally not associated with significant major organ toxicity [6]. Clinical experience supports this finding (with the exception of more recently recognized hormonal changes that will be discussed below) and certainly suggests significantly less GI, hepatic, and renal pathology related to opioid treatment than to chronic use of acetaminophen, aspirin, or NSAIDs. Hepatic dysfunction has been reported in patients on long-term methadone and in patients with comorbid alcoholism or viral hepatitis [7].

Cardiac Effects

Adverse cardiac side effects from opioids are not common although IV fentanyl has been associated with bradyarrhythmias and morphine has been associated with hypotension related to histamine release.

While reports conflict, there appears to be some association between higher doses of methadone causing prolongation of the QTc interval and torsades des pointes. Methadone should be used with caution in individuals who have or are at risk of cardiovascular disease, who suffer from a substance abuse-related cardiac condition, or who are currently using other medications that are known to extend the QTc interval (e.g., antipsychotics) as there is a significant increase in toxicity and mortality [49, 50]. In patients receiving more than moderate doses of methadone, it is recommended that the EKG be monitored during treatment [51].

It is also noted that medications inhibited by the cytochrome P450 3A4 enzyme system may also increase the risk of QTc prolongation [52]. Lists of these medications are readily available at the FDA's official Web site (www.fda.gov).

Endocrine Effects

There is considerable evidence to suggest that endocrine dysfunction in men and women may be directly related to chronic opioid use and is a problem that may be underdiagnosed and undertreated [53]. All opioids can cause some degree of endocrine dysfunction [54] and have a major impact on opioid receptors, located especially in the hypothalamus.

Screening for endocrine dysfunction should be considered at the initial pain evaluation and further evaluated at subsequent visits. Biochemical testing for assumed hypogonadism includes measuring total testosterone, free testosterone, SHBG, FSH, and LH. Despite age or cause of disease state, men with a total testosterone level of less than approximately 300 ng/dL often contract symptoms associated with hypogonadism.

Long-term opioid use can lead to hypogonadism, which is defined as the suppression of hypothalamic secretion of gonadotropin-releasing hormone. In males, low testosterone can lead to symptoms including decreased/loss of libido, erectile dysfunction, fatigue, anxiety, depression, infertility, loss of muscle mass, reduced analgesia, and osteoporosis. In females, LH, FSH, and estrogen can lead to amenorrhea and infertility [55]. Studies of opioid/heroin addicts on methadone maintenance treatment have documented the above hormonal changes and have also indicated that if these addicts are successful at getting off opioids, serum hormone levels generally return to normal. Untreated hormonal deficiencies may predispose perimenopausal women to osteoporosis and subsequent compression fractures [56]. For this reason, it is important that your patients have bone density studies and appropriate treatment for osteoporosis. There have been studies specifically focusing on the effects of intrathecal opioids. Christo noted, "Intrathecal opioids, even at low doses, can disrupt the hypothalamic-pituitary-gonadal axis, and thus cause reproductive and metabolic disturbances" [57].

If opioids are the suspected cause of hypogonadism, non-opioid pain management should be considered. If non-opioid options are inadequate, opioid rotation should be attempted, as hypogonadism may occur with varying severity depending on the agent. Hormone therapy should be instituted in patients requiring hormone replacement (unless there are medical contraindications), under the guidance of an endocrinologist if necessary [58]. Some men have demonstrated significant benefit from testosterone replacement therapy, and some women receiving hormonal therapy had more regular menses [57].

Daniell HW [59] noted up to 75 % of female patients on chronic opioid therapy suffer from hypogonadism. He reported the occurrence in women is significantly less than the occurrence in the male patient population. It has also been noted that the effects lead to changes in menstruation. Opioids may impede pituitary release of LH and FSH in women, subsequently obstructing the natural menstrual cycle [60]. The symptoms of such hormonal changes also include that of depression, reduced fertility osteoporosis, and hyperalgesia. Women also might need testosterone replacement therapy. In females, research reveals testosterone is secreted by the ovaries and adrenal glands and slowly declines with age [61]. After gonadal removal, testosterone declines by approximately 50 % within days after surgery [62]. Testosterone prescribed to a woman who has been oophorectomized is indicated when she develops a hypoactive sexual desire disorder (HSDD). This disorder is attributed to a lack of androgen. Results of two studies revealed a significantly higher percentage of women receiving testosterone patches reported the treatments as beneficial overall to their physical and psychosocial health [63]. These factors may have a direct influence on the prognosis of a chronic pain treatment scenario in our patient populations.

Reports from the Journal of Osteopathic Medicine reveal that both sexes present with the suppression of the hypothalamus (primary mechanism) causing opioid-induced hypogonadism [64]. The gonadotropins (LH and FSH) stimulate production of gonadal hormones. Decreased production generally results in erectile dysfunction, depression, and fatigue as well as associated hypersensitivity to pain.

Studies presented at *Pain Week 2014* revealed that men who take methadone, morphine, oxycodone, or fentanyl are more at risk for androgen deficiency than those maintained on hydrocodone-based substances. Studies reported by Daniell revealed patients treated with sustained action oxycodone, morphine, continuous transdermal fentanyl, and methadone of at least one month found DHEAS levels below normal in 67 % of the study population. Values of the DHEAS from Daniell's study may be a clinical marker for overall adrenal function for future baseline and follow-up DHEA androgen levels in opioid therapy patients [65].

Treatment

The first line of care in men with opioid-induced endocrinopathy is testosterone replacement following medical screening to assess risk factors for testosterone treatment. These supplements are available in creams, gels, buccal supplements, injections, and transdermal patches. Intramuscular treatment may cause fluctuating serum testosterone levels. Topical and buccal treatments provide relatively stable testosterone concentrations and are first lines of treatment. Baseline and follow-up testosterone and PSA levels must be monitored clinically in response to treatment. A prostate examination should be conducted prior to initiation of testosterone therapy. The Endocrine Society recommends that serum levels be taken 2–3 months after initiating therapy and subsequently adjusting doses as needed [66–68]. Physicians are to be mindful of the fact that the amount of time to obtain effective therapeutic levels of total T is longer in men treated with opioids than in those not treated with opioid analgesics. Guidelines also suggest that healthcare providers treating patients with chronic opioid therapy and utilizing long-term testosterone treatment should monitor hemoglobin, hematocrit, and liver function in addition to the testosterone concentrations.

Opioid Cognitive Effects

Folstein et al. reported a rate of 17–29 % [69, 70] of cognitive impairment during the initial phase of opioid treatment. This is often dose related and can be minimized by slow titration and beginning at low doses in at-risk patients. Most patients do not have clinically apparent cognitive dysfunction even at the onset of treatment.

Fortunately, those who do generally develop tolerance to cognitive effects. Although the perception of many practitioners and the lay public is that opioids significantly impair cognitive abilities, research data do not generally support this position in patients appropriately titrated. Vella-Brincat et al. researched the effects of intermediate- and long-term opioids on cognition in patients with chronic pain. The studies revealed that in cases where parenteral opiates are associated with significant dose-related cognitive impairment, oral opioids are associated with minimal mild impairment in opioid-naïve patients. Researchers concluded that most studies suggest that the greatest likelihood for cognitive impairment (if it is to occur) is during the initial several days of usage [71, 72]. A review of Payne's studies on the use of opioid analgesia noted very little effect not only on cognitive function but motor functioning as well, once a patient's opioids were stabilized [73]. O'Neill concluded that during the opioid-naïve stage, proper and slow titration of medications plays a significant part in reducing the probability of reduction in cognitive functioning. In my pain practice, I write on my opioid prescriptions (and in my progress note dictated in the presence of the patient) a warning for the patient not to drive or work unless fully alert with full mental capacity.

In 2005, as the senior author of a chapter, *Medication, Driving and Work (MDW)* [56], I focused my primary attention on opioids, while my colleagues commented on other medication classes such as benzodiazepines, sedating muscle relaxants, antihistamines, tricyclic antidepressants, and sedating psychotropic drugs. We were especially concerned about issues related to cognitive impairment that might adversely impact on work or driving. Highlights from the chapter noted:

- Our findings as well as evidence-based reviews have shown that many medications can impair psychomotor performance. Certain classes of medications, including benzodiazepines, muscle relaxants, sedating antihistamines, neuroleptics, anxiolytics, opioids, some non-opioid analgesics, and sedatives, have been shown to impair performance on driving tasks, at times to a similar degree as alcohol. Any of these could place the individual, his/her co-workers, or the public in danger.

- Studies suggest that benzodiazepine use increases accident risk up to 50 % with highest risk for increasing dose, day time use, initial therapy, or combined benzodiazepine use. Long-acting agents have greater effects than short-acting agents on function, including daytime function following nocturnal administration.

- Drowsiness and dizziness have been reported to occur in up to 30 % of patients taking muscle relaxants compared with placebos. Some agents (e.g., cyclobenzaprine, carisoprodol) may have greater effects on psychomotor performance than on less sedating medications.

- There is some evidence that patients habituate to the sedative and psychomotor effects of long-term opioids [74], permitting safe return to most work. While many HCPs restrict their patients from driving while on opioids, emerging research and opinion [75] suggests that some patients with normal mental status who are on stable doses of long-acting or sustained-acting time-released opioids may have acceptable risks for driving and work.

Some patients have mild cognitive impairment during the initial phase of opioid treatment. This is often dose related and can be minimized by slow titration and beginning at low doses in at-risk patients. Most patients do not have clinically apparent cognitive dysfunction even at the onset of treatment. Fortunately, those who do generally develop tolerance to cognitive effects. Although the perception of many practitioners and the lay public is that opioids significantly impair cognitive abilities, research data do not generally support this position in patients appropriately titrated.

Chapman et al. researched the effects of intermediate- and long-term opioids on cognition in patients with chronic pain [76]. They concluded that most studies suggest that the greatest likelihood for cognitive impairment (if it is to occur) is during the initial several days of usage. "In both cancer and non-cancer populations with chronic pain, comparisons between those patients with pain who are taking versus not taking opioids generally have failed to reveal significant differences."

Several other studies with patients on long-term opioid treatment found no significant adverse effects on attention, concentration, and memory or other problematic cognitive effects from the opioids [77].

Based upon review of the above studies and extensive clinical experience monitoring patients on chronic opioid therapy for driving and work, I monitor reaction time using the *Aronoff test of reaction time*. With a patient not anticipating the event, a soft rubber ball is thrown across the desk at the patient's face and the patient's reaction is observed. A normal response is for the patient to react appropriately and catch the ball (or reach for the ball to avoid being struck). The author feels that a patient sedated, with decreased mental acuity or impaired reaction time, will generally not be able to pass this test and will be struck by the ball or be unable to catch it. This has not been tested for scientific validity, nor is it being endorsed for widespread use at this time. However, this author believes that this test combined with a detailed mental status examination gives a good estimate of whether a patient has adequate reaction time to function in a number of situations, including driving and most work situations.

Risk of Addiction

The risk factors for addiction [78] include the following

- Personal past or current history of substance abuse problems;
- Family history of substance abuse problems;
- Prior treatment in a drug rehabilitation facility;
- Use of multiple drugs;
- IV drug use;
- Being a smoker;

- Significant comorbid anxiety, depression, personality disorders, and environmental stressors.

There is little evidence that opioid use in patients with painful conditions poses a significant risk for true addiction unless predisposing factors are present. Patients with a history of substance abuse or addiction, significant psychopathology, high family risk factors, or environmental stressors contributing to escalating pain and suffering in general should only cautiously, if at all, be maintained on opioids for non-malignant pain. Most chronic pain patients can be managed effectively without the regular daily use of narcotic analgesics. But addiction is rarely a clinical problem in patients carefully selected for opioid maintenance [79].

Use of Opioids with Patients Who Have a History of Substance Abuse [80]

Chronic pain clearly is a significant stressor that has been documented to bring about dysfunctional behaviors in vulnerable individuals. One can argue that patients with a history of substance problems or major psychopathology are such vulnerable individuals. The question is whether it is more likely that the patient with substance abuse in remission is more at risk for reactivation of the problem with prolonged unrelieved pain or the exposure to opioids. Some of these patients, as a result of past experiences or education, have been taught to never use opioids as it could rekindle their past addiction. They have learned the lesson well and are unwilling to consider a treatment approach that involves opioid usage. Their fears and wishes must be addressed, and if, after discussion of the risks and benefits, they continue to be resistant, opioids should not be used.

Other patients, however, will state that they no longer desire opioids, but the pain is so overwhelming that unless something can be done to alleviate it, they fear they will return to take drugs. These patients are at significant risk. Treatment approaches for all patients with a substance abuse history should involve others active in their health care or support network (family, sponsors, therapists, partners, friends, and other physicians) in the decision-making process. With the patient's consent, the decision to use opioids should be based on sound clinical principles and should involve appropriate consultants. While there are risk factors for addiction/abuse with this population, these risks may be acceptable given the alternative scenarios.

Some of these patients are abusing multiple substances for reasons other than their pain and efforts to get analgesia. Most have excuses to justify their dysfunctional behaviors. These patients should be considered for opioid pain treatment only if it is documented that their active medical condition warrants opioids and there are no acceptable alternatives. For some of these patients, it can be anticipated that their psychopathology will interfere with any type of therapeutic alliance with the treating physician or pain team. This population often demonstrates a high degree of sociopathic behavior, and it can be anticipated that they will be non-compliant, manipulative, and drug seeking throughout treatment. This does not mean that they should not be treated. However, physicians should not treat these patients without considerable experience in pain medicine and addiction medicine, and these patients should not be treated if they are unwilling to comply with treatment recommendations including participation in AA or NA, counseling or psychotherapy, and chemical dependency treatment.

To get a prescription, these patients must be present at the designated appointment time. All pain patients with active or remote substance problems must sign an opioid consent agreement noting that the potential risks of activating their substance problem were discussed with them and that the potential benefits justified the risks. As a general rule, I will not use short-acting opioids with this population regardless of their subjective complaints (however, some physicians are willing to do so). I also attempt to utilize sustained-acting or long-acting opioid analgesic medications formulated to be tamper deterrent, as well as careful use of adjuvant analgesics combined with non-pharmacological techniques of pain management in an attempt to decrease the opioid requirements [81].

Edema

It has been assumed that opioids cause peripheral edema. The mechanism that causes edema is uncertain, but theories suggest that opioids stimulate histamine release from mast cells causing amplified venous permeability leading to fluid retention or increased secretion of antidiuretic hormones causing fluid accumulation.

Peripheral edema occurs in 6.1–21.7 % of intrathecal opioid-treated cases. Research has identified intrathecal morphine to be the cause of edema in only 3 % of cases.

Edema is increasingly identified as a potential adverse effect of intraspinal opioid infusion treatment. Chronic leg edema is an identified precursor for cellulitis. Many physicians have controlled peripheral edema by titrating to lower opioid doses or by switching to non-opioid analgesia. Research has shown that studies of opioid infusion-related edema have been well controlled by intrathecal baclofen and clonidine, alternatively, to provide spinal antinociception in cases where intraspinal opioids fail due to intolerable pharmacological adverse effects.

Pruritus

Pruritus is another common adverse side effect, generally affecting the face and upper body and causing some patients significant distress. Most patients become tolerant, but some do not and require discontinuing the opioid or opioid rotation.

The majority of patients, however, will respond to hydroxyzine (Vistaril), to diphenhydramine (Benadryl) (both can be associated with significant sedation), or to other antihistamines, skin lotions, low-dose doxepin, other antihistaminic TCAs, or other histamine (H2) blockers.

Opioid-induced pruritus occurs in an estimated 2–10 % of patients and is disproportionately related to morphine use. The rate of pruritus is increased by IV administration. The itching associated with pruritus is due to the release of histamine from the mast cells. This release may cause erythema and/or swelling of the skin. Histamine release is not the only factor involved; this has been noted in patients that do not respond to antihistamine therapy for relief of their symptoms. In such cases, serotonin (5-HT) is released when platelets combine and stimulate serotonin receptors, and in such cases, $5\text{-}HT_2$ antagonists are the primary therapeutic agent used in treatment [81].

Pruritus should often be viewed as an adverse effect rather than an allergic reaction [82, 83].

This has been managed by the following: opioid rotation, dose reduction, antihistamines (diphenhydramine 25–50 mg po or IV is commonly used), cold compress application, and skin moisturizers [84].

Urinary Retention

Opioid-induced bladder dysfunction occurs in 3.8–18.1 % of patients receiving chronic opioid therapy. Symptoms occur more often after epidural injections of morphine rather than IM injections. Opioids are known to decrease detrusor tone and the force of contraction and in turn decrease the sensation of a full bladder or the urge to void and then restrain the void reflex [85]. Naloxone has been known to reverse these effects. Rosow et al. noted the changes in bladder function as being related to a peripheral opioid effect and being reversed by the application of methyl naltrexone (peripheral opioid agonist) [86]. Many clinicians have found that the rate of opioid-related urinary retention is increased in men with benign prostatic hyperplasia. Some have found it helpful to advise patients to double void or add pressure to the lower abdomen over the bladder during urination to help reduce the retention of urine. In more chronic cases, tamsulosin (Flomax) is added to medication regimens to relax bladder muscles and aid in the voiding process [87].

Hyperhidrosis

Opioids can effect thermoregulation. Hyperhidrosis can occur from the stimulation of mast cell degranulation with histamine release. This occurs commonly in 45 % of patients using methadone and has been a common adverse effect noted in transdermal fentanyl use [88–90]. In cases related to opioid discontinuation or withdrawal, hyperhidrosis is accompanied by the following:

- Low energy, irritability, anxiety, agitation, and insomnia.
- Runny nose and teary eyes.
- Hot and cold sweats and goose bumps.
- Yawning.
- Muscle aches and pains.
- Abdominal cramping, nausea, vomiting, and diarrhea.

Tramadol has a weak ɥ-receptor opioid antagonist allowing its properties to elevate the hypothalamic level inhibiting serotonin reuptake and norepinephrine in the spinal cord increasing hyperthermal and decreasing hypothermal response—reducing withdrawal effects.

Hyperalgesia

Chronic pain patients and physicians are faced with the dilemma of pain on a daily bases with the risk of opioid-induced pain sensitivity. Hyperalgesia is an enhanced pain response to a noxious stimulus, in this case, induced by opiate use. Recent studies indicate a distortion of pain perception in chronic opioid use as well as abuse in some cases [91]. Although still being debated, the presence of OIH could be a clinical challenge not only in chronic cancer pain management, but also in perioperative pain. Hyperalgesia may be related to increased tolerance, defined as a decreased response to the drug's analgesic effects over time, followed by loss of analgesic efficacy [92]. More recent studies indicate hyperalgesia as a probable starting point of pain sensitization and pain chronicity [93]. Mercandante indicated in his 2005 study that physicians should endeavor to prevent or treat OIH through modulatory or pharmacologic means based on an understanding of the likely mechanisms underlying OIH and these treatment means.

Opioid-induced hyperalgesia studies have identified decreased reuptake and enhanced nociceptive response as common mechanisms in etiology. Enhanced reaction of spinal neurons, β2-AR receptors signals, and neurotransmitters has been acknowledged as adaptive changes due to chronic opioid exposure [94]. Increased NMDA receptor activation is another proposed mechanism. Fishbain et al. described the pain found in hyperalgesia as a complex interaction of afferent sensitivity in conjunction with cognitive processing of this stimuli modulated on all levels of the neural axis [95]. Several brain studies reveal prefrontal brain regions are involved with inhibition of nociception. These systems are genetically influenced by catecholamine breakdown enzymes. A review of these brain studies revealed the reduced capacity to activate the µ-opioid system due to a reduced concentration of endogenous opioids has been shown to increase pain sensitivity in some individuals [96]. Studies also suggest the possibility of mechanisms such as pro-nociceptive stimulation and neuroplastic changes being responsible for hyperalgesia. Chronic opioid treatment relies, in part, on one's pain perception and the subjectivity of patients describing their pain experience. Hooten et al. studied the relationship between heat and pain perception in patients being tapered from opioids. They employed a quantitative sensory test to measure levels of sensitivity —results revealed suspicion of OIH being limited to patients who self-report inadequate relief. The problem with tracking OIH is that of patients switching providers, length of opioid therapies, agents of choice, and titration speeds of medications which if not documented accurately obscure the facts.

Management approaches to opioid-induced hyperalgesia as identified are as follows:

- Opioid dose reduction—which may in turn increase pain temporarily [97]
- Opioid rotation to induce the NMDA antagonist properties of some medications such as methadone
- Ketamine infusions (reinvigorating NMDA receptors) [98]
- Additions of alpha-2 adrenergic agonists
- IV lidocaine infusions [93]
- Low-dose naloxone infusions [93]
- Opioid rotation
- Use of partial agonists such as buprenorphine

Paradoxes providers face are not limited to self-reporting patient populations. It takes extreme patience on the part of the provider as well the chronic pain patient to treat OIH. Dose titration may increase pain sensitivity or induce mild withdrawal which can exacerbate pain ratings. Hyperalgesic effect may not be lessened until the proper opioid dose titration is reached, patients will become frustrated/discouraged at times during the process, and the subjective reporting may be misinterpreted as hyperalgesia. Proper titration may require more frequent office visits to ensure safety and efficacy during this time period. These factors must be explained effectively to patients before the therapeutic steps are taken in order to avoid patients requesting that their care be transferred. In accordance with proper patient care, one must try to determine the differences between hyperalgesia, tolerance, opioid dependence, and addiction. OIH is a less recognized and controversial adverse effect of chronic opioid therapy. Many new research papers have identified this as a factor that should be discussed at the onset of chronic opioid therapy in conjunction with discussion of the opioid agreement and treatment plan.

Myoclonus

Myoclonus, brief uncontrolled movements of the extremities, has been noted as an adverse effect in relation to several opioid medications. Research reveals the increased risk to be related to high opioid doses. The most frequent occurrence of opioid-induced myoclonus is related to meperidine (Demerol) and the accumulation of normeperidine (a neurotoxic metabolite of meperidine). In patients with hepatic dysfunction, oral morphine may also increase the occurrence of myoclonus [99]. Most individuals who experience myoclonus present with mild uncontrolled twitching, and in more severe cases, the presentation is in the form of involuntary movements of the limbs, spasms, or pain [100]. Opioid-induced myoclonus can be treated with the reduction of opioid doses, addition of muscle relaxants, and/or by increasing adjunctive/adjuvant analgesics.

Interactions with Marijuana and Safety Data

In my article published in Pain Medicine News in June 2013, I discussed the [101] "research with marijuana demonstrating efficacy with intractable nausea, anorexia and vomiting in cancer chemotherapy, HIV/AIDS, cachexia, as in other debilitating medical disorders [102–104]. There are multiple studies documenting efficacy with intractable pain disorders." Studies acknowledge the difference between medicinal marijuana in the form of Marinol at a therapeutic dose and THC from smoking marijuana. Such studies revealed that amounts of THC absorbed in Marinol are known dosages, and in contrast, the THC absorbed via smoking marijuana varies in terms of potency [105]. However, there have not been enough discussions on the long-term adverse effects of medical marijuana usage. Some of the most common secondary effects are respiratory distress, depression and anxiety, gastrointestinal complaints, and CNS disorders [106, 107].

In heavy marijuana smokers, opioid receptor blockade enhanced the subjective and cardiovascular effects of marijuana, suggesting that endogenous opioids dampen cannabinoid effects in this population. In conjunction with cardiovascular effects, clinicians face the challenges of altered perception, mental status changes, and the occasional dysphoria, hallucinations, and delusions associated with marijuana use in patients who may already have emotional disorders. When screening patients for risk in a chronic pain practice, the use of illicit substances is of concern to clinicians especially when the clinician needs to make decisions regarding writing for opioids or other controlled substances. In addition, even in states, cities, districts, and Indian reservations in which recreational marijuana is now legal, the use of recreational marijuana may often be in conjunction with a high-risk lifestyle pattern. In an observational study, Pesce et al. noted that up to 19 % of a chronic pain patient population used cannabinoids and this study showed roughly a fourfold incidence in the use of cocaine and methamphetamine among marijuana users in this population [108]. The use of marijuana may interfere with the therapeutic effect of pain medications or increase cognitive dysfunction. Therefore, for safety risks, in a pain practice, I strongly believe it is advisable that patients abstain from the use of marijuana or other psychoactive substances likely to adversely affect their mental status [109]. Consider the issue of risk to the individual smoking marijuana not only from immediate usage but from long-term effects among which is the possibility of substance abuse. Campbell et al. performed a qualitative systematic review revealing that cannabinoids were not more effective than codeine in controlling pain and often had a CNS depressant effect that limited their use in chronic pain control [110]. Campbell's review also noted the non-desirable physical effects of dry mouth, blurred vision, palpitations, tachycardia, and postural hypotension. The adverse effects were present in use of THC 10–20 mg. Many of the 222 patients displayed adverse effects after being administered THC; in this review, the cases reported one or more of the following dose–response-related adverse effects— mental clouding, ataxia, dizziness, numbness, disorientation, disconnected thought, slurred speech, muscle twitching, impaired memory, dry mouth, and blurred vision —and at 20 mg was sedating in 100 % of patients.

In my 2014 address to physicians attending the annual meeting of the American Academy of Pain Medicine, I strongly advised them to not write for any controlled substances including opiates to any patients testing positive for illicit drugs on urine drug screens drugs, even for regions noted above where THC is legal. I described what I feel to be a very possible legal and medical malpractice situation if they knowingly write these controlled substances for patients who they are aware are also concomitantly using marijuana. I gave them a hypothetical situation that very well could become a reality. Assume that their patient was using marijuana and that the physician was aware of this use and nonetheless wrote for an opioid, or another controlled substance. Now assume that their patient went through a stop sign or traffic light and killed a 6-year-old girl. Assume that their patient was taken in handcuffs to the police department and charged with vehicular homicide. Now assume that further urine screening or blood screening also found positive testing for not only the THC but also the opioid the physician was writing. Conceivably, it might be construed that it was not the THC that caused the accident resulting in the child's death, but possibly it was the opioid the physician was writing with the knowledge that the patient was also using marijuana. Potentially, that physician could be also charged with negligence or with malpractice [111–113].

I believe when writing for potent medications that we have an ethical responsibility to monitor patients very carefully to protect not only our patients, but other individuals who conceivably could be injured by the actions of our patients. For this reason, since 1999, I have frequently lectured and written on the importance of monitoring safety for driving and return to work when we write for controlled substances or any CNS active medication [101].

References

1. Chou R, Fanciullo GJ, Fine PG, et al. Clinical guidelines for the use of chronic opioid therapy in chronic noncancer pain. J Pain. 2009;10(2):113–30.
2. Fishbain DA, Gallagher RM. Comments on "prescription drug dependence and evolving beliefs about chronic pain management". Am J Psychiatry. 2006;163(12):2194–5.
3. Willy ME, Graham DJ, Racoosin JA, et al. Candidate metrics for evaluating the impact of prescriber education on the safe use of extended-release/long-acting (ER/LA) opioid analgesics. Pain Med. 2014;15(9):1558–68. doi:10.1111/pme.12459 Epub 2014 May 15.

4. Nersesyan H, Slavin KV. Current aproach to cancer pain management: availability and implications of different treatment options. Ther Clin Risk Manage. 2007;3(3):381–400.

5. Ballantyne JC. Opioid controls: regulate to educate. Pain Med. 2010;11(4):480–1, 2 p. doi: 10.1111/j.1526-4637.2010.00822.x.

6. Ballantyne JC. Safe and effective when used as directed: the case of chronic use of opioid analgesics. J Med Toxicol. 2012;8(4):417–23.

7. Dahan A, Overdyk F, Smith T, Aarts L, Niesters M. Pharmacovigilance: a review of opioid-induced respiratory depression in chronic pain patients. Pain Physician. 2013;16(2): E85–94.

8. Chou R, Turner JA, Devine EB, Hansen RN, et al. The effectiveness and risks of long-term opioid therapy for chronic pain: a systematic review for a national institutes of health pathways to prevention workshop. Ann Intern Med. 2015;162(4):276–86. doi:10.7326/M14-2559.

9. Wang L, Wei X, Wang X, Li J, Li H, Jia W. Long-term effects of methadone maintenance treatment with different psychosocial intervention models. PLoS ONE. 2014;9(2):e87931.

10. Salvi F, Marchetti A, D'Angelo F, et al. Adverse drug events as a cause of hospitalization in older adults. Drug Safety. 2012;35 Suppl:29–45. 17p.

11. Model policy for the use of controlled substances for the treatment of pain. Dallas, Tex: federation of state medical boards of the United States, Inc; 2004. Available at: http://www. fsmb.org/pdf/2004_grpol_Controlled_Substances.pdf.

12. Cepeda MS, Farrar JT, Baumgarten M, Boston R, Carr DB, Strom BL. Side effects of opioids during short-term administration: effect of age, gender, and race. Clin Pharmacol Ther. 2003;74:102–12.

13. Flake ZA, Scalley RG, Bailey AG. Practical selection of antiemetics. Am Fam Physician. 2004;69:1169–74.

14. Baldessarini RJ, Tarazi FI. Drugs and the treatment of psychiatric disorders. In: Goodman LS, Hardman JG, Limbird LE, Gilman AG, editors. Goodman and Gilman's the pharmacologic basis of therapeutics. 10th ed. New York, N.Y.: McGraw-Hill; 2001. p. 485–520.

15. Masui. Management of opioid-induced nausea and vomiting. 2013;62(7):829–35.

16. Ripamonti CI, Santini D, Maranzano E, Berti M, et al. Management of cancer pain: ESMO clinical practice guidelines. Ann Oncol October 1, 2012;23:vii139–54.

17. Laugsand EA, Kaasa S, Klepstad P. Management of opioid-induced nausea and vomiting in cancer patients: systematic review and evidence-based recommendations. Palliat Med. 2011;25:442–53.

18. Apfel CC, Korttila K, Abdalla M, Kerger H, Turan A, Veder I, et al. A factorial trial of six interventions for the prevention of postoperative nausea and vomiting. N Engl J Med. 2004;350:2441–51.

19. Sussman G, Shurman J, Creed MR, Larsen LS, Ferrer-Brechner T, Noll D, et al. Intravenous ondansetron for the control of opioid-induced nausea and vomiting. International S3AA3013 Study Group. Clin Ther. 1999;21:1216–27.

20. Canadian agency for drugs and technologies in health. Antiemetics for adults experiencing opioid-induced nausea: a review of clinical and cost effectiveness, benefits and harms and guidelines. [internet] Ottawa (ON): Canadian Agency for Drugs and Technologies in Health; 2014 Apr. CADTH Rapid Response Reports.

21. Apfel CC, Jukar-Rao S. Is palonosetron also effective for opioid-induced and post-discharge nausea and vomiting? Br J Anaesth. 2012;108(3):371–3.

22. Moon HY, Baek CW, Choi GJ, Shin HY, et al. Palonsetron and aprepitant for the prevention of postoperative nausea and vomiting in patients indicated for laparascopic gynaecologic surgery: a doble-blind randomized trial. BMC Anesthesiol. 2014;14:68. doi: 10.1186/1471-2253-14-68. eCollection 2014.

23. Yeh YC, Blouin GC, Reddy P. Evidence to support use of palonosetron over generic serotonin type 3–receptor antagonists for chemotherapy-induced nausea and vomiting. Am J Health-Syst Pharm. 2014;71:500–6.

24. Coluzzi F, Pappagallo M. Opioid therapy for chronic noncancer pain: practice guidelines for initiation and maintenance of therapy. Minerva Anestesiol. 2005;71:425–33.
25. Kolesar JM, Eickhoff Jens, Vermeulen LC. Serotonin type 3-receptor antagonists for chemotherapy-induced nausea and vomiting: therapeutically equivalent or meaningfully different? American Journal of Health-System Pharmacy. 2014;71(6):p507–10. 4p. 2 Charts. DOI: 10.2146/ajhp130653.
26. Swegle JM, Logemann C. Management of common opioid-induced adverse effects. Am Fam Physician. 2006;74:1347–54.
27. Marciniak CM, Toledo S, Lee J, Jesselson M, Bateman J, Grover B, Tierny J. World J Gastroenterol. 2014;20(43):16323–33. doi:10.3748/wjg.v20.i43.16323.
28. AGA technical review on constipation. Gastroenterology. 2000;119:1766.
29. Aronoff GM: eds. Carr, Thomas. Medication management of chronic pain: what you need to know: management of opiate-induced constipation. Indiana, Trafford, 2015.
30. Lawrence R. Schiller: treatment of constipation and diarrhea. In: Wolfe MM, editor. Therapy of digestive disorders: a companion to Sleisenger and Fordtran's gastrointestinal and liver disease. Philadelphia: WB Saunders; 2000. p. 747–55.
31. Fine PG. Treatment guidelines for the pharmacological management of pain in older persons. Pain Med. 2012;13 Suppl 2:S57–66.
32. Foley KM, Houde RW: Methadone in cancer pain management: individualize dose and titrate to effect. J Clin Oncol. 1998;16:3213–15, (editorial).
33. Slatkin N, Rhiner M. Treatment of opioid-induced delirium with acetylcholinesterase inhibitors: a case report. J Pain Symptom Manage. 2004;27:268–73.
34. Boyd KJ, Kelly M. Oral morphine as symptomatic treatment of dyspnoea in patients with advanced cancer. Palliat Med. 1997;11(4):277–81.
35. Dahan A, Aarts L, Smith TW. Incidence, reversal, and prevention of opioid-induced respiratory depression. Anesthesiology. 2010;112(1):226–38.
36. McEvoy T, Moore J, Generali J. Inpatient prescribing and monitoring of fentanyl transdermal systems: adherence to safety regulations. Hosp Pharm. 2014;49(10):942–9. doi:10.1310/hpj4910-942.
37. Zedler B, Xie L, Wang L, Joyce A, et al. Risk factors for serious prescription opioid-related toxicity or overdose among veterans health administration patients. Pain Med. 2014;15(11):1911–29.
38. Benyamin R, Trescot AM, Datta S, et al. Opioid complications and side effects. Pain Phys 2008 Opioid Spec Issue: 11:S105–20.
39. Gallagher R. Killing the symptom without killing the patient. Can Fam Physician. 2010;56(6):544–6, e210–12.
40. Boom M, Niester M, Sarton E, et al. Non-analgesic effects of opioids: opiod-induced respiratory depression. Curr Pharma Design. 5994–6004. http://www.eurekaselect.com/104017/article%20-%20sthash.b2qBpc8f.dpuf.
41. SAMHSA opioid overdose toolkit: information for prescribers. http://store.samhsa.gov/shin/content/SMA13-4742/Overdose_Toolkit_2014_Jan.pdf. Last accessed [February 23, 2015].
42. van der Schier R, Roozekrans M, van Velzen M, et al. Opioid-induced respiratory depression: reversal by non-opioid drugs. F1000Prime Rep. 2014;6:79. doi: 10.12703/P6-79. eCollection 2014.
43. Golder FJ, Hewitt MW, McLeod JF. Respiratory stimulant drugs in the post-operative setting. Resp Physiol Neurobiol. 2013;189:395–402.
44. Roozekrans M, van der Schrier R, Hoskins P, McLeod J, Dahan A. Doxapram reduces alfentanil plasma concentrations associated with an increase in cardiac output [abstract]. Anesthesiology. 2013;119:A3165.
45. Lötsch J, Skarke C, Schneider A, Hummel T, Geisslinger G. The 5-hydroxytriptamine 4 receptor agonist mosapride does antagonize morphine-induced respiratory depression. Clin Pharmacol Ther. 2005;78:278–87.

46. Oertel BG, Schneider A, Rohrbacher M, Schmidt H, Tegeder I, Geisslinger G, Lötsch J. The partial 5-hydroxytriptamine 1A receptor agonist buspirone does not antagonize morphine-induced respiratory depression in humans. Clin Pharmacol Ther. 2007;81:59–68.
47. Dahan A, Roozekrans M, van der Schrier R, Smith T, Aarts L. Primum non nocere or How to resolve drug-induced respiratory depression. Anesthesiology. 2013;118:1261–3.
48. Chidambaran V, Olbrecht V, Hossain M, Sadhasivam S, Rose J, Meyer MJ. Risk predictors of opioid-induced critical respiratory events in children: naloxone use as a quality measure of opioid safety. Pain Med. 2014;15(12):2139–49. doi:10.1111/pme.12575 Epub 2014 Oct 15.
49. Mujtaba S, Romero J, Taub CC. Methadone, QTc prolongation and torsades de pointes: current concepts, management and a hidden twist in the tale? J Cardiovasc Dis Res. 2013;4 (4):229–35. doi:10.1016/j.jcdr.2013.10.001 Epub 2013 Nov 16.
50. Stallvik M, Nordstrand B, Kristensen Ø, Bathen J, Skogvoll E, Spigset O. Corrected QT interval during treatment with methadone and buprenorphine—relation to doses and serum concentrations. Drug Alcohol Depend. 2013;129(1–2):88–93. doi:10.1016/j.drugalcdep. 2012.09.016 Epub 2012 Oct 16.
51. Price LC, Wobeter B, Delate T, Kurz D, Shanahan R. Methadone for pain and the risk of adverse cardiac outcomes. J Pain Symptom Manage. 2014;48(3):333–42. e1. doi: 10.1016/j. jpainsymman.2013.09.021. Epub 2014 Jan 28.
52. Baker JR, Best AM, Pade PA, McCance-Katz EF. Effect of buprenorphine and antiretroviral agents on the QT interval in opioid-dependent patients. Ann Pharmacother. 2006;40(3):392–6 Epub 2006 Feb 28.
53. Kim CH, Garcia R, Stover J, Ritchie K, Whealton T, Ata MA. Androgen deficiency in long-term intrathecal opioid administration. Pain Physician. 2014;17(4):E543–8.
54. De Maddalena C, Bellini M, Berra M, et al. Opioid-induced hypogonadism: why and how to treat it. Pain Physician. 2012;15(3):ES111–8.
55. Awwad JT, Farra C, Mitri F, Abdallah MA, Jaoudeh MA, Ghazeeri G. Split daily recombinant human LH dose in hypogonadotrophic hypogonadism: a nonrandomized controlled pilot study.
56. https://www.aace.com/files/osteo-guidelines-2010.pdf. ACCE Medical guidelines for clinical practice for the diagnosis and treatment of postmenopausal osteoporosis. [Last accessed 03/02/2015].
57. www.paulchristomd.com/wp.../flowhub/pdf/Opioid%20Effectiveness.pdf. [Last accessed 3/2/2015].
58. Gooren LJ, Bunk MC. Androgen replacement therapy: present and future. Drugs. 2004;64 (17):1861–91.
59. Daniell HW. Opioid endocrinopathy in women consuming prescribed sustained-action opioids for control of nonmalignant pain. J Pain. 2008;9(1):28–36.
60. Santen FJ, Sofsky J, Bilic N, Lippert R, et al. Mechanism of action of narcotics in the production of menstrual dysfunction in women. Fertil Steril. 1975;26:538–48.
61. Kingsburg S, Shifren J, Wkselman K, et al. Evaluation of the clinical relevance of benefits associated with transdermal testosterone treatment in postmenopausal women with hypoactive sexual desire disorder. J Sex Med. 2007;4(4 pt1):1001–1008.
62. North American Menopause Society. The role of testosterone therapy in postmenopausal women: position statement of The North American Menopause Society [published online ahead of print September 1, 2005]. Menopause 2005;12;496–511.
63. Palacio S. Advances in hormone replacement therapy: making the menopause manageable. BMC Womens Health. 2008;8:22.
64. Colameco S, Coren J. Opioid-induced endocrinopathy. J Am Osteopath Assoc. 2009;109:20–5.
65. Benefits of DHEA: the master normone. Life extension web site. Available at: http://www. lef.org/dhea/benefits_of_dhea.htm. Last accessed 02/02/2015.

66. Daniell HW, Lentz R, Mazer NA. Open-label pilot study of testosterone patch therapy in men with opioid-induced androgen deficiency.
67. Morales AJ, Haubrich RH, Hwang JY, et al. The effect of six months treatment with 100 mg daily dose of dehydroepiandrosterone (DHEA) on circulating sex steroids body composition and muscle strength in age-advanced men and women. Clin Endocrinol (Oxf). 1998;49:4201–432.
68. Katz N. The impact of opioids on the endocrine system. Pain Mange Rounds. 2005;1(9).
69. Folstein MF, Fetting JH, Lobo A, Niaz U, Capozzoli KD. Cognitive assessment of cancer patients. Cancer. 1983;53(suppl 10):2250–7.
70. Sjogren P, Thomsen AB, Olsen AK. Impaired neuropsychological performance in chronic nonmalignant pain patients receiving long-term oral opioid therapy. J Pain Symptom Manage. 2000;19:100–8.
71. Vella-Brincat j, Macleod AD. Adverse effects of opioids on the central nervous systems of palliative care patients. J. Pain Palliative Care Pharmacother. 2007;21(1):15–25.
72. Ersek M, Cherrier MM, Overman SS, Irving GA. The cognitive effects of opioids. Pain Manage Nurs. 2004;5(2):75–93.
73. Fishbain DA, Cutler B, Rosomoff HL, Rosomoff RS. Are opioid-dependent/tolerant patients impaired in driving-related skills? A structured evidence-based review. J Pain Symptom Manage. 2003;25(6):559–77.
74. Sabatowski R, Scharnagel R, Gyllensvärd A, Steigerwald I. Driving ability in patients with severe chronic low back or osteoarthritis knee pain on stable treatment with tapentadol prolonged release: a multicenter, open-label, phase 3b trial. Pain Ther. 2014;3(1):17–29. doi:10.1007/s40122-014-0025-3 Epub 2014 Apr 4.
75. Meijler WJ. Driving ban for patients on chronic opioid therapy unfounded. Ned Tijdschr Geneeskd. 2000;144:1644–5.
76. Chapman SL, Byas-Smith MG, Reed BA. Effects of intermediate- and long-term use of opioids on cognition in patients with chronic pain. Clin. J. Pain. 2002;18(4 Suppl):S83–90.
77. Højsted J, Kurita GP, Kendall S, de Lundorff L, Mattos Pimenta CA, Sjøgren P. Non-analgesic effects of opioids: the cognitive effects of opioids in chronic pain of malignant and non-malignant origin. An update. Curr Pharm Des. 2012;18(37):6116–22.
78. Zaaijer ER, Bruijel J, Blanken P, Hendriks V, et al. Personality as a risk factor for illicit opioid use and a protective factor for illicit opioid dependence. Drug Alcohol Depend. 2014;1(145):101–5. doi:10.1016/j.drugalcdep.2014.09.783 Epub 2014 Oct 14.
79. White KT, Dillingham TR, González-Fernández M, Rothfield L. Opiates for chronic nonmalignant pain syndromes: can appropriate candidates be identified for outpatient clinic management? Am J Phys Med Rehabil. 2009;88(12):995–1001. doi:10.1097/PHM. 0b013e3181bc006e.
80. Aronoff, GM eds. Bolen J. Medication management of chronic pain: use of controlled substances for pain management: a legal perspective Indiana: Trafford 2016.
81. Greaves MW, Wall PD. Pathophysiology of itching. Lancet. 1996;348:938–40.
82. McNicol E, Horowicz-Mehler N, Fisk RA, Bennett K, Gialeli-Goudas M, Chew PW, et al. Management of opioid side effects in cancer-related and chronic noncancer pain: a systematic review. J Pain. 2003;4:231–56.
83. Zylicz Z, Smits C, Krajnik M. Paroxetine for pruritus in advanced cancer. J Pain Symptom Manage. 1998;16:121–4.
84. http://www.merckmanuals.com/professional/neurologic_disorders/pain/treatment_of_pain. html. [Last accessed 2/24/2015].
85. Rosow CE, Gomery P, Chen TY, Stefanovich P, Stambler N, Israel R. Reversal of opioid-induced bladder dysfunction by intravenous naloxone and methylnaltrexone. Clin Pharmacol Ther. 2007;82:48–53.
86. Malinovsky JM, Le Normand L, Lepage JY, Malinge M, Cozian A, Pinaud M, Buzelin JM. The urodynamic effects of intravenous opioids and ketoprofen in humans.

87. http://www.merckmanuals.com/home/brain_spinal_cord_and_nerve_disorders/pain/treatment_ of_pain.html?qt=adverse%20effects%20opioids&alt=sh. [Last accessed 2/24/2015].

88. Ikeda T, Kurz A, Sessler DI, et al. The effect of opioids on thermoregulatory responses in humans and the special an tishivering action of meperidine. Ann NY Acad Sci. 1997;813:792–8.

89. Al-Adwani A, Basu N. Methadone and excessive sweating [letter]. Addiction. 2004;99:259.

90. Catterall RA. Problems of sweating and transfermal fentanyl. Palliat Med. 1997;11:169–70.

91. Mercadante S, Villari P, Ferrera P. Burst ketamine to reverse opioid tolerance in cancer pain. J Pain Symptom Manage. 2003;25:302–5.

92. Andrews HL. The effects of opiates on the pain threshold in post-addicts. J Clin Invest. 1943;22(4):511–6.

93. Mercadante S, Arcuri E. Hyperalgesia and opioid switching. Am J Hosp Palliat Care. 2005;22:291–4.

94. De-Yong L, Shi Xiaoyou, Li Xianggi, et al. The β2 adrenergic receptor regulates morphine tolerance and physical dependence. Behav Brain Res. 2007;181(1):118–26.

95. Fishbain DA, Cole B, Lewis JE, Gao J, Rosomoff RS. Do opioids induce hyperalgesia in humans? An evidence-based structured review. Pain Med. 2009;10(5):829–39. doi: 10.1111/j.1526-4637.2009.00653.x. Epub 2009 Jul 6. Review.

96. Zubieta JK, Heitzeg MM, Smith YR, Bueller JA, et al. COMT val158met genotype affects mu-opioid neurotransmitter responses to a pain stressor. Science. 2003;299:1240–3.

97. Lee M, Silverman S, Hansen H. A comprehensive review of opioid-induced. Hyperalgesia Pain Physician 2011;14:145–161.

98. Koppert W, Sittle R, Scheuber K, et al. Differential modulation of remifentanil-induced analgesia and post infusion hyperalgesia by S-ketamine and clonidine in humans. Anesthesiology. 2003;99(1):152–9.

99. Tiseo PJ, Thaler HT, Lapin J et al: Morphine-6-Glucuronide concentrations and opioid-related side effects: a survey in cancer patients. Pain. 1995;61(1):47–54. See more at: http://www.cancernetwork.com/oncology-journal/current-management-opioid-related-side-effects/page/0/3#sthash.j6HipfjC.dpuf.

100. McPherson ML. Strategies for management of opioid-induced adverse effects. Adv Stud Pharm. 2008;5(2):52–7.

101. Aronoff GM. Marijuana usage in chronic pain patients: driving and work guidelines for clinicians. Pain Medicine News. [epub]. 2013 June.

102. Marijuana as medicine: assessing the science base. National Academy Press, Washington, DC. 1999.

103. Jolly BT. Drugged driving—different spin on an old problem [Editorial]. Ann Emerg Med April 2000;35:399–400.

104. National Highway Traffic Safety Administration. Marijuana and alcohol combined severely impede driving performance. Ann Emerg Med. 2000;35:398–9.

105. Amar Ben. M. Cannaboids in medicine: a review of their therapeutic potential. J Ethnopharmacol. 2006;105:1–25.

106. Wang T, Collet JP, Shapiro S, et al. Adverse effects of medical cannaboids: a systematic review. CMAJ. 2008;178(13):1669–78. doi: 10.1503/cmaj.071178.

107. Ashton CH. Pharmacology and the effects of cannabis: a brief review. Br J Psychiatry. 2001;178:101–6.

108. Pesce, A, Ist, C, Rosenthal M, et al. Marijuana correlates with use of other illicit drugs in a pain patient population. Pain Physician. 2010;13(3):283–7.

109. Wang T, Collet JP, Shapiro S, et al. Adverse effects of medical cannaboids: a systematic review. CMAJ. 2008;178(13):1669–78. doi: 10.1503/cmaj.071178.

110. Campbell FA, Tramer MR, Carroll D, et al. Are cannabinoids an effective and safe treatment option in the management of pain? A Qual Syst Rev BMJ. 2001;323(7303):13–6.

111. Li G, Brady JE, Chenc Q. Drug use and fatal motor vehicle crashes: A case-control study. Accid Anal Prev. 2013;60:205–10.
112. Bolen, J. http://legalsideofpain.com/uploads/Marijuana-and-Your-Health-Just-The-Facts-Part-I.pdf.
113. Sehgal N, Manchikanti, L, Smith HS. Prescription opioid abuse in chronic pain: A review of opioid abuse predictors and strategies to curb opioid abuse. Pain Physician 2012;15:ES67–92.

Chapter 10
Risk Mitigation Strategies

Lynn R. Webster

Introduction

Controlled substances, including opioid analgesics, have a legitimate, recognized place in chronic pain management but are associated with significant risks to patients and society stemming from misuse, abuse, diversion, addiction, and overdose deaths. The health and societal consequences of opioid misuse and abuse are severe. Prescription opioids contribute to more than 16,000 drug-poisoning deaths per year [1]. Approximately 4.5 million Americans are current nonmedical users of opioids [2]. By one estimate, the economic costs of nonmedical opioid use reach $53.4 billion a year in lost productivity, criminal justice costs, drug abuse treatment, and medical complications [3], and the personal damage done to individuals and families is incalculable.

Opioids, though clearly potentially harmful, do reduce pain and restore functionality for some patients who suffer from severe, chronic pain that is unresponsive to alternative pharmacologic or nonpharmacologic therapies. Long-term effectiveness data are sparse but indicate a subset of patients benefit from opioid analgesics [4], and that periodic monitoring using clinical tools to reduce opioid misuse and abuse can improve patient outcomes and reduce costs [5–7].

This chapter discusses risk mitigation tools to track the clinical effect and patient adherence to medical direction in the use of therapeutic opioids and other controlled substances for pain. Aside from opioids, commonly prescribed medications in pain management include agents to treat depression, anxiety, sleep, and other psychiatric and medical comorbidities that frequently co-occur with pain. Newer abuse-deterrent opioid formulations are discussed, and clinical strategies in opioid rotation are presented to maximize analgesia and minimize risk.

L.R. Webster (✉)
Early Development Services, PRA Health Sciences, 3838 South 700 East, Suite 202, Salt Lake City, UT 84106, USA
e-mail: LRWebsterMD@gmail.com

© Springer International Publishing Switzerland 2016
P.S. Staats and S.M. Silverman (eds.), *Controlled Substance Management in Chronic Pain*, DOI 10.1007/978-3-319-30964-4_10

To aid clarity, this manuscript adheres to definitions of misuse and abuse reached by an expert panel as follows: Misuse is "use of a medication (for a medical purpose) other than as directed or indicated, whether willful or unintentional, and whether harm results or not [8]." Abuse is considered "any use of an illegal drug or the intentional self-administration of a medication for a nonmedical purpose such as altering one's state of consciousness, for example, getting high [8]."

The Essentials of Risk Mitigation

An essential step for clinical and medicolegal reasons is to diligently document risk mitigation strategies in the patient record. Good documentation practices help ensure timely and appropriate medical attention to any issues that arise and demonstrate to regulatory and law-enforcement authorities that prescribing is for a legitimate medical purpose within the usual course of professional medical practice [9].

Managing risk first entails careful assessment and risk stratification. Patients may be screened for degree of risk and triaged to determine the intensity, frequency, and type of risk mitigation strategies to follow. A strategy devised by Gourlay et al. [10] stratifies patients into three treatment groups:

- Group I contains patients without personal or family history of substance abuse and without major or untreated psychiatric or psychological disorder.
- Patients in Group II do not display active addiction but are at risk due to history of treated substance abuse, significant family history of substance abuse, past or comorbid psychiatric or psychological disorder, or some combination; they should be comanaged with the help of a specialist in pain, substance abuse, mental health, or some combination as appropriate.
- Patients in Group III are the most difficult to manage because of their active substance abuse or addiction or major untreated psychiatric or psychological disorder(s). Stringent follow-up or an opioid exit strategy should apply as appropriate. Recent data indicate recently released prisoners belong in this category [11].

Patients may be assessed using tools specifically formulated for opioid-treated patients, such as the Opioid Risk Tool (see Appendix C) [12] and the revised 24-item Screener and Opioid Assessment for Patients with Pain (SOAPP-R) (see Appendix D) [13]. These and additional available tools are not diagnostic of addiction nor are they intended to pinpoint whether a patient should be discharged from opioid therapy; rather, they assess the risk for aberrant drug-related behaviors by the patient, based on biological, social, and psychiatric risk factors, and are administered prior to beginning opioid therapy. Risk factors from the scientific literature include but are not limited to the following: [12–17]:

- Nonfunctional status due to pain;
- Exaggeration of pain;

- Unclear etiology for pain;
- Young age;
- Smoking;
- Poor social support;
- Personal history of substance abuse;
- Family history of substance abuse;
- Psychological stress;
- Psychological disease;
- Focus on opioids;
- Preadolescent sexual abuse.

Patients may not be honest when answering questions related to opioid abuse risk. Whether or not a formal tool is used, prescribers should be aware of risk factors and implement a clinical plan to assess patients based on them. Patients are monitored at a level in accordance with risk (Table 10.1) [18, 19]. However, patients may change

Table 10.1 Match monitoring to the patient's risk of opioid misuse/abuse[a] (adapted from [18] and [19])

Low risk (Routine)	Moderate risk	High risk
• Pain assessment	• More visits when appropriate	• Avoid opioids if possible
• Substance misuse/abuse assessment via validated tool	• More frequent prescriptions intervals when appropriate	• Use alternative therapies if possible
• Informed consent	• Regular prescription database check every 6 months or more often, depending on state regulations	• Weekly visits or more often as necessary
• Signed treatment agreement	• Verification via patient's family members/friends	• Weekly prescriptions (on attendance) or more often where possible
• Regular follow-up visits, prescriptions based on clinical need and behaviors	• Random UDT with any aberrant behavior or every 3–6 months	• Quarterly prescription database check or more frequent, depending on state regulations
• Initial prescription database check and every 6–12 months	• Evaluate for comorbid mental health disease	• Friend/family member controls medication
• Review previous medical records	• Consider psych/pain specialist evaluation	• UDT every visit
• Initial UDT and as directed by behaviors and state regulations	• Consider pill counts	• Consider blood screens
• Specialist consult as clinically determined	• Consider limiting RO analgesics	• Psych/addiction specialist evaluation
• Medication choices as clinically determined		• Consider pain specialist evaluation
• Document 4A's		• Limit RO analgesics
• Document clinical interactions		• Consider limiting SAO

[a]All recommendations from lower risk columns continue to apply as risk increases
UDT urine drug test
4A's analgesia, activities of daily living, adverse effects, aberrant drug-related behaviors
RO rapid onset
SAO short-acting opioids

risk categories over the course of treatment and require closer monitoring due to stress, increased pain, disease progression, social and familial difficulties, the onset or worsening of mental disease, and other factors. The toll chronic pain takes on family and social relationships, work, finances, and frequent struggles to obtain health insurance coverage significantly heighten stress and threaten adherence to the medication regimen. Tools are also available to assist with frequent reassessment and documentation to include the effects of opioid therapy on analgesia, daily activities, adverse effects, aberrant drug-related behaviors, cognition, and quality of life [20, 21].

Types of medication misuse and abuse occur in patients and nonpatients, and motivations manifest along a spectrum (Fig. 10.1) [22]. Reasons for patient medication misuse or abuse vary widely and include the following [23]:

- Misunderstanding between the patient and provider;
- Unauthorized self medication of pain, mood, or sleep problems;
- Desire to avoid symptoms of abstinence syndrome;
- Desire for euphoria or other psychoactive reward;
- Compulsive use due to addiction;
- Illegal diversion for financial gain.

Consider also that clinical manifestations of opioid-related substance abuse are more likely in a scenario of familial or social substance abuse. Talking about the issues with patients is critical. The physician can facilitate patient honesty by treating adherence to medical direction with opioid therapy as routine and by using an empathic rather than confrontational approach.

Although there is value in recognizing that patients do differ in their risk for medication misuse or abuse, clinicians should also meet a minimum threshold of

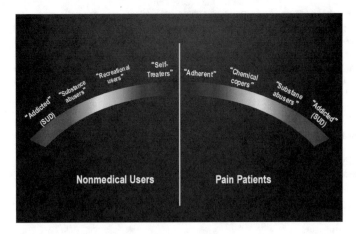

Fig. 10.1 Spectrum of medication misuse in nonmedical users and pain patients. *SUD* substance-use disorder. From Kirsh and Passik [22]

risk mitigation for every patient who receives treatment with opioids or other controlled substances for pain. Subjective evaluation of patient adherence is best when used in combination with objective measures. Because aberrant drug-related behaviors such as escalating doses or requesting early refills may be difficult to interpret, and consensus is lacking as to which types and frequencies of behaviors demand clinical action, quantifiable measures increase clinician control. Clinicians should track the effect of the therapeutic regimen on the patient's pain levels and functional, psychological, and social health throughout the course of therapy.

The discontinuation of opioid therapy may be necessary in some cases. Clinicians should have an exit strategy in place and be prepared to humanely taper patients and either treat or refer for treatment with alternatives to opioid therapy.

Clinical Monitoring Tools

Urine Toxicology

One of the most widely available, useful tools for monitoring adherence to the therapeutic regimen is the urine drug test (UDT) and one that is underutilized [24]. Results of a UDT are used to identify—within limitations—the presence of pre-scribed medications and the use of undisclosed, unauthorized prescription and illegal drugs. Compared with blood testing, it is less expensive, is less invasive, and has a longer window for detection of substances [25, 26]. In addition to ease of collection, turnaround time is quick and laboratories that provide the testing are accessible.

Urine toxicology is now an expected standard of practice in chronic pain management. As such, the UDT should be presented upfront to patients as a routine, consensual part of medical care, with a full explanation of why it is important.

Potential benefits of UDT include the following:

- Establishing routine medical practice akin to testing glucose levels in diabetes;
- Fostering communication between patient and clinician;
- Helping guide treatment decisions;
- Identifying early patients with potential substance-use disorders;
- Increasing safety;
- Allowing the clinicians to advocate on the patient's behalf;
- Discouraging drug misuse or recreational abuse;
- Heightening the chance for therapeutic success through patient adherence to the treatment regimen.

Two steps in testing are required in most instances: qualitative/presumptive and quantitative/definitive testing [26, 27]. The qualitative immunoassay is radioactive or enzyme mediated and can help quickly establish whether a new patient has recently ingested illegal drugs or other opioid and prescription drugs. It detects certain drug classes but typically cannot isolate specific opioids. If results from the initial, presumptive test are inconsistent with medical direction, a follow-up test is necessary. This second step is a quantitative evaluation, usually via gas chromatography/mass spectrometry (GC/MS) technology or liquid chromatography dual mass spectrometry (LC/MS/MS). These tests are more specific than immunoassay and can detect actual molecular structures of specific drugs. Although immunoassay followed by definitive testing historically has been the standard, some laboratories have begun to offer definitive testing via LC/MS/MS that can identify more drugs than conventional immunoassays and that may be given as the initial test [27].

The temperature of the sample should be measured at the point of collection. Laboratories can test for specific gravity. Both measures guard against tampering with the sample [19, 26].

Testing in a clinical setting with its emphasis on scientific data collection to inform medical decisions is different from that performed in forensic or workplace settings. Laboratories for definitive testing should be carefully selected and informed of pain management goals. Cutoff points for the detection of drugs during definitive testing vary, and clinicians should discuss clinically relevant cutoff points with personnel at the laboratory that is to perform the testing. Discuss, also, with laboratory personnel the importance of the presence or absence of the prescribed drug, which is equal in importance to the presence of unauthorized substances for mitigating abuse or diversion.

Drugs to test include illicit drugs, commonly prescribed opioids (i.e., morphine, hydrocodone, hydromorphone, oxycodone, oxymorphone, fentanyl, and buprenorphine), benzodiazepines, barbiturates, carisoprodol, tramadol, selective serotonin reuptake inhibitors, serotonin–norepinephrine reuptake inhibitors, anxiolytics, sleep medications, and other substances as necessary [19].

Best practices regarding the frequency of UDT in pain management are evolving and may vary by state. Clinical guidelines suggest a baseline UDT for every patient to be prescribed opioids or other controlled substances long term (in general, >3 months) to be followed by periodic tests in alliance with the patient's risk category or clinical signs of opioid misuse or abuse (Table 10.1) [18, 19, 28, 29]. A recent guideline from Peppin and colleagues recommends the possibility of periodic, random testing for every patient at every visit [19]. For patients at low risk, the same guideline recommends testing at least every 6 months and, if an immunoassay test is used, testing at least 1 time a year with GC/MS or LC/MS/MS. For moderate-to-high-risk patients, the recommendation is an immunoassay test every 3 months at minimum and definitive testing every 6 months. However, bear in mind, if a patient's risk is quite high or if problematic behaviors or clinical signs need to be addressed, a test during every clinic visit may be more appropriate.

Risk category should guide, to some extent, how often a patient is tested. However, it is not possible to identify beyond doubt who is adherent to medical direction and who is not. Therefore, every patient prescribed controlled substances is presumed to be at some risk and is thus subject to risk mitigation measures in line with universal precautions, which is modeled on the infectious disease paradigm [10].

The clinician must appreciate certain limitations of the UDT, caused by variables such as individual patient and drug metabolism and test unreliability. False

Table 10.2 Possible false positive results [26]

Substance ingested	Possible false result
Poppy seeds	Opiates
Quinolones (antibiotics)	Opiates
Quetiapine (antipsychotic)	Methadone
Trazodone (antidepressant)	Fentanyl
Venlafaxine (antidepressant)	Phencyclidine
Clobenzorex (diet pill)	Amphetamine
Fenproporex (diet pill)	Amphetamine
Promethazine (for allergies, agitation, nausea, and vomiting)	Amphetamine
l-methamphetamine OTC nasal inhaler	Amphetamine

OTC over the counter

positives (when a drug is absent though the test indicates it is present) and false negatives (when a drug is actually present though the test result says it is not) are possible, though far more common with immunoassay testing than with LC/MS/MS quantitative laboratory testing [30].

Some common causes of inaccurate UDT results are listed below.

Cross-reactivity with certain foods, over-the-counter (OTC) medications, and prescribed drugs may cause false positives (Table 10.2) [26]. It is important to know all prescribed and OTC medications a patient is taking and to inform the laboratory that will perform the testing.

Windows of detection are limited to 2–3 days after exposure for most substances [31], meaning a patient who misunderstands dosing directions or who metabolizes opioids faster than is typical due to genetic factors may have a false result.

Laboratory error or test insensitivity could skew results, particularly with immunoassays, which may not be sensitive enough to detect opioids at therapeutic levels. Follow-up with the laboratory is advised to ensure the personnel are testing the correct substances with the most sensitive test available.

Drug metabolism, as mentioned, varies among patients due to genetic factors [32], and those who are quick metabolizers may falsely appear to have failed to consume a prescribed drug. Pharmacogenetic testing is now available to identify genetic biomarkers that may influence a patient's response to medication, though it should be noted the clinical relevance of such biomarkers is still unclear with regard to supporting evidence [33].

Metabolites of prescribed drugs and manufacturing impurities may present as unexpected results [18, 34]. For example,

- Codeine is metabolized to morphine;
- Morphine is not metabolized to codeine, but small amounts of codeine may be a manufacturing by-product;
- Codeine is partially metabolized to hydrocodone;
- Hydrocodone is metabolized to hydromorphone;

- Morphine can produce the minor metabolite hydromorphone;
- Heroin is metabolized to 6-monoacetylmorphine (6-MAM) and morphine.

These limitations must be appreciated to help avoid errors in interpretation. One should understand, also, that the absence of a prescribed drug does not, in itself, prove hoarding or illegal diversion. Unexpected results should trigger a clinical discussion with the patient, which is then followed up in the medical record. Clinical decisions should only be made based on the most accurate test method, and all UDT results should be part of a broader risk mitigation strategy.

Prescription Drug-Monitoring Programs

Most states now operate electronic databases containing prescriber and patient data on dispensed prescriptions to enable healthcare, law-enforcement, and regulatory professionals to track clinically harmful or illegal activities involving controlled substances [35]. As of 2012, every state except Missouri either had a prescription drug-monitoring program (PDMP) or had plans to develop one, and systems were operational in 41 states [36]. A primary strength of state PDMPs is to identify quickly those who get opioids or other controlled substances from more than one medical source without authorization [36]. Newer systems offer real-time data and secure online access. The capabilities across states vary widely, however, and how effective the programs are in mitigating harm is still being assessed.

Some evidence indicates PDMPs do mitigate opioid-related harm in the general and treatment-seeking populations. Analysis of two data streams from the RADARS System showed reduced intentional exposures and substance-abuse treatment admissions involving opioids in states with PDMPs compared to states without [35]. The mechanism for the reduction is not completely clear. Another analysis found that states with proactive PDMPs, defined as those that generate unsolicited reports automatically, subsequently reported a reduced supply of prescribed opioids leading indirectly to less being available for misuse, abuse, and diversion [37]. Evidence pertaining to opioid-related mortality has, thus far, not shown a benefit from PDMPs, but additional research is necessary [38].

Discrepancies across state systems do limit the programs' effectiveness. According to a report funded by the Pew Charitable Trusts [36], this lack of uniformity and other limitations likely contribute to physician reluctance to use the databases. Suggestions in the report for improvements include the following:

- Increase the ability to share data across state lines;
- Standardize the data fields and move toward real-time collection;
- Collect data on all controlled substance schedules and some commonly abused drugs that are not scheduled;
- Better integrate data into patients' electronic health records (EHR);
- Establish criteria for identifying questionable activity;
- Generate automatic reports to guide prescribing decisions or investigations.

Overall, PDMPs appear to be beneficial and improving in quality, despite the need for further refining and better integration into daily practice. Most experts in the field of pain management and the Federation of State Medical Boards, on which many states base pain management guidelines, concur that PDMPs may help identify "doctor shopping" and provide information that may help make prescribing controlled substances safer for patients [25, 28]. In addition, some states are implementing requirements in regard to the timing and frequency of PDMP checks [39].

A prudent course is to check the state PDMP as follows:

- For every new patient;
- Periodically;
- Whenever medications or dosages are changed;
- When evidence of nonadherence to the therapeutic regimen occurs;
- When aberrant drug-related behaviors are observed.

The clinicians may identify harmful patterns of multiple unauthorized prescriptions, potential for drug–drug interactions, and early indications of substance-use disorders in the patient. However, as with UDT, results should be interpreted with caution. Results from a PDMP check are not diagnostic of the disease of addiction, and alternative causes of observed discrepancies are possible. For instance, recent reports indicate that drug shortages and regulatory efforts aimed at reining in illegal diversion of prescription drugs have brought about circumstances in which patients have been forced to visit multiple pharmacies to get legitimately issued prescriptions filled [40].

Pill Counts

Pill (or patch) counts are often recommended, usually in concert with other adherence monitoring strategies [24, 28]. A prospective study of 500 consecutive patients receiving controlled substances documented a 50 % reduction in signs of opioid misuse and abuse associated with adherence monitoring that included pill counts together with UDT and periodic evaluation of the patient [6].

Typically, pill counts are an intensified monitoring measure for patients who are at high risk or who have exhibited a pattern of behaviors that might indicate opioid misuse or abuse, such as frequent early refills, lost medications, or inconsistent UDT results. Pills may be counted on a random basis during regularly scheduled clinic visits, or patients may be called and given a time frame to come to the office with their original pill bottle. These tighter controls typically accompany closer prescribing intervals (e.g., monthly or weekly). A failed test is a no-show or a quantity of medication that is inconsistent with prescribed and expected consumption levels.

Documentation of this practice in the medical record may help demonstrate appropriate medical practice if questions about a clinician's prescribing practices should later arise with law-enforcement or regulatory authorities. Do note, however, that patients may circumvent the intent of pill counts through borrowing or purchasing medication so as to present the appropriate, expected quantity during the clinic visit. As with other objective risk mitigation measures, pill counts should be understood and implemented as part of an overall clinical strategy, not a single fix.

Abuse-Deterrent Formulations

The pharmaceutical industry is developing newer opioid formulations to maintain analgesia while reducing abuse liability. To date, the US Food and Drug Administration (FDA) has approved four products for labeling consistent with the agency's draft guidance on the properties required for abuse-deterrent formulations (ADFs) [41]. The agents are as follows: reformulated oxycodone hydrochloride (HCL) extended-release (ER) tablets, oxycodone HCL/naloxone HCL ER tablets, morphine sulfate/naltrexone HCL ER capsules (which were voluntarily recalled because of stability concerns; relaunched in 2015), and hydrocodone bitartrate ER tablets (Table 10.3) [42–47]. All are indicated for the management of pain severe enough to require daily, around-the-clock, long-term opioid treatment and for which alternative treatment options are inadequate.

Additional agents formulated to deter abuse but without abuse-deterrent labeling include the following: hydromorphone HCL ER tablets (EXALGO™), oxycodone HCL/acetaminophen ER tablets (XARTEMIS™ XR), oxycodone HCL tablets (OXECTA™), oxymorphone HCL ER tablets (OPANA® ER), and tapentadol HCL ER tablets (NUCYNTA® ER) [48–52].

Newer formulations work by blocking the physical or chemical manipulations through which a formulation may be improperly accessed and ingested via an

Table 10.3 Opioid products approved with abuse-deterrent labeling [42–47]

Formulation	Brand name	Company	Date labeling approved	Deterrence properties
Oxycodone ER	OxyContin™	Purdue Pharma L.P.	April 2013	Physicochemical barriers to crushing and dissolving
Oxycodone–naloxone	Targiniq™	Purdue Pharma L.P.	July 2014	Crushing, dissolving releases opioid antagonist
Morphine–naltrexone	Embeda™	Pfizer	October 2014	Crushing releases sequestered opioid antagonist
Hydrocodone ER	Hysingla™	Purdue Pharma L.P.	November 2014	Difficult to crush, forms a viscous gel

ER extended release

unintended route or method. Common methods and routes of opioid abuse include the following:

- Crushing and swallowing;
- Crushing and snorting;
- Crushing and smoking;
- Crushing and extracting for injection;
- Swallowing intact;
- Coingesting with alcohol or benzodiazepines.

The FDA classes the various properties of ADFs as follows [41]:

(1) *Physical or chemical barriers* to tampering with or altering the opioid product. Physical barriers, such as housing viscous gel, resist chewing, grinding, crushing, or grating; chemical barriers block extraction of active ingredient through dissolving in liquids such as water or alcohol.
(2) *Agonist/antagonist combinations* in which an agent such as naloxone or naltrexone is designed to remain inert during therapeutic use but is released so as to reverse the opioid effect if the formulation is altered.
(3) *Aversive agents* such as capsaicin that produce an unpleasant effect if used nontherapeutically.
(4) *Delivery systems* such as intramuscular depot injections or implants that are difficult to manipulate.
(5) *Prodrugs* that are activated for analgesic purposes only by the gastrointestinal tract, thus frustrating injection or intranasal routes.
(6) *Combinations* of the above methods.

Much research aims to deter abuse that is accomplished when long-acting opioid formulations are altered to access for immediate release (IR) an intended ER formulation. This principle of abuse potential associated with a drug is its *abuse quotient* (*AQ*), defined as the maximum serum concentration of the drug (C_{max}) divided by the time required to reach that maximum level (T_{max}) [53]. In general, tampering with ER formulations causes serum C_{max} to increase and T_{max} to decrease, as when a full dose of oxycodone ER is quickly released. Therefore, the larger the ratio, the greater the potential attractiveness of a drug to would-be abusers. The research focus on ER formulations is supported by the results that suggest that long-acting opioids, such as oxycodone ER, are more frequently abused than are IR, short-acting, and combination opioids once rates are normalized for the number of prescriptions written [54, 55].

People who misuse or abuse opioids may be patients or nonpatients. Patients who misuse opioids (i.e., any unauthorized use) may do so through error or for the medications' psychoactive effects due to the disease of addiction, to escape physical pain, or to escape emotional or psychological pain. Most patients will misuse or abuse an opioid orally by swallowing whole or chewing. Nonpatients, who divert opioids from legitimate prescribing channels in order to get high or to satisfy a drug

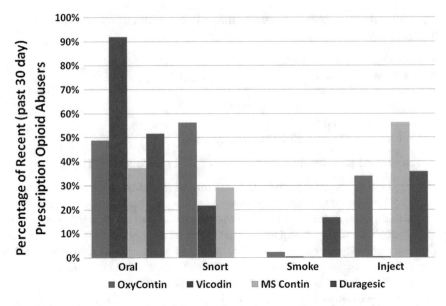

Fig. 10.2 Preferred routes of administration by patients entering substance-abuse treatment facilities [Population of individuals seeking substance-abuse treatment who indicated past 30-days abuse of prescription opioids ($N = 4807$)]. From Budman et al. [56]

craving, may swallow pills whole or chew them; however, this population is probably more likely to crush pills for intranasal or intravenous administration and to have set patterns of abuse based on their drug(s) of choice (Fig. 10.2) [56]. The technology of abuse deterrence is aimed principally at populations that alter the medications in order to abuse them.

Populations vary in their abuse of opioids. Three broad categories with over-lapping characteristics are as follows:

- Novices, experimenters, occasional users, typically but not necessarily young people;
- Nonaddicted, established users for whom prescription drug abuse is a recurrent activity;
- More severely substance-use-disordered or addicted users.

It appears ADFs have potential for deterring substance abuse with prescription opioids. The reformulated oxycodone ER developed by Purdue Pharma demonstrated reduced abuse compared with the conventional formulation in the first 20 months post-approval in an epidemiological sample of individuals at high risk for prescription opioid abuse, particularly for methods that involve tampering [57]. However, the science is evolving, and the ultimate impact of ADFs on the societal problem with prescription drug abuse is still uncertain. Another study demonstrated changes in oxycodone and heroin use after introduction of reformulated oxycodone [58].

The reformulated oxycodone showed a 36 % decrease in abuse exposures in two years after introduction with a 59 % decrease with 80 mg tablets. There was concomitant 20 % increase in abuse exposure with the original formulation of oxycodone ER and a 21 % increase in heroin exposure. Dart et al. [59] showed a concomitant increase in heroin use and decrease in reformulated oxycodone use via the RADARS System and from poison centers and substance-abuse treatment centers. Similarly, Cicero et al. [60] showed that reformulated oxycodone was associated with a significant reduction of past-month abuse after its introduction (45.1 % [95 % CI, 41.2–49.1 %]), apparently owing to a migration to other opioids, particularly heroin. However, this reduction leveled off, such that 25–30 % of the sample persisted in endorsing past-month abuse from 2012 to 2014.

Abuse of ADFs could still occur, particularly by the most common route: oral ingestion [41, 56]. Nor is there evidence as of yet that ADFs have any effect upon reducing rates of addiction, which is a chronic brain disease characterized by compulsive drug seeking and use despite adverse consequences [61]. What the evidence does suggest is that clinicians should not feel falsely secure when prescribing ADFs, but should consider them one part of a comprehensive pain management strategy in combination with other components of risk management.

The higher cost of ADFs compared to available generics currently may reduce the willingness of private and public insurance payers to offer coverage for them. However, given the potential for mitigating a public health problem with opioid abuse and associated cost reductions, payers would do well to keep current with ADF development and consider the possible role of newer formulations in a universal precautions approach to opioid prescribing [62]. Additional areas for coverage consideration could be reimbursement for patient risk assessment, provider training on best prescribing practices, including opioid-sparing multimodal therapy, and addiction treatment [62].

Opioid Rotation to Prevent Abuse

If one medication appears to have attractiveness for abuse, rotation to another opioid may prove safer and more beneficial. Rapid-onset opioids, for example, may be too rewarding for patients who have vulnerabilities to substance abuse because of the speed with which they enter the bloodstream and brain (Table 10.1). In addition, patients whose health insurance changes or is insufficient to cover a current opioid medication may, of necessity, need to be rotated to a different medication in the same class.

Caution and individual consideration for every patient are necessary when rotating from one opioid to another. Equianalgesic conversion tables are meant to provide guidance but are insufficient to determine the equivalent doses of different opioids [63, 64]. A published paradigm recommends decreasing one opioid slowly while slowly titrating the new opioid to effect using the following three steps [65]:

(1) Reduce the original opioid dose by 10–30 % while beginning the new opioid at the lowest available dose.
(2) Reduce the original opioid dose by 10–25 % per week while increasing the dose of the new daily opioid dose by 10–20 % based upon clinical need and safety.
(3) Provide sufficient IR opioid throughout the rotation to prevent withdrawal and keep pain levels down so the patient is not tempted to take too much medication.

In most instances, the complete switch can occur within 3 to 4 weeks. This process takes longer than most current opioid conversion practices suggest. Be sure to seek consultation with a more experienced prescriber of opioids when needed.

Rotation to methadone requires particular caution due to a long half-life (usually 8 to 59 h and up to 100 h) compared with the medication's analgesic effect, which usually lasts only 4–8 h [66, 67]. This unusual pharmacokinetic/pharmacodynamic profile can contribute to an unpredictable accumulation of methadone and toxicity. For this reason, patients should be treated as opioid naïve regardless of previous opioid dose when starting methadone: Consider starting patients (whether or not they are opioid naïve) on 15 mg or less per day in divided doses (q8h) and increase total daily dose by no more than 25–50 % no more frequently than weekly [68]. Again, seek expert consultation when necessary.

Clinical Considerations

When a treatment goal is to reduce the potential rewarding effect of a medication in a patient perceived to be at risk for opioid abuse, any and all of the following factors may contribute to substance abuse and should be considered [18, 56]:

- The drug (availability, cost, purity, mode of administration, speed of brain entry);
- The user whether patient or nonpatient (genetics, metabolism of drug, psychiatric symptoms, risk-taking behavior);
- The environment (social setting, community attitudes, availability of drug, employment, educational opportunities).

A patient perceived as being at risk for opioid abuse should be treated, when possible with nonopioid medications and nonpharmacological modalities, including cognitive behavioral therapy, physical rehabilitation, and other alternatives that encourage active participation by the patient. Combining therapies may help keep opioid doses low if an opioid is deemed necessary. For pain severe enough to warrant sustained, around-the-clock opioid analgesia, initiate using the lowest effective dose and titrate slowly. High-risk patients may require tight controls such as frequent clinic visits, smaller quantities per prescription, and medication choices with slower onset and slower entry into the brain and thus less chance of reward.

Conclusion

A number of risk management strategies are important for avoiding harm with controlled substances that are prescribed for pain, particularly opioid analgesics and comedications that also depress respiration. High-risk patients require more intense risk mitigation strategies; however, all patients who are prescribed controlled substances for pain should be monitored using universal precautions. A number of tools are available and include urine toxicology, prescription-monitoring databases, and pill counts to check for adherence to the therapeutic regimen. Opioid formulations designed to deter tampering and abuse have a place in current pain management strategies. Universal precautions may come to include ADFs with sufficient increased market availability, supporting post-marketing studies, and the willingness of insurance payers to extend coverage. A comprehensive strategy should incorporate a mix of objective and subjective monitoring measures to meet therapeutic goals and reduce adverse outcomes.

Acknowledgment   Beth Dove of Dove Medical Communications, LLC, in Salt Lake City, Utah, provided research and medical writing.

References

1. Chen LH, Hedegaard H, Warner M. Drug-poisoning deaths involving opioid analgesics: United States, 1999–2011. NCHS data brief, no 166. Hyattsville, MD: National Center for Health Statistics; 2014.
2. Substance Abuse and Mental Health Services Administration. Results from the 2011 National Survey on Drug Use and Health: Summary of National Findings, NSDUH Series H-44, HHS Publication No. (SMA) 12-4713. Rockville, MD: Substance Abuse and Mental Health Services Administration; 2012.
3. Hansen RN, Oster G, Edelsberg J, Woody GE, Sullivan SD. Economic costs of nonmedical use of prescription opioids. Clin J Pain. 2011;27(3):194–202.
4. Noble M, Treadwell JR, Tregear SJ, et al. Long-term opioid management for chronic noncancer pain. Cochrane Database Syst Rev. 2010;20(1):CD006605.
5. Manchikanti L, Manchukonda R, Pampati V, et al. Does random urine drug testing reduce illicit drug use in chronic pain patients receiving opioids? Pain Phys. 2006;9(2):123–9.
6. Manchikanti L, Manchukonda R, Damron KS, Brandon D, McManus CD, Cash K. Does adherence monitoring reduce controlled substance abuse in chronic pain patients? Pain Phys. 2006;9(1):57–60.
7. McCarberg BH. Chronic pain: reducing costs through early implementation of adherence testing and recognition of opioid misuse. Postgrad Med. 2011;123(6):132–9.

8. Katz NP, Adams EH, Chilcoat H, et al. Challenges in the development of prescription opioid abuse-deterrent formulations. Clin J Pain. 2007;23(8):648–60.
9. Dispensing Controlled Substances for the Treatment of Pain, DEA Policy Statement, 71 Fed. Reg. 52716, 52717, 6 Sept 2006.
10. Gourlay DL, Heit HA, Almahrezi A. Universal precautions in pain medicine: a rational approach to the treatment of chronic pain. Pain Med. 2005;6(2):107–12.
11. Binswanger IA, Blatchford PJ, Mueller SR, Stern MF. Mortality after prison release: opioid overdose and other causes of death, risk factors, and time trends from 1999 to 2009. Ann Intern Med. 2013;159(9):592–600.
12. Webster LR, Webster RM. Predicting aberrant behaviors in opioid-treated patients: preliminary validation of the opioid risk tool. Pain Med. 2005;6(6):432–42.
13. Butler SF, Fernandez K, Benoit C, Budman SH, Jamison RN. Validation of the revised screener and opioid assessment for patients with pain (SOAPP-R). J Pain. 2008;9(4):360–72.
14. Friedman R, Li V, Mehrotra D. Treating pain patients at risk: evaluation of a screening tool in opioid-treated pain patients with and without addiction. Pain Med. 2003;4(2):182–5.
15. Alturi S, Sudarshan G. A screening tool to determine the risk of prescription opioid abuse among patients with chronic non-malignant pain. Pain Physician. 2002;5(4):447–8.
16. Savage SR. Assessment for addiction in pain-treatment settings. Clin J Pain. 2002;18:28–38.
17. Dunbar SA, Katz NP. Chronic opioid therapy for non-malignant pain in patients with a history of substance abuse: report of 20 cases. J Pain Symptom Manage. 1996;11(3):163–71.
18. Webster LR, Dove B. Avoiding opioid abuse while managing pain: a guide for practitioners. North Branch, MN: Sunrise River Press; 2007. p. 126.
19. Peppin JF, Passik SD, Couto JE, et al. Recommendations for urine drug monitoring as a component of opioid therapy in the treatment of chronic pain. Pain Med. 2012;13(7):886–96.
20. Passik SD, Kirsh KL, Whitcomb L, et al. Monitoring outcomes during long-term opioid therapy for noncancer pain: results with the pain assessment and documentation tool. J Opioid Manag. 2005;1(257–66):423.
21. Butler SF, Budman SH, Fernandez KC, et al. Development and validation of the current opioid misuse measure. Pain. 2007;130:144–56.
22. Kirsh KL, Passik SD. The interface between pain and drug abuse and the evolution of strategies to optimize pain management while minimizing drug abuse. Exp Clin Psychopharmacol. 2008;16(5):400–4.
23. Savage SR. Multidimensional nature of pain: implications for opioid therapy. In: The 2014 international conference on opioids, Boston, MA, 8–10 June 2014.
24. Kahan M, Mailis-Gagnon A, Tunks E. Canadian guideline for safe and effective use of opioids for chronic non-cancer pain: implications for pain physicians. Pain Res Manag. 2011;16 (3):157–8.
25. Federation of State Medical Boards of the United States, Inc. Model policy on the use of opioid analgesics in the treatment of chronic pain. Washington, DC: Federation of State Medical Boards. 2013. Available at: http://www.fsmb.org/pdf/pain_policy_july2013.pdf. Accessed 22 Dec 2014.
26. Hammett-Stabler CA, Webster LR. A clinical guide to urine drug testing. Stamford: PharmaCom Group Ltd; 2008.
27. American Society of Addiction Medicine. Drug testing: a white paper of the American Society of Addiction Medicine (ASAM). Chevy Chase, MD; 2013.
28. Chou E, Fanciullo GJ, Fine PG, et al. American pain society-American academy of pain medicine opioids guidelines panel. clinical guidelines for the use of chronic opioid therapy in chronic non-cancer pain. J Pain. 2009;10(2):113–30.
29. Owen GT, Burton AW, Schade CM, Passik S. Urine drug testing: current recommendations and best practices. Pain Physician 2012;15(3 Suppl):ES119–33.
30. Manchikanti L, Malla Y, Wargo BW, Fellows B. Comparative evaluation of the accuracy of immunoassay with liquid chromatography tandem mass spectrometry (LC/MS/MS) of urine drug testing (UDT) opioids and illicit drugs in chronic pain patients. Pain Physician. 2011;14 (2):175–87.

31. Caplan YH, Goldberger BA. Alternative specimens for workplace drug testing. J Anal Toxicol. 2001;25(5):396–9.
32. Trescot AM, Faynboym S. A review of the role of genetic testing in pain medicine. Pain Phys. 2014;17(5):425–45.
33. Kitzmiller JP, Groen DK, Phelps MA, Sadee W. Pharmacogenomic testing: relevance in medical practice: why drugs work in some patients but not in others. Cleve Clin J Med. 2011;78(4):243–57.
34. Gourlay D, Heit HA, Caplan YH. Urine drug testing in clinical practice: dispelling the myths and designing strategies. Stamford, CT: PharmaCom Group, Inc.; 2006.
35. Reifler LM, Droz D, Bailey JE. Do prescription monitoring programs impact state trends in opioid abuse/misuse? Pain Med. 2012;13(3):434–42.
36. Clark T, Eadie J, Kreiner P, Strickler G. Prescription drug monitoring programs: an assessment of the evidence for best practices. The Prescription Drug Monitoring Program Center of Excellence, Heller School for Social Policy and Management, Brandeis University. Prepared for The Pew Charitable Trusts, 20 Sept 2012.
37. Simeone R, Holland L. An evaluation of prescription drug monitoring programs. Simeone Associates, Inc. 2006. Available at: http://media.timesfreepress.com/docs/2008/03/Federal_prescription_monitoring_report.pdf. Accessed 5 Dec 2014.
38. Paulozzi LJ, Kilbourne EM, Desai HA. Prescription drug monitoring programs and death rates from drug overdose. Pain Med. 2011;12(5):747–54.
39. National Alliance for Model State Drug Laws. Compilation of state prescription monitoring program maps. Charlottesville, VA, Current as of June 2014. Available at: http://www.namsdl.org/library/593BC7A6-1372-636C-DD7A83E6A8F6F0BC/. Accessed 22 Dec 2014.
40. Anson P. Pain patients forced to go 'cold turkey' from hydrocodone. National Pain Report. November 7, 2014. Available at: http://americannewsreport.com/nationalpainreport/pain-patients-forced-to-go-cold-turkey-from-hydrocodone-8825107.html. Accessed 5 Dec 2014.
41. US Food and Drug Administration (FDA), Center for Drug Evaluation and Research (CDER). Draft guidance for industry: abuse-deterrent opioids—evaluation and labeling. Published January 2013. FDA website. Available at: http://www.fda.gov/downloads/drugs/guidancecomplianceregulatoryinformation/guidances/ucm334743.pdf. Accessed 1 Dec 2014.
42. U.S. Food and Drug Administration (FDA). FDA approves abuse-deterrent labeling for reformulated OxyContin (News Release). Silver Spring, MD, 16 Apr 2013.
43. U.S. Food and Drug Administration (FDA). FDA approves new extended-release oxycodone with abuse-deterrent properties (News Release). Silver Spring, MD, 23 July 2014.
44. U.S. Food and Drug Administration (FDA). FDA approves labeling with abuse-deterrent features for third extended-release opioid analgesic [News Release]. Silver Spring, MD, 17 Oct 2014.
45. King Pharmaceuticals, Inc. Statement on voluntary recall of Embeda extended-release capsules CII. Published March 16, 2011. Available at: http://www.pfizer.com/files/news/embeda_recall_031611.pdf. Accessed 9 Dec 2014.
46. EMBEDA™ safety information. New York, NY: Pfizer, Inc.; 2014.
47. U.S. Food and Drug Administration (FDA). FDA approves extended-release, single-entity hydrocodone product with abuse-deterrent properties (News Release). Silver Spring, MD, 20 Nov 2014.
48. EXALGO (package insert). Hazelwood, MO: Mallinckrodt Brand Pharmaceuticals, Inc.; 2014.
49. Morton T, Kostenbader K, Montgomery J, Devarakonda K, Barrett T, Webster L. Comparison of subjective effects of extended-release versus immediate-release oxycodone/acetaminophen tablets in healthy nondependent recreational users of prescription opioids: a randomized trial. Postgrad Med. 2014;126(4):20–32.
50. OXECTA (package insert). New York, NY: Pfizer Inc.; 2014.
51. U.S. Food and Drug Administration (FDA). FDA statement: original Opana ER relisting determination. Published May 10, 2013. http://www.fda.gov/Drugs/DrugSafety/ucm351357.htm. Accessed 9 Dec 2014.

52. Vosburg SK, Jones JD, Manubay JM, Ashworth JB, Shapiro DY, Comer SD. A comparison among tapentadol tamper-resistant formulations (TRF) and OxyContin® (non-TRF) in prescription opioid abusers. Addiction. 2013;108(6):1095–106.
53. Webster LR. The question of opioid euphoria. Drug Discovery and Development. Published July 30, 2009. Available at: http://www.dddmag.com/Article-The-Question-of-Opioid-Euphoria-073009.aspx. Accessed 1 Dec 2014.
54. Butler SF, Black RA, Cassidy TA, Dailey TM, Budman SH. Abuse risks and routes of administration of different prescription opioid compounds and formulations. Harm Reduct J. 2011;8(29):1–17.
55. Cicero TJ, Surratt H, Inciardi JA, Munoz A. Relationship between therapeutic use and abuse of opioid analgesics in rural, suburban, and urban locations in the United States. Pharmacoepidemiol Drug Saf. 2007;16(8):827–40.
56. Budman SH, Grimes Serrano JM, Butler SF. Can abuse deterrent formulations make a difference? Expectation and speculation. Harm Reduct J. 2009;6:8.
57. Butler SF, Cassidy TA, Chilcoat H, et al. Abuse rates and routes of administration of reformulated extended-release oxycodone: initial findings from a sentinel surveillance sample of individuals assessed for substance abuse treatment. J Pain. 2013;14(4):351–8.
58. Coplan PM, Kale H, Sandstrom L, Landau C, Chilcoat HD. Changes in oxycodone and heroin exposures in the national poison data system after introduction of extended-release oxycodone with abuse-deterrent characteristics. Pharmacoepidemiol Drug Saf. 2013;22(12):1274–82.
59. Dart RC, Severtson SG, Bucher-Bartelson B. Trends in opioid analgesic abuse and mortality in the United States. N Engl J Med. 2015;372(16):573–4.
60. Cicero et al. Abuse-deterrent formulations and the prescription opioid abuse epidemic in the United States: lessons learned from OxyContin. JAMA Psychiatry 2015;72(5):424–30.
61. American Society of Addiction Medicine. Public Policy Statement: Definition of Addiction. 2011. ASAM website. Available at: http://www.asam.org/for-the-public/definition-of-addiction. Accessed 1 Dec 2014.
62. Katz NP, Birnbaum H, Brennan MJ, et al. Prescription opioid abuse: challenges and opportunities for payers. Am J Manag Care. 2013;19(4):295–302.
63. Knotkova H, Fine PG, Portenoy RK. Opioid rotation: the science and the limitations of the equianalgesic dose table. J Pain Symptom Manage 2009;38(3):426–39 (Review).
64. Webster LR, Fine PG. Review and critique of opioid rotation practices and associated risks of toxicity. Pain Med. 2012;13(4):562–70.
65. Webster LR, Fine PG. Overdose deaths demand a new paradigm for opioid rotation. Pain Med. 2012;13(4):571–4.
66. U.S. Food and Drug Administration. Information for healthcare professionals: methadone hydrochloride. U.S. Department of Health and Human Services. Silver Spring, MD, 2006.
67. Eap CB. BuclinT, Baumann P. Interindividual variability of the clinical pharmacokinetics of methadone: implications for the treatment of opioid dependence. Clin Pharmacokinet. 2002;41 (14):1153–93.
68. Webster LR. Methadone-related deaths. J Opioid Manage. 2005;1(4):211–7.

Chapter 11
Naloxone Treatment of Opioid Overdose

Sanford M. Silverman and Peter S. Staats

The prescription drug epidemic continues to plague the USA. In 2013, there were 16,235 opioid-related deaths in the USA. 83 % of these were considered unintentional. Although this represents a slight reduction from 2011 (17,000), the mortality rates continue to affect thousands of people, from relatives of patients to healthcare workers. Opioid-related deaths have a significant impact on the healthcare system [1–3].

There are a variety of strategies have been advocated to minimize risks of opioid-related deaths. Risk mitigation strategies that have been shown to minimize morbidity and to prevent deaths have included a detailed comprehensive evaluation, directed questionnaires, drug testing, and the accessing of prescription drug monitoring plans. However, not until recently has there been an effort to actually treat witnessed opioid overdose with pharmacologic agents known to reverse the respiratory depressant effects of opioids.

Providing a reversal agent to an individual who has overdosed on opioids is time sensitive. Once one has overdosed and developed respiratory depression, it is necessary to either reverse the opioid or provide artificial ventilation to the patient in order to avoid irreversible brain injury. If a patient cannot be immediately ventilated, the only other option is to reverse the respiratory depressant effect of opioids with a pharmacologic reversal agent.

It seems self-evident that providing an opioid reversal agent to patients and friends or family members, that can be safely administered, will improve the speed of the treatment and thus may improve the survival rate following a respiratory

S.M. Silverman (✉)
Comprehensive Pain Medicine, 100 E Sample Rd, Suite 200, Pompano Beach,
FL 33064, USA
e-mail: sanfordsilverman@cpmedicine.com

P.S. Staats
Department of Anesthesiology and Critical Care, Department of Oncology,
Johns Hopkins University, Baltimore, MD, USA

© Springer International Publishing Switzerland 2016
P.S. Staats and S.M. Silverman (eds.), *Controlled Substance
Management in Chronic Pain*, DOI 10.1007/978-3-319-30964-4_11

arrest. Others have argued, on the other hand, that the patient or person with an addiction disorder may take more drugs, with impunity, knowing that there is a reversal agent available should he/she have a respiratory arrest. Thus, improving the availability of a reversal agent inadvertently could cause an increase in the morbidity of respiratory depression. This, however, has not been demonstrated to date.

Naloxone is an opioid antagonist which has been traditionally utilized by emergency room physicians and paramedics to treat opioid overdose. Anesthesiologists routinely use naloxone in the operating suite to reverse opioid-related respiratory depression. Since naloxone is so effective in reversing opioid overdose, the concept has been promulgated to make this medication available to laypersons in the community. Studies have thus been done to demonstrate that patients who have access to a reversal agent have an increased survival. Community programs have been established and are referred to as opioid overdose prevention programs (OOPPs). A recent meta-analysis of 19 OOPPs was conducted and demonstrated efficacy in decreasing opioid-related deaths [4]. The demographics were analyzed with respect to the number of naloxone administrations, percentage of survival of victims receiving naloxone, barriers to naloxone administration, and changes in knowledge and attitudes of the community members with respect to opioid overdose. The current evidence from these nonrandomized studies suggests that bystanders (mostly opioid users) can and will use naloxone to reverse opioid overdoses when properly trained and that this training can be done successfully through OOPPs. Other examples of successful OOPPs include Project Lazarus [5] from North Carolina, which was endorsed universally by the state and in particular the North Carolina Medical Board. The idea behind these movements is that naloxone can be prescribed to relatives or significant others (other than the patient) to treat a possible overdose.

Unintentional overdose is not simply limited to the drug-abusing community. Patients with chronic pain who take opiates are at risk for unintentional overdose. The comorbidities and comedications associated with the treatment of chronic pain make this patient population particularly susceptible to unintentional overdose. Specifically, comorbidities include chronic respiratory disease, hepatic/renal impairment, psychiatric disorders, and prior substance-use disorders. The concomitant medications that increase overdose risk include CNS depressants (benzodiazepines) and medications that alter cytochrome P450 metabolism. Other opioid-related issues include morphine equivalent dose greater than or equal to 100 mg daily, initiation/titration/rotation/poly-opioid use, and the use of extended-release opioid preparations, transdermal fentanyl use, and intrathecal opioid administration [6–13].

Transdermal fentanyl may carry some specific untoward risks. 26 % of the overdose deaths occurred within four days of filling the prescription [14]. In a recent Veterans Administration study, it was shown that 73 % of the patients *did not* have a substance-abuse disorder diagnosis but did have significant risk factors for opioid overdose, which included morphine equivalent dose of greater than or equal to 50 mg per day, utilizing an extended-release opioid, and having a diagnosis of chronic pulmonary, kidney, or liver disease [15].

In 2014, the Substance Abuse and Mental Health Services Administration (SAMHSA) released its toolkit with recommendations regarding the treatment of opioid overdose [16]. Specifically, SAMHSA recommends prescribing naloxone along with the patient's *initial* opioid prescription. They identify candidates for naloxone (specifically injectable naloxone) who are as follows:

- Taking high doses of opioids for long-term management of chronic malignant or nonmalignant pain;
- Receiving rotating opioid medication regimens (and thus are at risk for incomplete cross-tolerance);
- Discharge from emergency medical care following opioid intoxication or poisoning;
- At high risk for overdose because of a legitimate medical need for analgesia, coupled with a suspected or confirmed history of substance abuse, dependence, or nonmedical use of prescription or illicit opioids;
- On certain opioid preparations that may increase risk for opioid overdose such as extended-release/long-acting preparations;
- Completing mandatory opioid detoxification or abstinence programs.

Naloxone

Naloxone (Fig. 11.1) is a short-acting reversal agent of an opiate. It is used to reverse the respiratory depressant and sedative effects of the opioid class of medication. When a patient has had a successful reversal of an opioid with an opioid antagonist, it is possible that the reversal agent will wear off. Accordingly, it is important that patients and caregivers be informed of this and to call 911 when a respiratory arrest occurs, even with a successful reversal.

Naloxone is synthesized from thebaine. Its chemical structure is related to that of oxymorphone, where the *N*-methyl group of oxymorphone is substituted with an allyl (prop-2-enyl) group. The name *naloxone* is derived from *N*-allyl and oxymorphone.

Fig. 11.1 Chemical structures of naloxone and oxymorphone

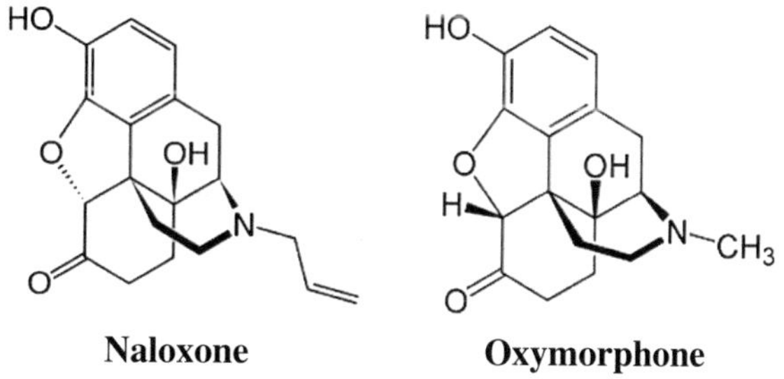

Naloxone   **Oxymorphone**

Pharmacokinetics

Distribution

Following parenteral administration, naloxone is rapidly distributed in the body and readily crosses the placenta. It is weakly bound by plasma proteins, albumin being the major binding constituent, but significant binding of naloxone also occurs to plasma constituents other than albumin. It is not known whether naloxone is excreted into human milk.

Metabolism and Elimination

Naloxone is metabolized in the liver, primarily by glucuronide conjugation with naloxone-3-glucuronide as the major metabolite. The serum half-life in adults ranges from 30 to 81 min. In a neonatal study, the mean plasma half-life was observed to be 3.1 ± 0.5 h. Naloxone is poorly absorbed orally, and only about 10 % sublingually, which makes it ideal for combination products (Suboxone® [Reckitt Benckiser Group, UK]) to deter parental abuse. After an intravenous dose, about 25–40 % of the drug is excreted as metabolites in urine within 6 h, about 50 % in 24 h, and 60–70 % in 72 h.

Pharmacodynamics

Naloxone has an extremely high affinity for μ-opioid receptors in the central nervous system (CNS). Naloxone is a μ-opioid receptor competitive antagonist, and its rapid blockade of those receptors produces rapid onset of withdrawal symptoms. Naloxone also has an antagonist action, though with a lower affinity, at the kappa κ-(KOR) and the delta δ-opioid receptors (DOR).

Naloxone is a pure antagonist with no agonist properties. If administered in the absence of concomitant opioid use, no functional pharmacological activity occurs. No evidence indicates the development of tolerance or dependence on naloxone. The mechanism of action is not completely understood, but studies suggest it functions to produce withdrawal symptoms by competing for opiate receptor sites within the CNS (a competitive antagonist, not a direct agonist), thereby preventing the action of both endogenous and exogenous opiates on these receptors without directly producing any effects itself.

Naloxone Preparations

Naloxone is available in a liquid form for parenteral use. It has been used for intranasal administration and most recently for FDA-approved autoinjector formulation (Evzio®, Kaleo Pharmaceuticals, and VA). The naloxone ampules can be adapted via an atomizer for any intranasal administration system [17]. As of 2015, the only FDA-approved formulation currently is the Evzio®, autoinjector.

Good Samaritan Laws

Currently, 19 states have Good Samaritan laws which protect prescribers and others who prescribe naloxone to treat opioid overdose. Specifically, the prescribers are protected for any untoward effects or accidental administration of the drug. Bystanders may fail to administer naloxone because of legal repercussions and may also fail to summon the police during a witnessed overdose secondary to their own fear of legal consequences. However, the law protects those individuals who administer naloxone for overdose with essentially "no questions asked."

Practical Considerations

The practitioner should consider prescribing a self-administered opioid reversal agent. This can be prescribed at the initial dose, or with significant dose escalation. The patient and caregiver should be counseled on how to administer the reversal agent and to call 911 when the respiratory arrest is recognized.

Summary

Patients receiving relatively high doses of opiates for chronic pain and patients with an opiate addiction disorder both are at risk of respiratory depression. The risks of patients with chronic pain who are at higher risk are receiving morphine equivalent dose of greater than 100 mg of morphine equivalent dose a day, have respiratory depression, are also receiving CNS depressants such as benzodiazepines, drink alcohol, have significant pulmonary dysfunction, or kidney disease, or have a psychiatric disorder characterized by impulsive behavior. In these settings, the practitioner should consider coadministering an opioid reversal agent should respiratory depression ensue and of course call 911 immediately.

References

1. Kochanek K, et al. National vital statistics report 2011. CDC vital signs. Prescription painkiller overdoses. Use and abuse of methadone as a painkiller. 2012;60:1–117.
2. Warner M, et al. Drug poisoning deaths in the United States, 1980–2008. NCHS data brief. Hyattsville MD: National Center for Health Statistics. 2011;81.
3. www.cdc.gov/homeandrecreationalsafety/rxbrief.
4. Clark et al. A systematic review of community opioid overdose prevention and naloxone distribution programs. J Addict Med. 2014;8(3).
5. Project Lazarus. http://projectlazarus.org/.
6. Bohnert A, et al. Association between opioid prescribing patterns and opioid overdose-related deaths. JAMA. 2011;305:1315–1321.
7. Paulozzi LJ, Logan JE, Hall AJ, McKinstry E, Kaplan JA, Crosby AE. A comparison of drug overdose deaths involving methadone and other opioid analgesics in West Virginia. Addiction (Abingdon, England). 2009;104:1541–1548.
8. Green TC, Grau LE, Carver HW, Kinzly M, Heimer R. Epidemiologic trends and geographic patterns of fatal opioid intoxications in Connecticut, USA: 1997–2007. Drug Alcohol Depend. 2011;115:221–8.
9. Dunn K, et al. Opioid prescriptions for chronic pain and overdose. Ann Intern Med. 2010;152:85–92.
10. Burrows D, et al. A fatal drug interaction between oxycodone and clonazepam. J Forensic Sci. 2003;48:683–6.
11. Zedler B, Xie L, Wang L, Joyce A, Vick C, Brigham Rands J, Kariburyo F, Baser O, Murrelle L. Risk factors for serious prescription opioid-related toxicity or overdose among veterans health administration patients. Pain Med. 2014.
12. Ruan X, et al. Respiratory failure following delayed intrathecal morphine pump refill: a valuable, but costly lesson. Pain Physician. 2010;13(4):337–41.
13. Coffey RJ, et al. Mortality associated with implantation and management of intrathecal opioid drug infusion systems to treat noncancer pain. Anesthesiology. 2009;111(4).
14. Jumbelic M. Deaths with transdermal fentanyl patches. Am J Forensic Med Pathol. 2010;31:18–21.
15. Zedler B, Xie L, Wang L, Joyce A, Vick C, Brigham Rands J, Kariburyo F, Baser O, Murrelle L. Risk factors for serious prescription opioid-related toxicity or overdose among veterans health administration patients. Pain Med. 2014.
16. Substance Abuse and Mental Health Services Administration. SAMHSA opioid overdose prevention toolkit. HHS Publication No. (SMA) 14–4742. Rockville MD: Substance Abuse and Mental Health Services Administration. 2014.
17. Wolfe TR. Bernstone T intranasal drug delivery: An alternative to intravenous administration in selected emergency cases. J Emerg Nurs. 2004;30(2):141–7.

Chapter 12
From Patient Evaluation to Opioid Overdose Prevention: Ten Steps to Make the Law Work for You and Your Patients

Jen Bolen

Introduction

The pain medicine community faces significant challenges every day—a blend of business, clinical, and legal hurdles, ranging from declining reimbursements to changing clinical perspectives on the use of opioids and intense law enforcement and regulatory scrutiny surrounding clinic operations and prescribing decisions. Practitioners and patients may feel as if they have targets on their backs and believe they are caught in the middle of the intense battle over the clinical value of opioids for treating chronic pain. Understandably, practitioners express concern that the clinical side of the practitioner–patient relationship is marginalized and often relegated to a checklist of "cop-like" questions designed to fulfill licensing board rules and meet law enforcement expectations that doctors detect abusers, addicts, and diverters prior to prescribing controlled medication. While most practitioners accept and embrace the obligation to evaluate patients carefully and prescribe controlled medication responsibly [1], the system does not yet uniformly encourage the full development of the practitioner–patient relationship. Thus, practitioners find themselves scrambling to protect their clinical decision-making and patient access to chronic opioid therapy in a system that lacks consistency in stakeholder approach to what constitutes "proper prescribing" of controlled medication in the context of chronic, non-terminal pain.

The federal government, through the US Department of Health and Human Services, Office of the Assistant Secretary for Planning and Evaluation (HHS-ASPE), recently announced [2] an initiative geared toward preventing opioid overdose deaths. The initiative is described in an issue brief entitled *Opioid Abuse in the U.S. and HHS Actions to Address Opioid-Drug Related Overdoses and Deaths* [2]. HHS-ASPE makes clear that it has secured funds and committed per-

J. Bolen (✉)
The Legal Side of Pain, 14875 Buttermilk Rd, Lenoir City, TN 37771, USA
e-mail: jbolen@legalsideofpain.com

© Springer International Publishing Switzerland 2016   187
P.S. Staats and S.M. Silverman (eds.), *Controlled Substance Management in Chronic Pain*, DOI 10.1007/978-3-319-30964-4_12

sonnel to focus on "three priority areas, grounded in the best research and clinical science available, to combat opioid abuse:

(1) Opioid prescribing practices to reduce opioid use disorders and overdose;
(2) The expanded use of naloxone, used to treat opioid overdoses; and
(3) Expanded use of medication-assisted treatment (MAT) to reduce opioid use disorders and overdose." [2]

HHS-ASPE cites three objectives associated with the above-stated priorities:

(1) Improve clinical decision-making to reduce inappropriate prescribing;
(2) Enhance prescription monitoring and health information technology (health IT) to support appropriate pain management; and
(3) Support data sharing to facilitate appropriate prescribing [3].

To effect the initiative, HHS-ASPE announced four immediate areas of focus:

(1) Enhancing prescription drug monitoring databases;
(2) Establishing opioid prescribing guidelines for chronic pain and working to ensure effective implementation of guidelines through information technology (IT) to ensure improved medical record documentation and clinical decision-making;
(3) Expanding utilization of naloxone, accelerating the development and availability of new naloxone formulations and user-friendly products, and identifying and disseminating best practice naloxone delivery models and strategies to help patients "at risk" of overdose; and
(4) Addressing barriers that hinder access to MAT, which includes methadone and buprenorphine, by addressing policy and regulation that limit eligible providers and supporting research that informs effective use and dissemination of MAT and accelerates development of new addiction treatment medications [2].

The HHS-ASPE initiative may help bring some uniformity to increasingly divergent state rules and guidelines on chronic opioid therapy. However, these initiatives must be well thought out or the problems will continue. For example, while making naloxone available to prevent opioid overdose, in the wrong hands this drug may be a gateway to "zeroing-out" receptors to allow for a greater high upon renewed opioid abuse. In addition, these initiatives must consider the various positions adopted by states with guidelines and/or rules on opioid dose triggers for consultations and referrals, such as California, which has a guideline referencing 80-mg morphine equivalent dose (MED) as a *trigger for considering* whether the patient needs a specialty evaluation [4], and Washington State, which uses 120-mg MED and *mandates a consultation, unless* the patient's case and physician meet certain criteria [5]. In all cases, initiatives led by the federal government may have desirable goals, but they must also recognize the impact they will have on medical practices, and ensure prescribers have the tools they need to fulfill clinical and regulatory expectations.

Changes are coming to this practice community, and practitioners and patients must strive to work together to understand their respective responsibilities toward the safe use of opioids and do so in a manner that minimizes the potential for adverse outcomes and further encroachment upon the sanctity of the practitioner–patient relationship. This chapter is designed to facilitate physician understanding of current medicolegal obligations relating to the prescribing of chronic opioid therapy to treat chronic, non-terminal pain. Frontline pain practitioners are encouraged to understand the professional licensing board directives on pain management clinic operational standards and chronic opioid therapy. The tone of this chapter is intentionally "how to" and designed to support the physician who wishes to perform a self-evaluation of his/her compliance with medicolegal obligations and to bring their respective practices current and ready for the changes coming through the HHS-ASPE initiative. The main body of this chapter contains ten "how to" suggestions related to patient education and provider self-assessment on specific aspects of controlled substance prescribing compliance. The end of this chapter contains a quick reference tool designed to facilitate the practitioner's understanding of licensing board directives through a short self-audit process. The quick reference tool focuses on key compliance areas, such as patient risk evaluation, stratification, and monitoring, as well as patient education on important topics such as learning the signs of an overdose and steps to prevent an overdose.

Not a day goes by without a reminder of the mounting number of overdose deaths, amended or newly filed legislation purportedly targeting only "pill mills," and political commentary on "how to" address the country's "reliance on opioids." Once again, practitioners and patients find themselves amid a swirling sea of change, wondering what happened and how to stay the course. What is the answer to balancing patient access to quality pain care while also taking reasonable steps to prevent abuse, diversion, and opioid overdose? There is no easy answer, but this chapter endeavors to provide some help to practitioners and patients on key topics of education and preserving the relationship through proper documentation of the medical record.

Then and Now

In 2002, the focus was treating pain—it had become a fifth vital sign. The DEA and 21 Healthcare Organizations were about to embark upon a joint effort to balance patient access to controlled medication with practitioner and other stakeholder efforts to reduce the abuse and diversion of these drugs [6]. Clinical drug testing was not a big emphasis at the time, but by 2006, the DEA would reference it as an example of a treatment agreement provision designed to prevent abuse and diversion [7]. Then, the focus was being "docs" instead of "cops" to the numerous patients suffering from debilitating chronic pain. In 2015, the "now" focus is on controlling much of the clinical decision-making related to medication quantity, MED limits, consult and referral requirements, and even the length of time for

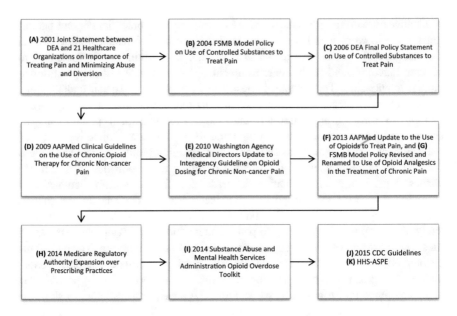

Fig. 12.1 Chronology of basic opioid prescribing policy [8]

overall chronicity of prescribing. Without question, these are important considerations, yet it is equally important to preserve practitioner discretion and patient choice about medication selection, dose, and chronicity of prescribing. Balance is required, and real objectivity should be the goal when third parties evaluate whether or not the underlying prescription was "legally" valid in the context of medical necessity and usual course of professional practice—the two critical elements of a valid prescription.

How did we get to where we are today? Figure 12.1 highlights some critical changes in key policy and professional guideline material between 2002 and 2015. It is important to remember that not all states follow the guidance offered by the American Academy of Pain Medicine (AAPMed), the Federation of State Medical Boards (FSMB), or Washington Agency Medical Directors Group (WA-AMDG). However, the materials published by and through these entities will continue to play an important role in the ongoing development of state regulatory material dealing with chronic opioid therapy and, likely, the Center for Disease Control and Prevention's (CDC) effort to universalize chronic opioid prescribing nationwide through the efforts of HHS-ASPE in reducing opioid overdose.

Practitioners therefore may wish to review the cited items and decide whether the suggestions contained within may be used to improve clinical practice and patient education. Similarly, practitioners may wish to chart out the evolution of pain management rules and guidelines within their states of licensure to better understand licensing board expectations. The last section of this chapter will facilitate a self-audit exercise and empower practitioners to take back some turf and make the law work for them and their patients.

Refresher—Basic Legal/Regulatory Framework

There are two basic levels of legal/regulatory authorities for controlled substance prescribing: federal and state governments and their agencies. Within the federal and state framework, there are three levels of legal/regulatory materials: laws, regulations, and guidelines/position statements (Fig. 12.2) [8].

Typically, *laws* are found in acts, codes, and/or statutes—federal or state. Examples include federal and state Controlled Substances Acts, and state Medical, Nursing, and Pharmacy Practice Acts, state Intractable Pain Treatment Acts, and state Electronic Prescription Monitoring Acts. Laws form the foundation of the legal/regulatory pyramid for prescribing controlled substances in general and for other legal/regulatory materials affecting pain management, such as controlled substance prescribing rules and regulations governing professional conduct.

Laws give permission to federal and state agencies to regulate the flow of controlled substances and, with respect to state licensing boards, to protect the public by setting minimum expectations/standards for the practice of medicine and use of controlled substances for pain management. Laws also contain penalty provisions (civil and criminal), which are enforceable through administrative or legal process.

Regulations and rules explain a corresponding law and set additional boundaries based specifically on the monitoring/sponsoring agency's interpretation of the law. Examples include the Code of Federal Regulations, which explains the Controlled Substances Act of 1970 and gives DEA oversight authority for the flow of controlled substances in the USA. Most states also have regulatory codes and publish rules explaining state controlled substances acts and medical practice acts.

Regulations and rules give agencies additional permissions to establish guidelines or position statements that further explain the regulations. Some state laws and regulations prohibit state licensing agencies from establishing "explanatory" or "interpretive" materials. Thus, some state medical licensing boards, like the medical boards in Illinois and Wisconsin, do not have expansive authority to adopt

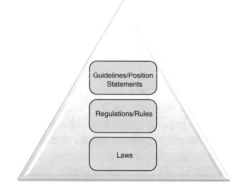

Fig. 12.2 Basic regulatory framework

controlled substance prescribing guidelines for pain management. In these states, practitioners often must look to area medical societies and to national organizations for references on opioid prescribing. Regulations and rules have the force of law, meaning violating regulations normally results in sanctions, such as licensing suspension or revocation, in addition to civil fines and penalties. Some states have both regulations and rules.

Guidelines (sometimes referred to as "position statements") contain an agency's explanation or interpretation of a particular subject. *Guidelines are not clinical care standards*. Rather, agencies use guidelines to establish *minimum* expectations of licensees related to the specific subject matter. Typically, those who fail to follow guidelines may face administrative sanctions (licensing restrictions or educational orders) unless one can show good (and often written) cause for the deviation from or failure to follow guidelines.

Despite these basic distinctions between laws, regulations, rules, and guidelines, lawyers use guidelines to establish the framework of civil and criminal lawsuits, including medical malpractice and wrongful death cases. Guidelines sometimes contain directives and language that are outdated and inconsistent with current clinical care standards. Practitioners located in states that lack or have outdated guidelines may find it useful to review the FSMB materials and materials published by mainstream organizations, such as a professional society or medical association. It is important to keep copies of any materials relied upon as a basis for clinical decision-making and regulatory compliance.

Refresher—What Makes a Controlled Substance Prescription Valid?

When an individual obtains a federal drug registration number, the DEA expects the registrant to follow federal controlled substances laws, regulations, and policies. The DEA expects clinicians to administer, dispense, and prescribe controlled substances for a *legitimate medical purpose while acting in the usual course of professional practice* [9]. The DEA also expects clinicians to *minimize the potential for the abuse and diversion of controlled substances* by adhering to applicable legal/regulatory boundaries and by following current, accepted clinical care standards [10].

A controlled substance prescription is therefore *valid* (1) when it is issued for a legitimate medical purpose, (2) by an individual practitioner who is acting in the usual course of professional practice, (3) while taking reasonable steps to prevent abuse and diversion [11]. Today, this obligation also likely includes "reasonable steps" to prevent opioid overdose, especially in those states with programs allowing easier access to address opioid overdose risk through increased access to naloxone [12]. States may lawfully impose stricter requirements to address state-specific challenges with controlled drugs. Figure 12.3 highlights the elements of a valid controlled substance prescription.

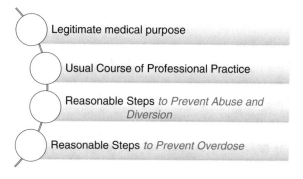

Fig. 12.3 Basic elements of a valid controlled substance prescription

In 2006, the US DEA published a Final Policy Statement on Dispensing Controlled Substances for the Treatment of Pain [7]. This publication, while dated, contains additional insight into the DEA's perspective on the three elements of a valid prescription and includes the following valuable comment about taking "reasonable steps to prevent abuse and diversion":

> Moreover, as a condition of being a DEA registrant, a physician who prescribes controlled substances has an obligation to take reasonable measures to prevent diversion. The overwhelming majority of physicians in the United States who prescribe controlled substances do, in fact, *exercise the appropriate degree of medical supervision—as part of their routine practice during office visits—to minimize the likelihood of diversion or abuse*. Again, each patient's situation is unique and the nature and degree of physician oversight should be tailored accordingly, *based on the physician's sound medical judgment and consistent with established medical standards* [13].

The DEA also publishes online information on cases against physicians [14]. The DEA categorizes this information into criminal and administrative case reports, and practitioners will find value in reviewing the information made public by the agency. In particular, the administrative case opinions offer a look at how government-retained medical experts talk about whether a practitioner acted in the usual course of professional practice when evaluating and monitoring patients using chronic opioid therapy. The true challenge is in the law enforcement and the medical expert interpretation of "usual course of professional practice" and "reasonable steps to prevent abuse and diversion." A discussion of the case law on these topics is beyond the scope of this chapter. Nevertheless, it is fair to say that while a medical expert's assessment of a controlled substance prescription and the clinical underpinnings is supposed to be "objective," the case reports tend to show that medical experts insert their subjective opinions regarding dose, quantity, chronicity, risk evaluation tools and frequency of use, drug testing methods and frequency, and other topics related to use of chronic opioid therapy. Some of the subjectivity may be due to a void in the evidence-based research in this area, leaving room for the expert's personal practices and preferences to supplant those chosen by the defendant-registrant.

Refresher—Breach of the Duty of Trust

In *USA, v. Schneider* [15], the trial judge sentenced Dr. Schneider to a thirty (30) year imprisonment, and the sentence included an enhanced penalty for healthcare fraud "if the violation results in death." 18 U.S.C. § 1347(a). The trial judge also found Dr. Schneider "abused his position of trust" over his patients, meaning when the prescriber does not act as a "reasonably prudent practitioner" (or act in the usual course of professional practice) when issuing a controlled substance prescription, the patient may be harmed (or is harmed) and the prescriber is viewed as abusing his/her position of trust over the patient; harsh penalties may apply, including the potential for a significant term of imprisonment. Similar concepts apply at the state licensing board level, where boards consider aggravating and mitigating informa- tion surrounding controlled substance prescribing decisions and practices, and penalties may include revocation of professional licenses as well as referral to law enforcement authorities for further investigation, including criminal prosecution.

Recently, a federal judge sentenced an Akron, Ohio, physician, to five years' imprisonment following a guilty plea to conspiracy to illegally distribute drugs and twenty (20) counts of illegal distribution [16]. The physician was registered with the State of Ohio Medical Board as a medical doctor specializing in family medicine, obstetrics, and gynecology. In court, the physician entered a guilty plea, admitting he distributed and dispensed more than 30,000 tablets of oxycodone, Oxycontin, and Opana, to various individuals without a legitimate medical purpose. He also admitted he *did so by acting outside the usual course of professional practice, because he prescribed the controlled medication without*:

(1) Adequate verification of the patient's identity or medical complaint;
(2) Adequate and reliable patient medical history;
(3) Performance of a complete or adequate examination;
(4) Establishment of a true diagnosis; and
(5) The use of appropriate diagnostic or laboratory testing, among other methods.

The physician and his staff used presigned blank prescription forms to facilitate their controlled substance prescribing to patients. The government asked the court to apply a two-point increase to the physician's overall sentence potential, agreeing with the government's claim the physician used a special skill to accomplish the crime and abused his position of trust relative to his patients and the public [17].

There are many more examples of cases against physicians, but it is not the purpose of this chapter to focus on these bad actors. It is, however, important to understand the "position of trust/special skill" argument and how violating the trust associated with medical degrees and controlled substance prescribing registrations may lead to enhanced penalties and terms of imprisonment in administrative and criminal prosecutions. Cases against prescribers often reference expert opinions about prescriber action or inaction [18] constituting activity outside the usual course of professional practice—activity that constitutes the breach of trust and misuse of a special skill. Such references to what a prescriber did or failed to do may be helpful to the practitioner seeking to compile a checklist for use during a self-audit of prescribing habits and medical record documentation, and ultimately turned into a risk management work plan to support their good faith prescribing of controlled medication. Those wishing to know more about "Cases Against Doctors" will find many examples on the DEA's Web site [19]. Criminal prescribing [20] is a slap in the face to all the practitioners who work hard to do it right and legitimately prescribe controlled medication to treat pain.

Shall and Should, and the Reasonably Prudent Practitioner

So what is it that a "reasonably prudent" practitioner does to meet the "usual course of professional practice" standard for a valid prescription? DEA regulations do not give much insight as to what the agency means by "usual course of professional practice." There are federal case opinions that attempt to explain what is meant by this element of a valid prescription, and most acknowledge the relevance of state licensing board rules and guidelines in making the determination. Once again, a discussion of the legal analysis associated with the "usual course of professional practice" standard is beyond the scope of this chapter.

State licensing boards use "directive" language in rules and guidelines, such as the practitioner "shall" perform a task or document certain information, and the practitioner "should" take certain steps when re-evaluating a patient. These terms are often associated with the board's explanation of how it intends for its licensees to use a rule or guideline. For example, the Texas Medical Board (TMB) has a rule (Chapter 170) on pain management, and the rule also contains the board's policy for "proper" pain management. A guideline within a rule usually means the document is replete with "directive" language on what the board thinks the physician is required to do and what he/she should do absent a good and documented reason to do otherwise. Here is the relevant language from the TMB's Chapter 170:

> The intent of these guidelines is not to impose regulatory burdens on the practice of medicine. *Rather, these guidelines are intended to set forth those items expected to be done by any reasonable physician involved in the treatment of pain.* The use of the word "shall" in these guidelines is used to identify those items a physician is required to perform in all such cases. The word "should" and the phrase "it is the responsibility of the physician" in these guidelines are used to identify those actions that a prudent physician will either do and document in the treatment of pain or be able to provide a thoughtful explanation as to why the physician did not do so [21].

Understanding the state licensing board's policy for proper pain management is critical to a comprehensive compliance program—clinical and regulatory. As the next section reveals, a solid working knowledge of licensing board expectations is critical in light of Medicare's expanded authority to examine prescribing patterns of its enrolled providers or provider applicants.

Expanded Agency Authority—CMS and Prescribing Patterns

Healthcare professionals, facilities, and equipment suppliers must be enrolled in the Medicare program to receive payment for covered items and services. In 2006, the Centers for Medicare & Medicaid Services (CMS) adopted a comprehensive set of enrollment rules purposed to protect the Medicare fund and to ensure payments are made only to qualified providers and suppliers [22]. In 2014, CMS took additional steps to revise and supplement enrollment regulations to further protect the integrity of program payments, and several other rules take effect throughout 2015. This section focuses on CMS's expanded authority to review the prescribing practices of Medicare program enrollees and to take action against those who are believed to be "inappropriately prescribing" controlled medications under Medicare Part D.

CMS references an Office of the Inspector General (OIG) report that highlights instances in which physicians and eligible professionals prescribed "inordinate amounts" of drugs to Part D beneficiaries in 2009, as well as prescribers of high percentages of Schedule II and III drugs [23]. In the same report, OIG recommends that CMS exercise greater oversight of the Part D program. Consequently, CMS added a new provision to its enforcement regulations allowing the agency to deny an enrollment application if the prescriber's DEA Certificate is suspended or revoked or if the prescriber's ability to prescribe drugs has been suspended or revoked by the state licensing or administrative body in which the prescriber practices [24]. CMS's rationale for expansion of its authority here pertains to its belief that the loss of the ability to prescribe drugs via a suspension or revocation of a DEA Certificate or by state action is a "clear indicator" that a physician or eligible professional may be misusing or abusing his or her authority to prescribe such substances.

CMS also has authority to initiate action against an enrollee if it determines that a physician or eligible professional has engaged in improper prescribing practices [25]. One way CMS might make such a determination is if the agency finds that the prescribing pattern or practice is abusive or represents a threat to the health and safety of Medicare beneficiaries or both. Another way CMS might use its expanded authority is when the agency finds the pattern or practice of prescribing fails to meet Medicare requirements. Figure 12.4 shows the "criteria" CMS may use to make its determinations, and provides support for the self-audit proposed at the end of this chapter.

Clearly, CMS's expanded authority to evaluate prescribing practices, and to do so under these vague terms, suggests the time is ripe—whether or not you are an enrolled Medicare provider—to ensure clear documentation of practitioner prescribing rationale matched against the facts of each individual patient's medical situation.

Abusive Prescribing and/or Presents a Threat to the Health and Safety of Medicare Beneficiaries

- Whether there are diagnoses to support prescribing.
- Evidence of fraudulent prescribing.
- Prescribing of excessive dosages that are linked to patient overdoses.
- Disciplinary actions taken against the prescriber and details.
- History of "final adverse actions".
- Malpractice suits related to prescribing that have resulted in a final judgment against the prescriber OR a settlement of same.
- Has any program restricted, suspended, revoked, or terminated prescriber's ability to prescribe medications, and why?
- Any other relevant information provided to CMS.

The pattern or practice of prescribing fails to meet Medicare requirements

- Whether the physician or eligible professional has a pattern or practice of prescribing without valid prescribing authority.
- Whether the physician or eligible professional has a pattern or practice of prescribing for controlled substances outside the scope of the prescriber's DEA registration.
- Whether the physician or eligible professional has a pattern or practice of prescribing drugs for indications that were not medically accepted—that is, for indications neither approved by the FDA nor medically accepted under section 1860D-2(e)(4) of the Act—and whether there is evidence that the physician or eligible professional acted in reckless disregard for the health and safety of the patient

Fig. 12.4 Medicare criteria for abusive prescribing and problematic patterns

Self-Assessment of Prescribing Compliance—Ten Steps

Prescribing compliance is generally not something one can self-assess in a single setting. Similarly, the patient's clinical need for controlled medication is not easily evaluated in a single visit, as the patient's full history and medical condition may not known be until several months into the practitioner–patient relationship. The tension here is obvious: Regulatory authorities view prescribing practices in a silo, but the development of a treatment plan and the prescriber's rationale develops over a series of visits and a constant filter of information—incoming and outgoing. Practitioners need time to gather facts, identify boundaries, and apply knowledge to the task at hand.

This section describes the basic self-assessment process for evaluating whether the practitioner is "acting in the usual course of professional practice," as a reasonably prudent practitioner, when prescribing controlled medication. Intentionally omitted are points about the more technical aspects of issuing a controlled substance prescription, such as how to properly date and sign a prescription or what type of information is required to be on the prescription pad or how e-prescribing works. It is the author's hope that practitioners will incorporate the following ten suggestions into their overall plan to minimize the potential of a "hit-and-run" patient experience. The self-audit process is intended to help the prescriber improve his or her documentation of the prescriber–patient experience and better situate the medical record in the event of an audit.

The Ten Steps You Can Do to Take Back Your Turf

The goal of a self-audit is to develop and protect your position as a "reasonably prudent" practitioner. The ten-step process will also facilitate interaction with legal counsel, should you be in that position (Fig. 12.5) [26].

It will take time to accomplish the ten-step review described below; there really is no way to shortcut these tasks, as each of them is critical to a complete self-assessment. If, however, you already have a prescribing compliance notebook (Step 1) and you have reviewed your state licensing board materials in the past three months (Step 2), you may wish to start at Step 3 or Step 4. Whatever the case, the steps outlined below will contribute to the overall success of your efforts to perform a complete self-audit and ultimately create a comprehensive compliance program for controlled substance prescribing in the medical practice.

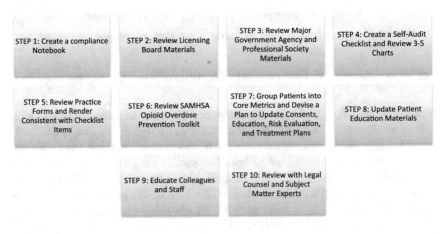

Fig. 12.5 Ten-step summary

Step 1—Create and Keep a Compliance Notebook—Hardcopy or Virtual

Goal: *To create a go-to resource for major clinical and regulatory resources on controlled substance prescribing; to create a resource for use in practitioner self-audit and with legal counsel when working on risk management policies and protocols or an active legal matter.*

Rationale: The body of clinical and legal materials governing controlled substance prescribing is large, and compiling a notebook proactively can minimize stressors associated with the task and avoid panic should the need for the information arise in connection with legal proceedings.

Considerations and Recommendations: Obtain and label a three-ring binder "Prescribing Compliance Handbook," or create a virtual binder online in a Dropbox or basecamp-type solution. Assign someone on your staff to take responsibility for organizing the binder and making sure it stays current. Use this binder: when you have questions about compliance; when you host internal education for your staff; if you face a payor inquiry about your prescribing policies, or; if you come under investigation by your licensing board or DEA. You may find that your business attorney does not have a solid working knowledge of all of the clinical and regulatory material governing pain management and controlled substance prescribing; thus, the binder may be useful in communications with your business attorney. While the handbook is not a substitute for good legal counsel and consulting expert input, having it will facilitate everyone's understanding of current expectations for the "reasonably prudent" pain practitioner.

Step 2—Review Your Licensing Board Materials; Keep the Most Relevant Items in your Notebook

Goal: *To ensure your compliance handbook contains relevant licensing board materials on prescribing controlled medications, pain management—acute, chronic, and palliative—medical office-based treatment of opioid addiction, pain clinic registration and operation, prescription drug monitoring databases, and use of naloxone to prevent opioid overdose.*

Rationale: This one is obvious: You need to fill your notebook with relevant licensing board materials and take steps to ensure you have the most current material relating to your licensing board's expectations when controlled medications are part of the treatment plan.

Considerations and Recommendations: Go online and search for your licensing board's home page. If you are licensed and treat patients in more than one state, then you will need to repeat the process for each licensing board and create a separate notebook for each state. Most licensing board Web sites offer a search feature, so enter common search terms such as "opioid guidelines," "pain management," and "treatment of addiction." Some licensing boards are better than others at providing licensees with easy access to pain management and addiction treatment materials. A good example is the State Medical Board of Ohio [27], which publishes its own prescriber resources page for licensees. When you search your licensing board's Web site, look for the following commonly grouped items: (1) Practice Act (medical, nursing, pharmacy); (2) Pain Clinic Registration Act (most states do not have these, but several southern states do, including, but not limited to, Florida, Georgia, Kentucky, Mississippi, Tennessee, and Texas); (3) Controlled Substances Act (more about authority to schedule and control the flow of drugs within the state, but often supplying information about criminal acts related to controlled substances); (4) Prescription Drug Monitoring Database Act and Data Monitoring Program Rules (PDMP), relating to your responsibilities to look up and handle information about patient pharmacy utilization for controlled medications; (5) Licensing Board Rules, including those specific to unprofessional conduct, pain management, addiction treatment, and pain clinic operation; and (6) Licensing Board Guidelines and Position Statements, again specific to pain management, addiction treatment, PDMP, and pain clinics. There are many more areas of licensing board and state regulatory material that may impact controlled substance prescribing, so check with your legal counsel to ensure you have all the material that contains rules and guidelines governing your daily medical practice operations and controlled substance prescribing standards.

Step 3—Identify and Review Major Government and Professional Organization/Society Materials on Chronic Opioid Therapy, Office-Based Treatment of Addiction, and Opioid Overdose Prevention; Keep Highly Relevant Documents in Your Notebook

Goal: *To identify and review, as well as maintain copies of, major government and professional organization/society articles, guidelines, and tools related to chronic opioid therapy, office-based treatment of opioid addiction, and opioid overdose prevention, including material on pain management decision-making, patient risk evaluation and monitoring, opioid selection, and the use of naloxone with patients at risk for opioid overdose.*

Rationale: Licensing boards and medical experts often refer to major clinical articles and publications released by government and major professional organizations when evaluating a practitioner's controlled substance prescribing practices and related treatment practices. Licensing boards also use this material to create licensing board rules and guidelines. A review of these materials will facilitate the practitioner's goal of creating a comprehensive checklist for a self-assessment of controlled substance prescribing practices and overall adherence to "reasonably prudent" practitioner standards for the area of practice. This review will help the practitioner identify common threads between licensing board rules and guidelines, and mainstream clinical literature, on using chronic opioid therapy to treat chronic pain, delivering addiction treatment in the medical office, and opioid overdose prevention. The exercise will also facilitate the creation of written practice protocols and common tools for gathering patient information and documenting the medical record.

Considerations and Recommendations: Start with major federal agencies, such as the DEA, the FDA, and SAMHSA. Use agency Web sites [28] for easy access to DEA Registrant Manuals, FDA REMS Material, the CDC Guidelines, and SAMHSA Opioid Overdose Prevention Toolkits and related items. When reviewing professional organizations/societies, you may wish to first consider the Model Policy documents published by the FSMB [29]. You may also find helpful material through the AAPMed [30], the American Society of Pain Educators (ASPE) [31], and the American Academy of Pain Management (AAPMgmt) [32].

The pool of materials in Step 3 is significant, and you may wish to narrow it down a bit by focusing first on FSMB materials and then turning to educational items derived from the federal agencies and professional societies. Some may find it helpful to include copies of DEA regulations, all of which are available through the DEA Office of Diversion Control's Web site [33].

Step 4—Create a Basic Self-Audit Checklist and Perform an Internal Review of Three to Five Medical Charts; Review the Results with Practice Managers and Legal Counsel

Goal: *To create a checklist of items the prescriber can use to evaluate his/her adherence to state licensing board rules and guidelines on the use of chronic opioid therapy for pain management.*

Rationale: Practitioners like to know that when they provide treatment with controlled substances, they are doing so in a way that maximizes benefits to the patient and minimizes the potential of a bad outcome—for both the patient and the practitioner. Licensing boards provide some sense of the "board's" idea of what is expected when chronic opioid therapy is part of the treatment plan. It is important to understand that a licensing board's expectations are often described as "minimum standards" to maintain licensing in the state, meaning practitioners will be expected to meet the minimum standards and then some to demonstrate that they have acted in a "reasonably prudent" fashion when prescribing controlled medications.

Considerations and Recommendations: To create a checklist tool focused on your licensing board's materials (or FSMB materials if you are in a state that lacks licensing board guidelines/rules), divide a piece of paper (or create three columns in a computer document) into three columns: Column 1—topic area; Column 2—shall/must; and Column 3—should/may. As you read each article/item, highlight and write down any directive language and specific instructions from your licensing board. Ultimately, you will use this checklist in Step Five, below.

Sample Self-Audit Checklist

Though simplified, Table 12.1 contains a sample checklist on the seven basic elements of most licensing board rules and guidelines on the use of opioid analgesics for the treatment of chronic pain.

Table 12.1 Sample self-audit checklist [45]

Topic area	Shall/Must	Should/May
Patient history	*Shall* obtain a medical history of the patient—general and specific to the pain complaint.	*May* wish to contact prior treating practitioners to fill in any gaps related to medical records of the patient's history.
Physical examination	*Shall* perform a physical examination prior to prescribing a controlled substance.	The examination *may* be focused and tailored to the patient's specific complaint of pain.
Treatment plan	*Shall* create a written treatment plan, containing (a) the goals for treatment, (b) diagnostic test orders, and (c) orders for non-drug treatment, as appropriate, and identifying the terms of an opioid trial, if this course of treatment is selected. An opioid trial *shall* be for a reasonable period commensurate with the patient's specific pain needs and be explained and fully specified in the medical record. The treatment plan *shall* also include a written plan for discontinuing the opioids.	*Should* document specifically other treatments tried and failed (or inappropriate) prior to prescribing opioid therapy.
Informed consent	*Shall* discuss the risks and benefits of opioid therapy with the patient (or caregiver/guardian), along with special issues for the use of this medication and treatment alternatives, if any.	*Should* document the informed consent process in the medical record and revisit consent issues as dose changes, medication adjustments are made, including the addition of other controlled medication.
Treatment agreement	*Shall* use a written treatment agreement outlining the patient's responsibilities when treatment involves controlled substances, *including* the responsibility to use only one provider for controlled substance prescribing, to fill prescriptions at a single pharmacy, and to provide a urine (or other) specimen for drug testing when asked to do so by the practitioner, etc. *This agreement shall* (a) contain provisions for monitoring the patient's compliance with the treatment plan, including notification to the patient that the practitioner will check and use information from the state's prescription drug monitoring	*The practitioner should* review the terms of the agreement prior to prescribing controlled substances to the patient. *The practitioner should* allow the patient sufficient opportunity to ask questions about the agreement and the specifics of treatment with controlled substances, and document the questions asked and the answers given in the medical record to ensure understanding between the parties.

(continued)

Table 12.1   (continued)

Topic area	Shall/Must	Should/May
	program; (b) contain notification of the consequences if the patient does not keep his/her promises as made in this document; (c) be reviewed, signed by the patient, and kept in the medical record; and (d) be updated at least annually, and when monitoring circumstances change.	
Drug testing	*The practitioner shall* drug test patients placed on chronic opioid therapy, and such testing shall take place (a) prior to issuing the first prescription for a controlled medication and (b) periodically thereafter at least twice every twelve (12)-month period, or more if the patient's medical history and risk level warrant. *The practitioner shall* document test orders, test results, and clinical decision-making following the review of test results in the medical record.	*The practitioner should* test for common drugs of abuse, including illicit drugs, and consider whether to add or subtract drugs from the test panel based on the individual patient's medical history and properly evaluated risk potential for drug abuse, addiction, diversion, and overdose.
Periodic review	*The practitioner shall* periodically review the patient's progress under the treatment plan and make adjustments, as necessary, to evaluate whether controlled medication remains indicated in the patient's individual case. "Periodically" means the practitioner shall evaluate the patient at least every twelve (12) weeks, or more frequently if warranted by existing or developing clinical and/or risk factors. All follow-up evaluations shall include a written assessment of activity, analgesia, adverse events, aberrant behavior, and affect.	*The practitioner should* carefully monitor the patient's opioid use using medication counts, database checks, drug testing, behavioral health evaluations, and referrals to specialty resources.
Morphine equivalent dose (MED)	*Not all states have a mandate on this topic, so no example is provided to avoid confusion on this very hot topic.*	***Example from California Guidelines Only***: *The practitioner should consider a consult with or a referral to an appropriate specialist as the patient approaches a MED value of **80 mg**.* [46]

(continued)

Table 12.1 (continued)

Topic area	Shall/Must	Should/May
Consultations and referrals	*The practitioner shall use consultations and make referrals as necessary to accomplish the directives in these rules and to ensure the patient's initial and ongoing use of controlled medication is for a legitimate medical purpose and appropriate in the usual course of professional medical practice.*	*The practitioner should document all consultations and referrals and relate them to the ongoing treatment plan and medical decision-making.*

You may wish to perform this same exercise using government or mainstream professional organization/society materials. If you decide to do so, you may need to alter the table slightly when you do as these groups do not typically use "shall" and "must" terminology to describe recommendations to practitioners. In any case, the point of the exercise is to create a checklist by which you can measure your own practices and make any necessary improvements. Very recent government publications on preventing opioid overdose are likely to lead soon to changes in licensing board guidelines on the same topic. For example, the SAMHSA Opioid Overdose toolkit [34] contains a recommendation that practitioners *consider* prescribing naloxone to patient's "at risk" of opioid overdose. If a practitioner faces a legal challenge related to an opioid overdose, it is very likely that the medical expert for the opposing party would testify "a reasonably prudent practitioner would consider whether naloxone is appropriate for his/her patients and discuss the matter during office visits." This same medical expert would also likely state "a reasonably prudent practitioner would prescribe naloxone to patients identified in an "at-risk" category, even if ultimately the patient does not fill the prescription because of cost (the government is working hard to drive down costs associated with equipping patients "at risk" of opioid overdose with a naloxone kit)" [2]. Of course, much back-and-forth battle would take place over the challenges associated with identifying "at-risk" patients, and the realities associated with supply of these kits, but the damage is often done when the prescriber failed to address the matter at all.

The overall goal in creating this self-audit checklist is to facilitate a practitioner's ability to create a framework for controlled substance prescribing due diligence and the practitioner's ability to demonstrate "good faith" compliance with published guidelines and rules—the ability to demonstrate "reasonable prudence" with the prescription pad.

Step 5—Review Your Forms and Make Necessary Changes to Render Them Consistent with Your Self-audit Checklist

Goal: *To align common practice forms with licensing board rules and guidelines on opioid prescribing and pain management; to ensure consistent use of terminology used in licensing board rules and guidelines.*

Rationale: When practice forms, such as informed consent and treatment agreement documents, contain words and phrases used by state licensing boards in rules and guidelines on opioid prescribing and pain management, documentation tends to demonstrate your familiarity with the rules and guidelines and help prescribers and practice staff set boundaries consistent with board expectations. Additional benefits are realized when documentation lines up with licensing board expectations and terminology in current, peer-reviewed literature. Proper documentation is also critical to overcoming an investigation tied to inappropriate prescribing.

Considerations and Recommendations: Gather standard patient forms, including informed consent and treatment agreement documents. Print out a copy of current state licensing board rules and guidelines on the use of chronic opioid therapy to treat pain (or similar). If you practice in a state lacking such rules and guidelines, consider using the FSMB's 2013 Model Policy Statement on the Use of Opioid Analgesics to Treat Chronic Pain and compare the language in your forms to the language used in the FSMB document. The major focus of your review will be a comparison of your licensing board's terminology with the terminology in your practice forms. If you start with your treatment agreement document, your review will go like this: compare the language of your state board's rule/guideline (or the FSMB 2013 Model Policy) on "treatment agreements" with the language used in your "treatment agreement."

Ideally, your treatment agreement should include and track the language used by your state licensing board to refer to this concept. Pay special attention to whether the board's rule/guideline refers to the patient agreement as a "treatment agreement" or "narcotic contract." Most states use the phrase treatment agreement, but some may use "informed consent." Similarly, compare the actual terms of your treatment agreement provisions with the terms set forth in the board's rule or guideline. Your treatment agreement should contain the same provisions used by your licensing board. If your board's materials are outdated, use the treatment agreement provisions cited by the FSMB in its 2013 Model Policy, so you have a nationally recognized resource to cite if questioned on your treatment agreement (or similar document). The FSMB's 2013 Model Policy, as well as most state medical licensing boards, more clearly differentiates between the concepts of informed consent and treatment agreement, even though the FSMB suggests it may be acceptable to combine the provisions or terms of each concept into a single document for convenience purposes [35]. Figure 12.6 contains the language from the FSMB Model Policies from 2004 and 2013 on the subject of "treatment agreement." Figure 12.7 contains the language from these two resources on the subject of "informed consent."

From a legal perspective, it may not be wise to combine the concepts and specific provisions of informed consent with the specific provisions of a treatment agreement; patients may claim a failure of a true informed consent process, and practitioners may be tempted to relegate the informed consent process to a piece of paper, which further increases the potential for legal exposure. Remember, if you are investigated or prosecuted, most of your prescribing-related documentation will

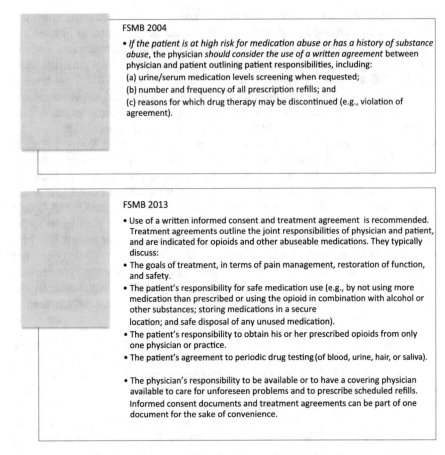

FSMB 2004

• *If the patient is at high risk for medication abuse or has a history of substance abuse*, the physician *should consider the use of a written agreement* between physician and patient outlining patient responsibilities, including:

(a) urine/serum medication levels screening when requested;

(b) number and frequency of all prescription refills; and

(c) reasons for which drug therapy may be discontinued (e.g., violation of agreement).

FSMB 2013

• Use of a written informed consent and treatment agreement is recommended. Treatment agreements outline the joint responsibilities of physician and patient, and are indicated for opioids and other abuseable medications. They typically discuss:

• The goals of treatment, in terms of pain management, restoration of function, and safety.

• The patient's responsibility for safe medication use (e.g., by not using more medication than prescribed or using the opioid in combination with alcohol or other substances; storing medications in a secure
location; and safe disposal of any unused medication).

• The patient's responsibility to obtain his or her prescribed opioids from only one physician or practice.

• The patient's agreement to periodic drug testing (of blood, urine, hair, or saliva).

• The physician's responsibility to be available or to have a covering physician available to care for unforeseen problems and to prescribe scheduled refills.
Informed consent documents and treatment agreements can be part of one document for the sake of convenience.

Fig. 12.6 Basic evolution of treatment agreement language in policy statements and licensing board rules

end up literally on a courtroom wall making it very easy to see whether you put some thought into patient boundaries and obligations or simply copied a document from someone else without first considering whether it followed licensing board rules/guidelines. If you use a document supplied by a medical society or other professional organization, it is advisable to compare the terminology in the document with the terminology contained within your state board's pain guideline or rule. A professional society's silence in a sample treatment agreement on controversial issues, such as marijuana use with opioids, alcohol and opioids, and drug testing frequency, may not offer you much protection. Your position may be more defensible in that situation, but be sure to consider community standards and your licensing board's position.

In any case, pay close attention to the emphasis your state licensing board places on the process of informed consent and make sure you take your cues from your

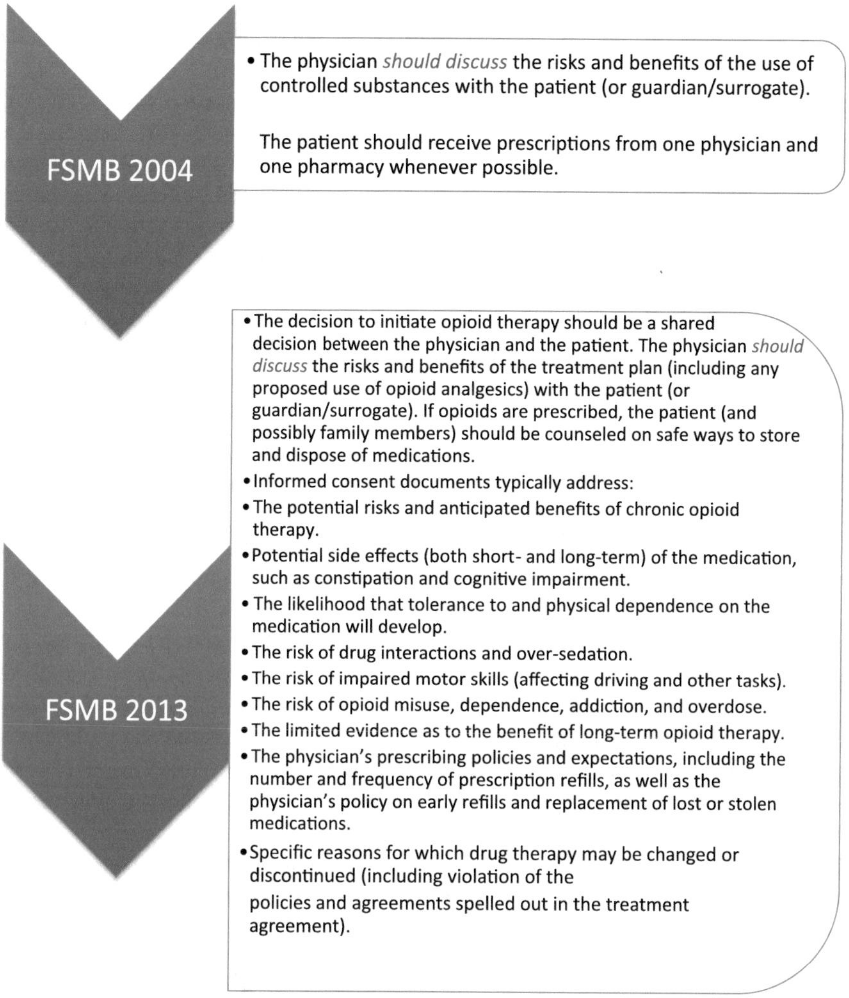

FSMB 2004

- The physician *should discuss* the risks and benefits of the use of controlled substances with the patient (or guardian/surrogate).

  The patient should receive prescriptions from one physician and one pharmacy whenever possible.

FSMB 2013

- The decision to initiate opioid therapy should be a shared decision between the physician and the patient. The physician *should discuss* the risks and benefits of the treatment plan (including any proposed use of opioid analgesics) with the patient (or guardian/surrogate). If opioids are prescribed, the patient (and possibly family members) should be counseled on safe ways to store and dispose of medications.
- Informed consent documents typically address:
- The potential risks and anticipated benefits of chronic opioid therapy.
- Potential side effects (both short- and long-term) of the medication, such as constipation and cognitive impairment.
- The likelihood that tolerance to and physical dependence on the medication will develop.
- The risk of drug interactions and over-sedation.
- The risk of impaired motor skills (affecting driving and other tasks).
- The risk of opioid misuse, dependence, addiction, and overdose.
- The limited evidence as to the benefit of long-term opioid therapy.
- The physician's prescribing policies and expectations, including the number and frequency of prescription refills, as well as the physician's policy on early refills and replacement of lost or stolen medications.
- Specific reasons for which drug therapy may be changed or discontinued (including violation of the policies and agreements spelled out in the treatment agreement).

Fig. 12.7 Basic evolution of informed consent language in the FSMB 2004 and 2013 Model Policy

licensing board and the FSMB, so you have something to point to if someone challenges your informed consent process. Informed consent directives have similarly changed over time and merit review.

Step 6—Review SAMHSA Opioid Overdose Toolkit

Goal: *To gather current educational information related to opioid overdose prevention, along with current data on patients believed to be "at risk" of potential overdose; to understand how the use of naloxone kits (injectable or intranasal) may fit into an overall risk management strategy to minimize the potential of overdose in all patients.*

Rationale: Opioid overdose is a major problem in this country. "At-risk" patients go well beyond the traditional abuser and addict population, and include patients using high doses of extended release/long-acting opioid formulations [36], patients with medical conditions that cause some sort of respiratory distress [12], and patients undergoing rotation from an opioid, like hydrocodone or morphine, to methadone [36]. Practitioners should assess all patients who are or will be receiving opioid analgesics, especially when prescribing involves chronic opioid therapy— for more than 90 consecutive days. Once assessed, practitioners should consider whether the patient is a candidate for a naloxone overdose prevention kit. The use of naloxone in combination with chronic opioid therapy is a relatively new concept. Proactive prescribing of naloxone kits may not be fully embraced by state medical and nursing boards; it may not even be legal in some states. Practitioners should actively seek more information from licensing boards and professional medical organizations.

Considerations and Recommendations: Those who prescribe controlled substances to treat pain have always been held accountable for preventing opioid overdose, but not to the same degree seen today in media headlines, federal and state law enforcement efforts, and courtrooms nationwide. Opioid overdose prevention is now among one of the most talked about topics when it comes to addressing the prescription drug abuse problem in the US. Federal agencies, such as the Substance Abuse Mental Health Services Administration (SAMHSA) and the CDC, are now actively pursuing a universal approach to stemming the tide of overdose deaths associated with prescription medication misuse, especially opioid misuse. Practitioners should read the documents shown in Fig. 12.8 to facilitate understanding of the federal government's position on preventing overdose and professional licensing board involvement in adopting more localized guidelines for licensees.

Note, the SAMHSA Opioid Overdose Toolkit contains several versions—one each for practitioner, patient, community, family member, and first responders. At the

Fig. 12.8 Add to your library
—federal and state opioid
overdose prevention materials

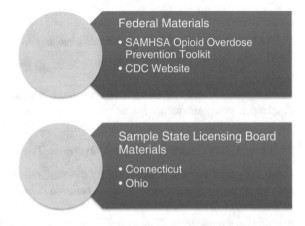

OPIOID OVERDOSE

The risk of opioid overdose *can be minimized* through adherence to the following clinical practices, which are supported by a considerable body of evidence.

ASSESS THE PATIENT. Obtaining a history of the patient's past use of drugs (either illicit drugs or prescribed medications with abuse potential) *is an essential first step* in appropriate prescribing.

Such a history *should include very specific questions.* For example:
1. "In the past 6 months, have you taken any medications to help you calm down, keep from getting nervous or upset, raise your spirits, make you feel better, and the like?"
2. "Have you been taking any medications to help you sleep? Have you been using alcohol for this purpose?"
3. "Have you ever taken a medication to help you with a drug or alcohol problem?"
4. "Have you ever taken a medication for a nervous stomach?"
5. "Have you taken a medication to give you more energy or to cut down on your appetite?"
6. "Have you ever been treated for a possible or suspected opioid overdose?"

Fig. 12.9 Basic "at-risk" questions from SAMHSA Opioid Overdose Toolkit. From Substance Abuse Mental Health Services Administration [37]

very least, read the practitioner and patient versions. Look for "should" directives within the practitioner version and make a list of SAMHSA's recommendations for assessing patients for "risk of overdose" and taking preventative action by prescribing naloxone kits and through other boundaries, such as visit frequency and other monitoring tools. Make a list of these "directives" and use the list to evaluate your current practices. Figure 12.9 contains a sample set of patient assessment questions excerpted from the SAMHSA prescriber's opioid overdose toolkit [37] to help determine whether a patient might be "at risk" of an opioid overdose based on their past relationship with medication.

Your assessment should also include a specific review of the other characteristics SAMHSA designates as placing a patient "at risk" of opioid overdose, as reflected in Fig. 12.10.

The language of the SAMHSA Opioid Overdose Toolkit encourages practitioners to make naloxone kits available to patients who fall into one of these "at-risk" groups [34], and failure to properly consider and document medical decision-making on this issue may give rise to potential for legal liability.

State materials are not as widely available on the topic of opioid overdose prevention as one might think. The first large-scale opioid overdose prevention project began in Wilkes County, North Carolina, with an initiative now widely known as Project Lazarus [38], the first program designed to distribute naloxone kits to at-risk patients and caregivers/family members. The North Carolina Medical Board was the first licensing board to adopt an opioid overdose prevention position statement [39]. More recently, Ohio took action to adopt one of the first (and most comprehensive) joint guidance documents on opioid overdose prevention through its medical, nursing, and pharmacy boards. The Ohio guideline contains a broader set of "at-risk" patient groups [12] than does the SAMHSA toolkit, as illustrated in

CONSIDER PRESCRIBING NALOXONE ALONG WITH THE PATIENT'S INITIAL OPIOID PRESCRIPTION

Naloxone competitively binds opioid receptors and is the antidote to acute opioid toxicity. With proper education, patients on long-term opioid therapy and others at risk for overdose may benefit from having a naloxone kit containing naloxone, syringes and needles or prescribing Evzio® which delivers a single dose of naloxone via a hand-held auto-injector that can be carried in a pocket or stored in a medicine cabinet to use in the event of known or suspected overdose.

Patients who are candidates for such kits include those who are:

Taking high doses of opioids for long-term management of chronic malignant or non- malignant pain.

Receiving rotating opioid medication regimens (and thus are at risk for incomplete cross-tolerance).

Discharged from emergency medical care following opioid intoxication or poisoning.

At high risk for overdose because of a legitimate medical need for analgesia, coupled with a suspected or confirmed history of substance abuse, dependence, or non-medical use of prescription or illicit opioids.

On certain opioid preparations that may increase risk for opioid overdose such as extended release/long-acting preparations.

Completing mandatory opioid detoxification or abstinence programs.

Recently released from incarceration and a past user or abuser of opioids (and presumably with reduced opioid tolerance and high risk of relapse to opioid use).

It also may be advisable to suggest that the at-risk patient create an "overdose plan" to share with friends, partners and/or caregivers. Such a plan would contain information on the signs of overdose and how to administer naloxone (e.g.: using a FDA-approved preparation of naloxone, a naloxone auto-injector or other FDA approved devices as they become available) or otherwise provide emergency care (as by calling 911).

Fig. 12.10 SAMHSA "at-risk" patient populations and overdose prevention recommendations. From Substance Abuse Mental Health Services Administration [37]

Fig. 12.11. Practitioners may wish to consider the Ohio guideline if practicing in a state lacking opioid overdose prevention guidelines [12]. It is important to stay current in this developing area, and you can do so by assigning someone in your practice to check your licensing board's Web site monthly to determine whether opioid overdose prevention rules or guidelines have been adopted.

When a state licensing board lacks a rule or guideline on opioid overdose prevention, practitioners should consider the "at-risk" patient populations named in

Patients with the Risk Factors Below May be in Danger of an Opioid Overdose

These risk factors may be indicators for prescribing or personally furnishing naloxone directly to the patient or to a third party that is in a position to assist an individual who meets these risk factors. The factors include, but are not limited to:

1. Recent medical care for opioid poisoning/intoxication/overdose

2. Participant in Medication-Assistance Treatment (MAT) for opiate addiction

3. Suspected or confirmed history of heroin or nonmedical opioid use

4. High-dose opioid prescription (≥80mg/day morphine equivalence)

5. Any Methadone prescription for opioid naïve patient

6. Recent release from jail or prison with a history of opioid abuse

7. Recent release from mandatory abstinence program or drug detoxification program

8. Enrolled in Methadone or buprenorphine detoxification or maintenance program (for either addiction or pain management)

9. Any opioid prescription, known or suspected: smoking, COPD, emphysema, asthma, sleep apnea, or other respiratory system disease, renal or hepatic disease, alcohol use, concurrent benzodiazepine use or any concurrent sedating medication use, concurrent antidepressant prescription, remoteness from or difficulty accessing medical care, voluntary patient request for naloxone, or any other factor that makes the patient at high-risk for opioid overdose.

Fig. 12.11 Ohio factors for "overdose risk." From State of Ohio, Regulatory Statement [12]

both the SAMHSA and Ohio documents and adopt their own "at-risk" criteria. Carefully evaluate patients for their opioid overdose risk status and, at the very minimum, educate them about the possibility and signs of overdose. Use the SAMHSA patient and family member portion of the opioid overdose prevention toolkit as an educational handout, and consider prescribing a naloxone kit if the patient presents with any of the "at-risk" criteria or makes a supportable request for a kit. Failure to take these steps may be viewed by licensing boards and controlled substance authorities, including the DEA, as acting outside the usual course of professional practice when prescribing opioids.

Patient education is crucial to a proper informed consent process. The SAMHSA Opioid Overdose Prevention Toolkit for Prescribers contains a discussion of informed consent topics related to opioid overdose prevention. Consider giving copies of the toolkit to clinical staff and designate someone in your practice to serve as a patient education coordinator. Decide how you will go about educating your patients on this important topic. Will you give your patients their own copies of the toolkit? Will you make available waiting room copies? Will you take excerpts from the toolkit and turn them into posters for your examination rooms? How will you handle medical record documentation of your educational efforts here? Naloxone kits are not presented here as the be-all and end-all solution to opioid overdose prevention, and the kits certainly present their own risks, as they may precipitate severe withdrawal symptoms in patients physically dependent on opiates, and present other challenges to practitioners attempting to properly use them with patients [40]. Despite potential side effects and safe use challenges, both federal and state governments have seen fit to use them on the front lines in the fight to stop opioid overdoses and save lives.

Step 7—Prepare a Work Plan Using Core Risk Metrics to Improve your Practice Protocols on Critical Risk Issues

Goal: *To identify and use core risk metrics, such as dose, drug combinations, risk level associated with opioid use and potential for opioid overdose, need for consult/referral (or internal peer review or consult with peer if specialist), visit frequency, and various aspects of risk monitoring, to create a more universal approach to setting boundaries in chronic opioid therapy.*

Rationale: Licensing board material (rules, guidelines, enduring educational material), DEA Administrative Case Opinions and Federal Appellate Court Opinions, and a developing body of clinical literature discuss various risk metrics used to evaluate whether the prescriber acted "within the usual course of professional practice" when prescribing controlled medications to patients. A review of the 2013 FSMB Model Policy on the Use of Opioid Analgesics to Treat Chronic Pain, reveals core risk metrics, including the potential relevance of dose, drug combinations, patient risk level, visit frequency, risk monitoring, including the use of prescription drug monitoring databases, medication counts, and drug testing, among other measures, and all play a role in the proper and safe prescribing of opioids [41]. Therefore, the practitioner should identify as many of these core risk metrics as possible through review of licensing board material and current clinical literature, at a minimum, and perform an analysis of his/her integration of the same into daily, routine medical practice. After identifying core risk metrics, the practitioner should use the checklist in Table 12.2 and build upon it during the self-audit process.

Considerations and Recommendations: Use the checklist in Table 12.2 to begin the process of organizing and assessing your prescribing of opioids to treat pain and risk management of your patients on chronic opioid therapy. Consider your overall patient population and pick a patient demographic, such as MED, to use as a sorting factor when identifying which charts to assess first during your self-audit process. I recommend you keep action steps associated with each file reviewed so you are able to return to each chart assessment and determine what, if anything, needs to be done to render the chart complete and sufficient such that a peer could review it and discern your clinical rationale for the prescribed treatment and opine that you prescribed for a "legitimate medical purpose" while acting within the "usual course of professional practice" and taking "reasonable steps to prevent abuse and diversion, as well as opioid overdose." Remember, Table 12.2 contains just a few examples of the considerations relevant to each core evaluation area. Keep track of

Table 12.2 Examples of core areas of patient groupings to address during self-audit

Core evaluation area	Other/related	Next steps
Risk evaluation tools	Do I use a validated risk assessment questionnaire? Am I appropriately assessing patients who are potentially "at risk" of opioid overdose?	Do I have a process by which to confirm proper assessment of questionnaire results? Do I have a process by which to ensure I am using the most current and validated risk assessment tool? Am I permitted to prescribe a naloxone kit proactively if my patients are "at risk" of opioid overdose? How will I educate my patients on overdose and naloxone?
Risk stratification and keeping track	Low, moderate, high risk (or similar)	Do I have a process by which to ensure patients are properly risk stratified? Do I have a protocol for ensuring patients are not skipped around inappropriately between risk categories?
Current informed consent	Does my informed consent process include proper documentation of state licensing board provisions or specific terms of informed consent?	Create a true process of informed consent.
Current treatment agreement	Does my treatment agreement track my state licensing board rule or guideline and include specific terminology and provisions used by my licensing board?	Do I have a protocol for ensuring my office documents interaction with clinical decision-making?
Dose levels (markers for next steps or board-required steps)	Consider where you need to set boundaries for patient risk levels associated with morphine equivalent doses of opioid (MED values). For example, consider using 80-mg MED or less as one boundary; 80-mg MED to 120 mg as the next boundary, and 120-mg MED or above as your final dose-related boundary.	Use these boundaries as a starting point for chart selection associated with your self-audit. Start auditing charts with the patients on 120-mg MED or more.
Drug testing	Have you matched your drug testing protocols with your patients and their risk potentials? Am I using proper patient testing profiles tied to risk potentials?	Consider what the licensing board says about drug testing. Adopt a drug testing protocol. Practitioners may also need to consider payor coverage determinations and, if applicable, discuss with the patient the potential that drug testing may not be covered.

(continued)

Table 12.2 (continued)

Core evaluation area	Other/related	Next steps
Prescription drug monitoring program database	Am I using my state's database as my professional licensing board intended?	Develop a protocol to avoid confusion and inappropriate disclosures and use of personal health information associated with database checks.
Consultations and referrals	Keep track of patients referred to you; Specialists you consult with for patients where consults are needed.	Develop a protocol to track incoming and outgoing consultation and referral paperwork. Be sure to track outcomes—did the patient follow-through on the referral you made? If no, why not? A decision tree may be helpful here, especially when the patient skips referrals, but not their medication appointments.
Older adults	Older adults may be at higher risk of adverse events relating to opioids, especially when opioids are prescribed to an older individual using benzodiazepines. Check out the California Board of Medicine Guidelines on Prescribing Controlled Substances to Treat Pain [47] and the comments relating to prescribing this therapy to older persons.	Consider whether you should adopt protocols for prescribing opioids to older adults, including boundaries related to initiating opioid therapy with lower starting doses, slower titration, longer dosing intervals, and more frequent patient monitoring. Also, consider whether tapering of benzodiazepines is indicated to reduce the potential for respiratory depression. All of these suggestions and more may be found in the California Board of Medicine's 2014 controlled substance prescribing guideline cited in the previous column.
Patients using opioids and benzodiazepines	What, if anything, does your licensing board say about prescribing opioids to patients using benzodiazepines? Does your licensing board impose any special requirements if patients are on chronic benzodiazepine therapy?	Review current clinical literature relating to the potential for increased risks associated with chronic opioid therapy and prescribing benzodiazepines. Consider whether additional protocols are necessary for your practice.

(continued)

Table 12.2 (continued)

Core evaluation area	Other/related	Next steps
High-dose therapy —identification and monitoring	Review current literature on "high-dose" opioid therapy, and determine how this literature may impact your MED boundaries mentioned above.	Determine whether and what type of additional monitoring is recommended for patients on high-dose opioid therapy. Determine whether your state requires you to make an attempt to taper the patient down from the high doses or something similar. Consider discussing these more difficult boundaries with legal counsel and experts in opioid risk management. Make sure your documentation adequately reflects clinical decision-making associated with long-term, high-dose opioid therapy.

other considerations under each core area, and add your own at the end so you have a comprehensive checklist for future audits.

Step 8—Update Patient Education Materials

Goal: *To ensure the practitioner is supplementing the informed consent process with the most current patient education material, and to facilitate improved communication between the practitioner and the patient regarding common patient education issues.*

Rationale: Informed consent is a process not just a piece of paper. Informed consent involves the ongoing education of the patient in a manner that allows the patient to make "informed" healthcare choices. Many informed consent documents confuse the elements of informed consent (risks, benefits, expected treatment alternatives, and special issues associated with the prescribed medication or treatment) with the elements of a treatment agreement (patient obligations when the treatment plan involves controlled substances and consequences for failing to follow the treatment plan and medication safety requirements). While an argument can be made for the convenience of combining these concepts into one document, the practitioner must never lose site of the fact the informed consent requirement is not met by paper alone, but instead requires a true process by which the patient is educated and informed, and allowed to seek clarity on treatment recommendations, risks, benefits, alternatives, and special issues, before and during treatment. During today's litigation over controlled substance prescribing practices, it is highly unlikely that the prescriber accused of inappropriate prescribing will survive to practice another day unless he/she has a true informed consent process—one that includes regular patient education.

Overall, your goal in Step 8 is to adopt an informed consent process robust enough to allow the prescriber to show they did more than hand the patient a piece of paper with informed consent terminology contained within. The informed consent process should contain high-profile educational items published by the US Food & Drug Administration (FDA) and SAMHSA, such as the 2007 FDA consumer piece on "Safe Use of Pain Medication" [42] or the 2014 SAMHSA Opioid Overdose Toolkit for Patients [43]. It is helpful to compile a list of key patient educational topics and to develop a process by which to use cited items to educate patients on a regular basis. Not only will you improve your informed consent *process*, but your efforts will also serve to put the patient on notice that they too have important responsibilities when seeking out medical treatment that involves controlled medication.

Considerations and Recommendations: If you have not already done so, review your state's informed consent requirements and make sure you have the most current opioid education published by the FDA and SAMHSA. Check your state licensing board for additional recommended patient educational material. Identify someone in your practice to serve as an educational coordinator. This person should have authority to research, review, and make recommendations about patient educational material on a variety of topics, especially safe use, safe storage, and safe disposal of opioids and other controlled medication, along with opioid overdose prevention. Patient education should be routine and documented in each patient's file. Tailor education to the extent possible. For example, it is okay to educate every patient on the safe storage and disposal of medication, but not every patient needs education on benzodiazepine use. Patient education does not have to be expensive or time-consuming. Patient education should take place at every visit in some small way. On the first visit, your education might consist of a "Dear Patient" Letter, welcoming the patient to your practice and giving them basic boundaries about how you run your practice, how patient evaluations are conducted, and when and why opioids might prescribed or not. You might find it more useful to adopt a policy of not prescribing opioids on the first visit and to save the review of the written treatment agreement with the patient for the second or third visit. You may also wish to obtain copies of the FDA's "Safe Use of Pain Medication" publication and frame them for hanging in examination rooms; you may also give them out to patients and obtain each patient's signature on the last page of the document and save it in the patient file. Some patients may be at increased risk of overdose, and you may wish to provide them with a copy of or guidance on how to access the SAMHSA Opioid Overdose Toolkit for Patients and Family Members. Similarly, some patients may require education if they fail to uphold the treatment agreement and put you in a position of having to change their treatment plan (more frequent visits, change in medication, discontinuation of medication, or even discontinuation of care) because of their inappropriate or unacceptable conduct or failure to abide by the terms of your plan of care.

Patient education has always been an important aspect of a sustainable business platform for a medical practice. Patient education is also critical to a sound informed consent policy, especially when treatment involves controlled medication. Today, patient education goes a long way to ensuring the patient bears part of the burden of responsibility when it comes to safe use, storage, and disposal of controlled medication; patient education also facilitates the understanding regarding the potential for and symptoms of a drug overdose. For these reasons and more, practitioners may wish to evaluate their plan for educating patients about controlled medication. Proper documentation of educational efforts goes a long way toward supporting the prescriber and his/her quest to balance patient access to controlled medication with the prescriber's responsibility to prevent abuse, diversion, and overdose. Informed consent is largely about patient education.

Whatever you decide, educate your staff on the importance of consistent patient education and take the necessary steps to ensure each staff member understands his/her role in the patient education process. If you take these steps, both your patients and your staff will be better prepared to speak up about your educational efforts if interviewed during a licensing board or DEA/law enforcement investigation of your prescribing practices. Education counts!

The Ethics of Informed Consent

Practitioners have an ethical obligation to ensure that competent patients (or patient caregivers/guardians) are made aware of and understand enough about the intended benefits and possible risks of proposed treatment to make an informed decision, e.g., to use or not use an opioid. The American Medical Association (AMA) publishes the Code of Medical Ethics. Most, if not all, medical licensing boards in the country have adopted and incorporated the AMA Code of Medical Ethics into its state's Medical Practice Act, meaning the subject matter of the code and guidance is relevant to ensuring a compliant practice. Specifically, the AMA has also published an Opinion on Informed Consent, and it is set forth in detail below.

Opinion 8.08–Informed Consent

According to the AMA Code of Medical Ethics, Opinion 8.08—Informed Consent, "the patient's right of self-decision, can be effectively exercised only if the patient possesses enough information to enable an informed choice. The patient should make his or her own determination about treatment. The physician's obligation is to present the medical facts accurately to the patient or to the individual responsible for the patient's care and to make recommendations for management in accordance with good medical practice. The physician has an ethical obligation to help the patient make choices from among the therapeutic alternatives consistent with good medical practice. Informed consent is a basic policy in both ethics and law that physicians must honor, unless the patient is unconscious or otherwise incapable of consenting and harm from failure to treat is imminent. In special circumstances, it may be appropriate to postpone disclosure of information, (see Opinion E-8.122, "Withholding Information from Patients").

Physicians should sensitively and respectfully disclose all relevant medical information to patients. The quantity and specificity of this information should be tailored to meet the preferences and needs of individual patients. Physicians need not communicate all information at one time, but should assess the amount of information that patients are capable of receiving at a given time and present the remainder when appropriate." [44]

Patient education is part of a valid informed consent for medical treatment, including controlled medication. The challenge of informed consent in connection with the prescribing of controlled medication is reviewing and narrowing down the possible educational tools to facilitate the informed consent process when chronic opioid therapy is part of the treatment plan.

Step 9—Educate Colleagues and Staff

Goal: *To educate practice partners and clinical staff on the topics within this chapter and to create an internal process for ongoing education and peer review on these matters.*

Rationale: If your staff is with you on the clinical and regulatory boundaries associated with controlled substance prescribing, you will more likely have support if your prescribing practices are challenged. In most administrative and criminal cases, the medical staff is interviewed and often called to testify against the prescriber. Staff testimony typically focuses on the prescriber's overall routine for evaluating, treating, and monitoring patients. Very often, staff members are asked to testify about the prescriber's amenability toward and role in patient and staff education on critical topics, such as safe use, storage, and disposal of medication, and opioid overdose prevention. Staff members may also be asked about existing protocols for handling patient assessment, including risk evaluation, and monitoring, including any internal process for handling patients who violate the treatment plan and treatment agreements. Investigators typically interview staff members about, or even explore in an undercover capacity, the internal processes for handling complaints about patients, drug testing and test results, doctor-shopping allegations, medication count problems, etc. Practice staff who do not believe their voices are reasonably heard on these important topics typically become whistle-blowers—directly or indirectly. Thoughtful education of medical staff will not only minimize the potential of creating internal strife and adverse witnesses, but it will also help you determine whether someone on your staff has a different opinion regarding chronic opioid therapy.

Considerations and Recommendations: When creating an educational program for practice staff, ask all staff members to provide input and opinion on educational topics. Give each staff member a voice and seek their "buy-in" on patient education topics as well, as active staff member participation may make the difference in the overall outcome of any controlled substance prescribing inquiry or investigation, and may result in patient lives saved. An educated staff may also help when DEA representatives visit your practice or irate family members or reluctant pharmacists call over your prescribing decisions.

Whatever the challenge, do your best to involve your staff in the educational process, which starts with their education and access to you to express ideas and opinions on these challenging topics. You will need to select a staff member to (a) take the lead on organizing a survey for staff member input, (b) keep track of your checklists and collection of Internet resource material, (c) put together educational handbooks for staff members, and (d) organize and keep track of patient education material, among other related tasks. This staff member should be well respected by the majority, if not all, of your staff. Determine whether you are able to make participation in educational sessions mandatory and part of the staff member's performance review, especially at the administrative, clinical, and practitioner levels.

Step 10—Consult Outside Experts—Legal and Medical—To Ensure a Sufficient Self-audit and to Address Specific Risk Management Issues

Goal: *To identify when it might be time to consult with outside experts—legal or medical—to ensure a proper self-audit and overall approach to controlled substance prescribing risk management, and to tackle specific risk management issues.*

Rationale: Without question, there are times when you should consult with outside legal and even experienced medical experts to address scope and sufficiency issues associated with your self-audit, and to tackle specific risk management issues. Legal and medical experts may offer improved insight into licensing board expectations and standard of care questions. Similarly, legal and medical experts may have input on recent cases—administrative and criminal—and thereby be in a better position to offer supplemental detail to the items raised in this chapter about self-audit areas. If you (a) face notices of over payment, especially from Medicare contractors, (b) are under a licensing board audit, or (c) have had a recent visit from the DEA or other federal or state law enforcement authority, it may help to discuss the need for and scope of a self-audit with your legal counsel and perhaps even a risk management expert. The main purpose of the visit would be to ensure your proactive action plan is supportive of your reactive action plan tied to your response to any of the three circumstances listed above.

Considerations and Recommendations: There are many considerations associated with the selection of outside legal counsel and medical experts, and most of these are beyond the scope of this chapter. Suffice it to say, you want to select legal counsel and medical experts who are truly experts on the subject matter (or are willing to engage subject matter experts). It will not do you any good to engage counsel and experts who do not understand the challenges brought about by a financial or prescribing audit related to the prescribing of controlled substances to treat pain. The stakes are high whether you face a financial inquiry or a direct challenge to your prescribing practices. Perhaps, one of the best reasons to walk through the exercises in this chapter is to ready a handbook for use with your legal counsel or medical expert. Many lawyers and medical experts do not stay current with changing rules and guidelines specific to the use of controlled substances to treat pain; some lack familiarity with them altogether, which likely means they are not true experts on the subject matter. Save yourself some time and money by keeping the notebook referenced in Step One, above. Take notes when you speak with legal counsel or medical experts. Interview them, just as they will interview you. Take the time you need to decide whether legal counsel truly understands the complexity of the issues associated with the prescribing of controlled substances to treat pain. If they do not, explore whether they are truly willing to work with a subject matter expert of your choice without feeling as if their role in the case (or financial gain) is threatened. Good lawyers welcome the opportunity to work with subject matter experts. Good medical experts welcome the opportunity to work with other clinical experts and should have familiarity with the courtroom and arguments on both sides of the opioid issue. Good legal counsel and medical experts cost money, but they can save you a great deal of aggravation and money in the long run, and they typically have (or should have) good relationships with third parties undertaking your investigation and prosecution. Even if you only consult with legal counsel a couple of times per year to ensure you are on the correct path for practice risk management protocols and educational efforts, your money will be well spent. Finally, do not hesitate to engage physicians as mentors or practice reviewers. Input from a true medical expert may make the difference between a letter of reprimand and medical license suspension. It helps to get medical experts on your team early and keep them engaged proactively to minimize the potential for a bad legal outcome.

Summary

This chapter was intended to provide practitioners with a few tools to facilitate a self-audit of controlled substance prescribing practices. This chapter was not intended to be a comprehensive source on each of the topics raised within or all of the legal issues a prescriber may potentially face in an administrative audit or criminal investigation of his/her prescribing practices or financial underpinnings of the medical practice. The landscape for the use of opioids to treat chronic pain is rapidly changing, and federal and state agencies are focused on opioid overdose prevention. Much of this chapter is likewise focused on opioid overdose prevention through patient and staff education, and proper patient evaluation for overdose risk and receipt of a naloxone overdose prevention kit.

Practitioners should make time to perform a self-audit of their prescribing practices and to educate patients and practice staff on critical issues associated with the use of opioids to treat pain. The checklists referenced in this chapter will help practitioners accomplish a self-audit and improve risk management programs tied to controlled substance prescribing. Practitioners should strive to stay current with changing licensing board rules and guidelines, as well as clinical standards of care, and focus on accurately and completely documenting clinical rationale and decision-making to ensure there is no question as to whether there exists a legitimate medical reason for the use of a controlled substance and whether prescribing took place within the usual course of professional practice. Practitioners are held in a position of trust over the patient and must exercise good faith when prescribing controlled medications to all patients. Federal and state laws, as well as clinical standards of care, play a role in defining what constitutes "reasonable measures to prevent abuse and diversion" or a controlled medication; the same applies to the evaluation of "reasonable measures to prevent opioid overdose." While this chapter was not intended to provide an in-depth legal analysis of "reasonable measures," the self-audit tools will facilitate the prescriber's demonstration of "good faith" fulfillment of his/her clinical and legal obligations, and will also facilitate improved dialogue with local legal counsel and medical experts who are cast in risk management and litigation roles. Our country depends on practitioners like you who are willing to be proactive in the effort to combat prescription drug abuse, diversion, and overdose deaths, while at the same time remaining committed to providing quality pain management.

References

1. U.S. Drug Enforcement Administration. Final policy statement on dispensing controlled substances for the treatment of pain, Vol. 71(172), 6 Sept 2006, as published in the Federal Register, pp. 52716–23. Available at http://wais.access.gpo.gov (DOCID:fr fr06se06-139).
2. US Department of Health and Human Services, Office of the Assistant Secretary for Planning and Evaluation, press release 26 Mar 2015, entitled Opioid Abuse in the U.S. and HHS actions to address opioid-drug related overdoses and deaths. Available online at http://aspe.hhs.gov/sp/reports/2015/OpioidInitiative/ib_OpioidInitiative.cfm.
3. HHS-ASPE Executive Briefing on Opioid Overdose Prevention Initiative. Available online at http://aspe.hhs.gov/sp/reports/2015/OpioidInitiative/es_OpioidInitiative.pdf.
4. Medical Board of California. Guidelines for prescribing controlled substances for pain, Nov 2014. Available online at http://www.mbc.ca.gov/Licensees/Prescribing/Pain_Guidelines.pdf. Accessed 31 Mar 2015.
5. Washington State Department of Health. Frequently asked questions regarding the morphine equivalent dose rules associated with consultation requirement. Available online at http://www.doh.wa.gov/ForPublicHealthandHealthcareProviders/HealthcareProfessionsandFacilities/PainManagement/FrequentlyAskedQuestionsforPractitioners/MorphineEquivalentDosageMed. Accessed 31 Mar 2015.
6. For a copy of the US Drug Enforcement Administration's Press Release on the Consensus Statement, see http://www.deadiversion.usdoj.gov/pubs/advisories/newsrel_102301.pdf. For a copy of the final consensus statement, see University of Wisconsin, Pain & Policy Studies Group, http://www.painpolicy.wisc.edu/sites/www.painpolicy.wisc.edu/files/Consensus2.pdf. Accessed 31 Mar 2015.

7. U.S. Drug Enforcement Administration. Final policy statement on dispensing controlled substances for the treatment of pain, Vol. 71(172), 6 Sept 2006. Federal Register; 2006. p. 52716–23. Available online at www.deadiversion.usdoj.gov or www.gpo.gov.

8. Adapted from Bolen J. Taking back your turf: understanding the role of law in medical decision making in opioid management (Part I—overview). J Opioid Manage. 2005;1(3):125–9.

9. 21 CFR 1306.04. Available on-line at www.deadiversion.usdoj.gov.

10. U.S. Drug Enforcement Administration. Interim policy statement on dispensing controlled substances for the treatment of pain, Vol. 60(220), 16 Nov 2004, as published in the Federal Register, p. 67170–2. Available at http://waisaccess.gpo.gov (DOCID:fr16no04-82). Accessed 10 Jan 2006. Although the DEA used the term "dispensing" in the IPS, the DEA will apply its interpretation to other conduct, including administering and prescribing controlled substances to treat pain.

11. 21 CFR 1306.04, available online at http://www.deadiversion.usdoj.gov/21cfr/cfr/1306/1306_04.htm.

12. State of Ohio, Regulatory Statement. Prescription of naloxone to high risk individuals and third parties who are in a position to assist an individual who is experiencing opioid-related overdose, updated Sept 2014. Available online at http://www.dw.ohio.gov/med/pdf/NEWS/Naloxone-Joint-Regulatory-Statement-2014.pdf. Accessed 31 Mar 2015.

13. U.S. Drug Enforcement Administration. Final policy statement on dispensing controlled substances for the treatment of pain, Vol. 71(172), 6 Sept 2006. Federal Register; 2006. p. 52723. Available online at www.deadiversion.usdoj.gov or www.gpo.gov.

14. Available online at http://www.deadiversion.usdoj.gov/crim_admin_actions/index.html.

15. *United States v. Schneider*, 594 F.3d 1219 (10th Cir. 2010), specifically Document 525 (Sentencing Memorandum).

16. *US v. Brian Heim*, et al. DEA press release dated 16 Mar 2015. Available online at http://www.dea.gov/divisions/det/2015/det031615.shtml.

17. *US v. Brian Heim*, et al. Case: 5:14-cr-00412-DAP, Doc #: 11, Sentencing Memorandum, Filed: 03/16/15, available through the United States Court System known as PACER, see https://pacer.login.uscourts.gov (subscription required).

18. In 2015, following a hearing and expert testimony, a DEA Administrative law judge issued a decision with an extensive opinion finding against the DEA Registrations for Reynolds BD, Killebrew TL, Stout DR. Federal Register, Vol. 80(96) (Tuesday, 19 May 2015), p. 28643–67, available online via the Government Publishing Office [www.gpo.gov] [FR Doc No: 2015-12038]. This case involved inappropriate controlled substance prescribing by three Tennessee-licensed Nurse Practitioners (NPs), who were each authorized to prescribe controlled medications. The government engaged an advanced practice nurse expert to review patient files and present expert testimony on a variety of facts and findings related to the issue of whether the NPs prescribed outside the usual course of professional practice. Focusing in on the role of drug testing in chronic pain management, the government's expert made the following statements during the revocation hearing: The Expert noted the attending practitioner properly ordered a Urine Drug Screen (UDS) for patient "N.S." According to the Expert, a UDS is a particularly useful tool when the practitioner is presented with a red flag indicating the patient may not be in compliance, such as when the patient presents at the office exhibiting the behaviors N.S. did on this visit. As the Expert explained, a UDS can assist the practitioner in determining whether the patient has been taking the drug(s) prescribed and if the patient was ingesting non-prescribed controlled substances, including illicit substances. Thus, UDS results help practitioners to determine whether a patient is abusing and/or diverting controlled substances. While this other practitioner appropriately ordered a UDS, according to the Expert, **he then inappropriately issued to N.S. another prescription for thirty tablets of** 60 mg of [a long-acting morphine product] at this visit. As the Expert found, at this visit, N.S.'s file still lacked any information of her prior treatment history and substance abuse history. **According to the Expert, in the absence of this information, and in light of the fact N.S. presented at this visit demonstrating slurred speech and somnolence, the issuance of the**

[morphine] prescription was below the standard of care in Tennessee and outside the usual course of professional practice and actually medically contraindicated given the mental status changes documented in her record. The Expert further explained under the circumstances presented by N.S., the standard of care and usual course of professional practice required the patient's referral for a comprehensive evaluation (the emergency room) to determine the underlying cause of the symptoms of her increased heart rate, slurred speech, and somnolence. Moreover, the patient should not have received prescriptions (of any type) at this visit until medical clearance was provided, confirming she was not experiencing drug intoxication or an acute neurologic event. … [B]ecause N.S. was not referred or transferred for further evaluation, she should not have received any controlled medications until the urine drug screen results were available to the provider. Nearly three months later (on September 29, 2004), N.S. returned … for her next visit and was seen by [another NP]. Prior to this visit, the practice had received the report of the results of the UDS administered to N.S. at her July 7, 2004 visit. According to the Expert, on the date of the UDS, N.S. should have had [morphine] left from the prescription issued at her first visit and should have still been taking the drug. However, the UDS was negative for opiates, positive for benzodiazepines, and positive for cocaine. According to the Expert, these results should have been a "huge red flag of abuse and diversion" for [the NP] because not only did N.S. test positive for cocaine, she also tested positive for three different benzodiazepines, none of which had been prescribed to her at her first visit. The Expert further explained … the presence of the three benzodiazepines, in addition to the presence of cocaine, were consistent with the somnolence, slurred speech, and increased pulse rate documented during the July 7, 2004 visit. The Expert also noted … N.S. tested negative for opiates, when she should have tested positive for the [morphine], which she should have still been taking. This case contains many additional points of discussion, all of which support the proactive self-assessment of practice routines to ensure compliance with applicable standards of care and regulatory prescribing requirements.

19. U.S. Drug Enforcement Administration, Office of Diversion Control, *Cases Against Doctors*, available online at http://www.deadiversion.usdoj.gov/crim_admin_actions/.

20. In 2006, DEA made the following comment in its Final Policy Statement: "DEA recognizes that the overwhelming majority of American physicians who prescribe controlled substances do so for legitimate medical purposes. In fact, the overwhelming majority of physicians who prescribe controlled substances do so in a legitimate manner that will never warrant scrutiny by Federal or State law enforcement officials." U.S. Drug Enforcement Administration. Final policy statement on dispensing controlled substances for the treatment of pain, Vol. 71(172), 6 Sept 2006. Federal Register; 2006. p. 52716–23. Available online at www.deadiversion.usdoj.gov or www.gpo.gov.

21. Texas Medical Board Rules. Chapter 170 (Pain management, starting at p. 55). Available online at http://www.tmb.state.tx.us/idl/21CF17CA-9AAB-05B9-E924–01227E0694E1. Accessed 31 Mar 2015.

22. 42 CFR § 424 (2006).

23. HHS-Office of the Inspector General. Prescribers with questionable patterns in medicare Part D, June 2013, OEI-02-09-00603. Available online at http://oig.hhs.gov/oei/reports/oei-02-09-00603.pdf. Accessed 31 Mar 2015.

24. 42 CFR §424.535 Revocation of enrollment in the Medicare program. In (13) *Prescribing authority*. (i) The physician or eligible professional's Drug Enforcement Administration (DEA) Certificate of Registration is suspended or revoked; or (ii) The applicable licensing or administrative body for any state in which the physician or eligible professional practices suspends or revokes the physician or eligible professional's ability to prescribe drugs. (14) *Improper prescribing practices.* CMS determines whether the physician or eligible professional has a pattern or practice of prescribing Part D drugs that falls into one of the following categories: (i) The pattern or practice is abusive or represents a threat to the health and safety of Medicare beneficiaries or both. In making this determination, CMS considers the following factors: (A) Whether there are diagnoses to support the indications

for which the drugs were prescribed. (B) Whether there are instances when the necessary evaluation of the patient for whom the drug was prescribed could not have occurred (for example, the patient was deceased or out of state at the time of the alleged office visit). (C) Whether the physician or eligible professional has prescribed controlled substances in excessive dosages linked to patient overdoses. (D) The number and type(s) of disciplinary actions taken against the physician or eligible professional by the licensing body or medical board for the State or States in which he or she practices, and the reason(s) for the action(s). (E) Whether the physician or eligible professional has any history of "final adverse actions" (as the term is defined in §424.502). (F) The number and type(s) of malpractice suits filed against the physician or eligible professional related to prescribing and which have resulted in a final judgment against the physician or eligible professional or in which the physician or eligible professional has paid a settlement to the plaintiff(s) (to the extent this can be determined). (G) Whether any State Medicaid program or any other public or private health insurance program has restricted, suspended, revoked, or terminated the physician or eligible professional's ability to prescribe medications, and the reason(s) for any such restriction, suspension, revocation, or termination. (H) Any other relevant information provided to CMS. **(ii) The pattern or practice of prescribing fails to meet Medicare requirements. In making this determination, CMS considers the following factors**: (A) Whether the physician or eligible professional has a pattern or practice of prescribing without valid prescribing authority. (B) Whether the physician or eligible professional has a pattern or practice of prescribing for controlled substances outside the scope of the prescriber's DEA registration. (C) Whether the physician or eligible professional has a pattern or practice of prescribing drugs for indications generally viewed as medically unacceptable—that is, for indications neither approved by the FDA nor medically accepted under section 1860D-2(e)(4) of the Act—and whether there is evidence the physician or eligible professional acted in reckless disregard for the health and safety of the patient.

25. 42 CFR § 424.530(14).
26. The author recognizes licensing board rules and standards of care vary and often differentiate obligations for prescribing controlled medication to treat acute from those associated with prescribing these medications to treat chronic pain of a non-terminal origin. While the ten steps listed in the chapter are limited to controlled substance prescribing in the context of chronic, non-terminal pain, readers may wish to delve further into licensing board and professional organization material to determine whether there are additional rules and guidelines governing the use of controlled medication in the acute or palliative settings.
27. State Medical Board of Ohio, Prescriber Resources Webpage, http://med.ohio.gov/ PrescriberResources.aspx.
28. DEA Diversion website http://www.deadiversion.usdoj.gov, FDA REMS website http://www. fda.gov/Drugs/DrugSafety/PostmarketDrugSafetyInformationforPatientsandProviders/ ucm111350.htm, SAMHSA Opioid Overdose Toolkit website http://store.samhsa.gov/ product/Opioid-Overdose-Prevention-Toolkit-Updated-2014/SMA14-4742, and the CDC website http://www.cdc.gov/primarycare/materials/opoidabuse/index.html.
29. FSMB website, http://www.fsmb.org/.
30. AAPMed website, http://www.painmed.org/.
31. ASPE website, http://www.paineducators.org/.
32. AAPMGMT website, http://www.aapainmanage.org/.
33. U.S. Drug Enforcement Administration, Office of Diversion Control, website available at http://www.deadiversion.usdoj.gov/.
34. Substance Abuse Mental Health Services Administration. Opioid overdose prevention toolkit (Updated 2014), at p. 6. Available online at http://store.samhsa.gov/product/Opioid-Overdose-Prevention-Toolkit-Updated-2014/SMA14-4742. Accessed 31 Mar 2015.
35. See Figs. 6 and 7, and Federation of State Medical Boards. Model policy on the use of opioid analgesics for the treatment of chronic pain. 2013. Available online at http://www.fsmb.org/ Media/Default/PDF/FSMB/Advocacy/pain_policy_july2013.pdf. Accessed 1 June 2015.

36. Substance Abuse Mental Health Services Administration. Opioid overdose prevention toolkit (Updated 2014), at p. 3. Available online at http://store.samhsa.gov/product/Opioid-Overdose-Prevention-Toolkit-Updated-2014/SMA14-4742. Accessed 31 Mar 2015. See also State of Ohio, Regulatory Statement. Prescription of naloxone to high risk individuals and third parties who are in a position to assist an individual who is experiencing opioid-related overdose, updated Sept 2014. Available online at http://www.dw.ohio.gov/med/pdf/NEWS/Naloxone-Joint-Regulatory-Statement-2014.pdf. Accessed 31 Mar 2015.
37. Substance Abuse Mental Health Services Administration. Opioid overdose prevention toolkit (Updated 2014), p. 3. Available online at http://store.samhsa.gov/product/Opioid-Overdose-Prevention-Toolkit-Updated-2014/SMA14-4742. Accessed 31 Mar 2015.
38. http://projectlazarus.org/. Project Lazarus is a secular public health non-profit organization established in 2008 in response to extremely high drug overdose death rates in Wilkes County, North Carolina (four times higher than the state average). In 2007, Wilkes County had the third highest drug overdose death rate in the nation, according to the Centers for Disease Control and Prevention (CDC). Project Lazarus kits are now in numerous states, and the success of the project has led to new state legislation and licensing board rules and guidelines.
39. The September 1. 2008, North Carolina Medical Board position statement on opioid overdose prevention may be found online at http://www.ncmedboard.org/position_statements/detail/drug_overdose_prevention/, and contains the following statement by the board: The Board is concerned about the rise in overdose deaths over the past decade in the State of North Carolina as a result of both prescription and non-prescription drugs. The Board is encouraged by programs attempting to reduce the number of drug overdoses by making available or pre-scribing an opioid antagonist such as naloxone to someone in a position to assist a person at risk of an opiate-related overdose. The prevention of drug overdoses is consistent with the Board's statutory mission to protect the people of North Carolina. *The Board therefore encourages its licensees to cooperate with programs in their efforts to make opioid antagonists available to persons at risk of suffering an opiate-related overdose.*
40. Substance Abuse Mental Health Services Administration. Opioid Overdose Prevention Toolkit (Updated 2014). Available online at http://store.samhsa.gov/product/Opioid-Overdose-Prevention-Toolkit-Updated-2014/SMA14-4742. Accessed 31 Mar 2015. See also, Drugs.com Narcan Monograph, available online at http://www.drugs.com/monograph/narcan.html; Beletsky L, Rich JD, Walley AY. Prevention of fatal opioid overdose. JAMA. 2012; 308 (18):1863–4. doi:10.1001/jama.2012. Available online at http://www.ncbi.nlm.nih.gov/pmc/articles/PMC3551246/pdf/nihms-431424.pdf.
41. Federation of State Medical Boards. Model policy on the use of opioid analgesics for the treatment of chronic pain; 2013. Available online at http://www.fsmb.org/Media/Default/PDF/FSMB/Advocacy/pain_policy_july2013.pdf. Accessed 1 June 2015.
42. U.S. Food and Drug Administration. A guide to safe use of pain medication, 23 Feb 2009. Available online at http://www.fda.gov/ForConsumers/ConsumerUpdates/ucm095673.htm.
43. Substance Abuse Mental Health Services Administration. Opioid overdose prevention toolkit (Updated 2014). Available online at http://store.samhsa.gov/product/Opioid-Overdose-Prevention-Toolkit-Updated-2014/SMA14-4742. Accessed 31 Mar 2015.
44. American Medical Association. Opinion 8.08—informed consent. Available online at http://www.ama-assn.org/ama/pub/physician-resources/medical-ethics/code-medical-ethics/opinion808.page.
45. The language in this table is a blend of directives from several different sources, including: FSMB Model Policy on the Use of Opioid Analgesics for the Treatment of Chronic Pain (2013), Texas Medical Board Practice Rule, Chapter 170, Pain Management (2015); Washington State Area Medical Directors Guidelines on Chronic Opioid Therapy (2010 to present); California Guidelines on Chronic Opioid Therapy (2014); Georgia Composite Board, Pain Management Rule (2012, as updated); and Tennessee Department of Health Related Boards, Chronic Opioid Therapy Guidelines (2014). Some of the directives have been modified for educational purposes, and the table is not intended to cover every possible aspect

of a state guideline analysis. To ensure complete understanding of prescriber legal obligations, consult with qualified legal counsel in an attorney-client setting.

46. The 80 mg MED value is derived from the California Medical Board's November 2014 Opioid Prescribing Guidelines, available online at http://www.mbc.ca.gov/Licensees/ Prescribing/Pain_Guidelines.pdf. The value is included in Table 12.1 only as an example of how a medical board may insert dose and MED levels into licensing standards and guidelines. Note, in its 2014 guidelines, the California Medical Board makes clear the 80 mg MED value DOES NOT represent a ceiling dose. Rather, the California Medical Board uses the value to identify "yellow flag" issues for its licensees, and to urge caution with dose increases and the overall treatment plan, including the decision to seek consultations and make referrals as opioid doses increase. In fact, the California Medical Board encourages physicians to carefully evaluate whether a consult is appropriate for patients at or near the 80 mg MED level. Other states, such as Washington, use the 120 mg MED value as a "trip wire" for the use of a consult. Practitioners are encouraged to review licensing board material and check for a MED value tied to a directive to obtain consults and referrals, or to take other steps to minimize potential for adverse outcomes and reevaluate the risk-to-benefit aspects of the patient's ongoing use of opioids.

47. California Board of Medicine. Guidelines for prescribing controlled substances for pain, Nov 2014. Available online at http://www.mbc.ca.gov/Licensees/Prescribing/Pain_Guidelines.pdf.

Chapter 13
Treating the Difficult Patient

Hans Hansen and Judith Holmes

Ride tall in the saddle you take more arrows.

John Wayne (maybe).

Introduction

The challenging patient is a fact of life and part of our practice. The clinic that understands the complex issues of dealing with difficult patients and responds to threats appropriately will minimize risks. Risk can come in the form of malpractice claims, board of medicine complaints, Employee Equal Opportunity Commission (EEOC) charges, employee whistle-blowers, and patient allegations that lead to a financial and time drain.

Interventional techniques are sophisticated, medications are complex, and pain medicine involves treating a rainbow of complex patients. We as medical providers love to talk to our "good" patients; patients that are difficult, angry, needy, threatening make us cringe. How do healthcare practitioners navigate through the myriad of ill will thrust our way? Offering the latest treatment is of little value if conflict leads to disciplinary action and poor patient satisfaction.

There are many factors involved in dealing with patients with difficult personalities. Difficult personalities are in the office or hospital, or around the corner. Difficult people thrive on conflict. Land mines are abundant, and government agencies exist for the sole purpose of rendering recourse to the provider or employer that does not give the outlier a good day.

Challenging people may manifest personality disorders that may be ready to erupt. A physician's office is a building of *accommodation* and expected to service

H. Hansen (✉)
Pain Relief Centers, 1224 Commerce St. SW, Conover, NC 28613, USA
e-mail: hhansen@painreliefcenters.com

J. Holmes
The Compliance Clinic, LLC, 991 Mt. Rose Way, Golden, CO 80401, USA

© Springer International Publishing Switzerland 2016
P.S. Staats and S.M. Silverman (eds.), *Controlled Substance Management in Chronic Pain*, DOI 10.1007/978-3-319-30964-4_13

a broad range of problems and people [1]. Expect conflict. React with appropriate professional integrity, and you will inevitably defer the next stages of drama.

It is the purpose of this chapter to assist the provider with the most difficult part of the medical process—not patient management, but people risk management. Risk management prevents loss of time, money, professional status, and a calm sense of self-being. The ever-changing temperament and conflict that surrounds the daily practice of medicine cannot be avoided, but it can be managed. There are 400 physician suicides a year and underreported death by substance abuse, all preventable and tragic [2]. It is important to keep the issues in perspective and not allow those with personality disorders to ruin the practice of medicine. This chapter strives to be practice-protective and provides strategies to keep the practitioner happy.

Vignette

> Patient—"I've heard about you, people in the waiting room said that you had an attitude. They also complain about your bedside manner. They said you also judge. I am not an addict and you make me feel like an addict. You are rude."

Physician response—Incredibly, common terms are used commonly by difficult people. It seems that the term "rude" is used as an accepted polite way to say that they don't like you and you're not acting their way. This type of interaction is a personal affront. The first response you might have is one of anger and desire to confront. As we shall see, this is not our best approach. We shall see that people act as a reactionary. I'm going to call this behavior based on emotion. Neurobiologically, there are pathways that become altered or diminished in the difficult patient, particularly the patient that is suffering from pain, situational depression, anxiety, reliance on opioids, and other controlled substances (the alprazolam band aid…). Your communication skills are your best defense. For example, you might respond with "I am sorry that you feel that way. I hope to convince you that what you have heard is not accurate and we can establish a fruitful doctor–patient relationship."

Introduction to Communication

There is a difference between hearing and listening.

Communication skills are not an exact science and neither is the practice of medicine. Over the course of the day, the provider is expected to extract a history, define medical decision making, apply a care plan, and then repeat this over and over in the course of a daily practice. The process might involve a minor care issue, or an experience that an individual will consider life altering. The provider is a source of inspiration and hope, or a point of conflict. All the while, the extraneous factors that include nurses, administration, ancillary personnel, and ever more burdensome regulatory requirements are forever perpetuating a background noise that can't be ignored. The day can be good, or it can be driven by distraction. It all points to the leadership the provider offers and that requires communication skills.

Providers are paid less and less, with the expectation of more skill sets and time given to the practice of medicine. The regulatory burden is relentless, and the paperwork is endless. Patients want a perfect outcome, and, of course, always want to retain the right to litigate if imperfection results in an unforeseeable outcome. Most providers want an uneventful day and rewarding experiences, because a career in medicine should be fulfilled for all. If communication skills are robust, it's odds on that the day will end without consequence. Unfortunately, providers are frequently poorly trained in communication skills. Communication skills, however, are as important as any healing tool the physician has; no laboratories, scans, X-rays are more important.

The physician, or provider, that lacks fundamental communication skills will not be able to manage difficult people and patients. Difficult people often see themselves as *victims*. They believe their priorities are foremost, and they are posed to retaliate if their immediate needs are not met. There is no more dangerous consequence in medicine, that is of higher risk to the provider and the care environment, than the breakdown of communication between an angry person who perceives themselves as a victim.

Vignette

Patient—"I'm here because my doctor sent me here. I don't want to be one of those "pain patients." Those people are out for drugs. I'm not here for drugs. I just want to be honest with you; I am a person of religious conviction. It's not that I don't want to give you a urine screen, but I just want to be honest with you. I think honesty is the best policy. My mother was seeing me suffer so she gave me her Percocet."

Provider—It is your unfortunate burden to utilize patient care agreements, extra documentation, and practice-protective language to ensure that there is "no barrier to communication." In other words, these people are sure that you didn't tell them something, or they didn't hear it. They didn't read it, they didn't understand it. They just got what they wanted. The difficult person, or patient, requires a level of documentation, and practice policy that will be known as the *rules*. You or your staff ensure they understand the terminology and received adequate informed consent. It is labor intensive, takes time, but it is worth it [3]. An appropriate response to this patient might be "I understand your concerns regarding the urine drug test, but is a policy for all our patients, and I assure you that you are not being singled out."

Types of People We Meet

Our mothers told us not to judge others and place labels. That is exactly the opposite of how we are trained as medical professionals. The differential diagnosis is full of labels, and ICD-10 has about 150,000 of them. If the ICD-10 defines an injury from a burning water ski (they do; V91.07), then we're all a label waiting to happen. There exists a medical diagnosis for everyone. So it makes sense that having a label is not so bad. The types of people we meet can be described, and labeled, into a few distinguishable types. There may be variants, but generally speaking, patients and people in general don't deviate too far from basic personality foundations.

Personalities

There are four temperaments dating from Hippocrates' day, felt to be present in humans [4]. Hippocrates believed humans humorous. They were felt to be affected by body fluids, behaviors, and their environment. Hippocrates observed human moods, emotions, and behaviors and felt they were caused by excess fluids in the body, thus "bodily humors." These included blood, bile, and phlegm. They were believed to keep a body in balance. Adding on this theme are the four "temperaments" defined by Galen [5].

1. Sanguine
2. Choleric
3. Melancholic
4. Phlegmatic.

The Sanguine is a lively, talkative, pleasure-seeking individual, but flighty. These people are chronically late, forgetful and have trouble with tasks.

Choleric is ego-centric, task-oriented, and strong willed. They often have a strong work ethic.

The Melancholic is introverted and paranoid. They are, however, conscientious trying to get the job done, but unsociable.

The Phlegmatic is retrospective, very private, thoughtful, and pensive. Fast forward through multiple philosophers and generations of pundits, and we have a new generation of personality types.

These are defined by culture, experience, social demand, and the recently unrestrained environment of the Internet and social media.

Personality Disorders Have More Recently Been Defined by the Diagnostic and Statistical Manual of Mental Disorders (DSM-5)

Narcissistic Personality Disorder

The only difference between you, your employees, and your patients is that your patients are usually Axis II.

Difficult people understand that you will be working in your comfort zone, by intellect and reason, whereas they are operating on *instincts* and *emotion*. The narcissistic personality is manipulative and demands that you give them what they want, not what they need [6]. This is where you will find a black and white personality that is best handled by policy over policing. Dialectic over confrontation. Communication skills require restraint, because people with this personality disorder desire conflict. Policies avoid these misunderstandings. Most people understand that part of their day has to have something upset, and no day is perfect. The patient with a **narcissistic personality** believes they are never wrong, utopia is right around the corner, and every day should be on their terms.

Many times the narcissistic personality may become more than a neurosis, but a bonafide personality disorder (axis II) and they attempt to transfer their emotional issues to you. They want to draw you into their world and expect a reaction. The narcissist understands that they are best served when they elicit a reaction from you. They will challenge the rules, and anything that exists in the way of their construed expectations. A narcissistic personality will walk into a room and expect to be first and foremost the center of attention and make no distinction between your office and the cocktail party. They are goal-oriented and will insist that all eyes be on them. Not a lot else exists, only their needs (for example, if it is opiates they desire). Some of the most successful, and unsuccessful, people in history have had narcissistic personalities. There is not a person or group that will continually forgive their intrusions and demands, and they will eventually self-destruct.

Borderline Personality

The borderline personality is impulsive and often unable to remain stable when disappointed or refused a desire. The borderline personality is at risk for substance abuse [7]. The narcissist and borderline personality often coexist peacefully with each other within a chronic disease state, such as pain, addiction, and depression. They are rarely observed alone.

Vignette

> Patient—"I really want to thank you for being the world's best doctor. You seem to understand me and we have an understanding that your care model is in my best interest. Thank you so much for getting me that Percocet. Oxycodone of course is the only thing that helps."

Provider—"We have other medications that work better, that are pharmacokinetically more correct, and I don't have to worry about so many side effects. Oh, and that acetaminophen, we have to be careful because you have Hepatitis C."

Patient—"What? You're not going to give me oxycodone? Are you kidding me?" (Escalating voice.) "You are a horrible doctor. I am going to report you to the medical board and I will call my attorney" (borderline).

A Narcissistic personality might say: "I have been diagnosed by several people and have come to the conclusion that I have this condition which can only be managed by oxycodone." As an opioid stress test, you suggest other options. Push back is common, and anger followed by threats is the norm, not the exception.

Solution—The *narcissistic and borderline personalities* are individuals who do not understand "no." This is where the concept of *script* comes into your daily routine. Staying predictable, you respond "this treatment course is in your best interest and safety." If escalation is occurring, they likely will exhibit their borderline personality. Document and state your course. This is your clinic, and this is how you practice. You are the one that is trained.

Narcissistic and borderline personalities are many things, and from a risk management perspective, they also may be retaliatory. When they feel they are wronged, there must be justice. Some of the successful narcissists find safe haven in a profession, where bold individualism is tolerated, even respected. Professions are replete with narcissists found in medicine, law, and, of course, politics. We've all met them. We all know them. The problem is, when they are a patient, and they are expecting a treatment course, they will not see any other way than their perception, making it your problem. Using the dialectic technique, and reflective interviewing, the narcissist receives what he/she needs, not what they want [8].

An example of reflective interviewing is when the patient asks a question, and you ask the patient that question [9]. "So why do you think you need Percocet?" "Because nothing else works." "What do you mean by work?" "What is your ideal outcome?" "What are your benchmarks at 3, 6, 9, and 12 months?" "Of course there is an exit strategy to opioids, isn't there?" "You don't want to be on these the rest of your life do you?" Let the narcissist believe they are controlling the interview, and confrontations will melt away. Direct confrontation and the fight to nowhere is what the narcissist craves, consciously desired or not, and you have effectively taken it away.

Types of People We Meet and the Concept of Risk Shift

What is the secret to success? Right decisions. How do you make right decisions?
Experience. How do you get experience? Wrong decisions.

John Wayne

The concept of credibility and risk shift is real. The everyday reality is that a website, patient, or even an anonymous source creating a rating online has more credibility than the provider. Gone are the days of the highly respected physician rendering advice and the patient (and/or significant other) who nod in agreement and acquiescence. Many are suspicious of our intent and retain the 1980s mind-set that doctors do things to get rich. There is better advice on YouTube® than you are giving. You don't practice in a major metropolitan area where good doctors practice so they need a referral to the big city. "Your online reviews were not very good, you know, and those are always right." Just like Craigslist. Our care is judged the same as a plumber when rated on Angie's list (no offense to plumbers, just an illustration). We meet all kinds and must be agreeable to most, or we're out of business.

Let's start our day.

The Agreeable Type

You must know your enemy. To know your enemy is to also know your friends.
The Art of War.

Sun Tzu

Our travels through the Web describe different personalities by cute names or acronyms and provide trite explanations of difficult people, which are dumbed down and not useful. Examples are Angry Andy, Bashful Bob, Gregarious Gary, or whatever. Psychiatrists spend careers trying to figure these people out, and the Web leads us to think that most are benign, when they are not. The personality is a complicated inter-relationship of environment, genetics, life experiences, and emotion—not to mention the personality altered too easily by what medications are consumed. The proliferation of benzodiazepines, antipsychotics, antidepressants, opioids, and sedatives leaves little doubt that a personality is often altered by external influences. Patients are stressed. And in the pain clinic environment, these tones spill over to the front desk, nurses, and even the back office. The entire clinical environment can be caught up in the complexities of a personality that can't be touched, felt, or measured, only experienced. The fact that the provider must control the interview cannot change. Patients are not your friends, and friends are not your patients. The most vulnerable patients feel almost powerless in a clinical environment. So they agree. It's easy and effective. The agreeable patient/person will agree with everything you are saying and have a personal agenda waiting to be released. An agreeable type is often suppressing a personality disorder. There will never be a push back, and they are happy to be overwhelmingly supportive of your decision making, but plan to do nothing that you recommend. In fact, lurking behind the curtain may even be a "you never told me that" attack. I will be agreeable until you don't suit me. These people will never be loyal or safe.

The Bully

Bullying is a new media favorite. Bullying is a process. These people are rarely dangerous because they're so obvious, and you can protect yourself. The caveat is the potentially explosive personality with poor impulse control, such as those with traumatic brain injuries, or the addict. They are out there and easy to see coming. A bully will impose his/her values on the environment of care, without boundary or restraint. They seek out and manipulate people whom they feel are vulnerable. If a patient, or coworker, feels that you are easily bullied, and you do not have a direct response to their aggressions, the bullying will continue. This is a case where the patient or individual that postures can be called out. Never raise your voice, do not argue. You have more control over your emotions than they do, so you will always own the conversation. A word of warning. The physical bully is another story, and workplace violence is more common than most believe.

Mr./Ms. Negativity

These people are exhausting. You should have very few patients and employees that are always downers. You don't have the energy for these people. They are joy drainers. Reflective conversation and interviewing will keep the time and emotional drivel to a minimum. Reflective interviewing—"what do you mean by that remark?" "You feel everyone is out to get you?" etc. You get it.

Difficult patients are teachers in the value of strong communication skills. They often cannot control their reactions, but want to control yours. They often operate on emotion, and not logic. Many are only happy when you are unhappy. The negative person is ultimately telling you they are unhappy. Once again, they are a victim and you are responsible.

Dealing with Challenging People

People don't care how much you know, until they know how much you care.
Teddy Roosevelt

During the process of communicating, there is input and output. Many patients are just tired of being tired. Whatever problem they have, it is magnified by the fact that they do not perceive themselves as getting well. Those with a chronic condition often do not believe you are helping them get well, but they understand that you are charging them. Techniques to teach the wellness and keep the positive momentum forward include behavior modification, such as the dialectic technique. A dialectic approach is a standard therapy for solving communication and interview problems. Too often, chronic pain care devolves to a prescription per month plan instead of a real plan. Where are you going to be 3, 6, 9 months from now? These are benchmarks. If they aren't realized, questions should follow.

Vignette

Provider—"Let's be clear on our benchmarks. I think these are very important. It just doesn't make sense for us to see each other every month to obtain a prescription. Same old story. The frustrations you are experiencing I think are because we haven't clearly outlined our goals."

What to do—This is one of the simplest and most often ignored parts of pain practitioner's daily routine. The provider and patient forget about goals. A goal can be set in months, weeks, or years. It depends on the pathology. That is up to you, and your patients' diagnosis. Clearly, somebody with fibromyalgia will respond to exercise, increasing function, and working on quality-of-life indices such as smoking cessation, weight loss, etc. Benchmarks can be set for those ideals. Somebody with post-laminectomy syndrome may need other solutions, such as interventional procedures, and proper selection of optimized medications. If function is not enhanced, it doesn't make any sense to continue the current course of care. Pain is not an opioid deficiency. If opioids aren't helping, they are an item of risk and we acknowledge the patient's best interest by finding alternative ways to address their pain. This may include adjunctive medication and techniques such as cognitive behavioral therapy [10]. Both are powerful tools that are often underutilized.

Humans add an emotional component to a chronic therapeutic plan. As part of your therapeutic goal, it is necessary to present the premise that you are working with the individual instead of against them. Developing a good dialectic technique is something every provider eventually matures to varying degrees, and these communication skills are the cornerstone to a wellness plan. We would expect a psychiatrist or internist to be very good at this, and the family practice doctor that is taking care of the individual for years to be the best. Some specialties, especially those that heal pain from an anesthesia background, may not be as adept at such techniques. Anesthesiologists will have limited training in long-term emotional management. Remember, some people you can't help. You are there to help heal, not cure.

Communicating—The Pain Chronicles

You're short on ears, and long on mouth.

John Wayne

Challenging people will often hear when you are speaking, but they will not necessarily listen. The active process of listening assumes that the recipient understands. In medicine, this is not always the case. Patients, in particular, are overwhelmed by the clinical environment and the medical experience. To you, it is a daily and repetitive event. Walking into a room, time pressured and efficiency driven, you are often multitasking. Then there's your action. The story is presented to the listener, an expectation of action is assumed by the patient, and you reference your conclusion as a gesture. For example, writing medications is an expected point of reference. The communication that follows is perception of understanding. Often our communication experience is received, and sometimes it is not. Challenging people's expectations are driven by an action. If they don't get what they want, they act on emotion, become demanding, and intimidating the environment of care. You cannot avoid patients that will not cooperate, will not follow medical advice, or will not keep appointments. Patients that are disruptive and abusive to the provider and staff seem to be on the rise. We all have them, so script your response based on logic. Logic trumps emotion. Good communication skills reduce conflict.

Vignette

> Patient—"I called your office six times at least and got no response. I almost went into withdrawal, and I didn't know what to do. I went to the Emergency Room, and they wouldn't give me anything because they said I was under a contract with you. You are negligent, and you don't have good office practices. I don't know how you stay in business."

What to do—In this situation, your communication skills will suppress a progressively angry encounter. Remember every one or two patients that are unhappy with you, will message 10–15 others. It might be in your waiting room, it might be in the community, quite probably posted online. The point is, your best offense is a reflective moment, and to step back. "I see that this is something I may need to look into." "Do you have the names of people that you have talked to in this office?" "I do have somebody that you can talk to and I want to make sure you have that contact information." "Let's make sure you have a good experience here." "Certainly we're all busy, but we are interested in you first and foremost."

Consider the process of transference, defined as unconscious redirection of feelings from one person to another, which is a deficit in personal security and results in one-way communication [11, 12]. Challenging people feel their opinion can only be understood when they are aggressive and posturing. A feeling that control must remain with them, and they feel they are in a position of power.

Particularly in medicine, and especially in pain medicine, personalities can clash. These challenging patients come with the territory. The practice of pain medicine is expected to be a unique and challenging specialty and is a high-risk experience. Often patients come to you exhausted, having seen multiple providers, with multiple encounters, of which many are not good. Patients know that you are suspicious of them, and developing a patient/physician relationship is very difficult when trust is fractured. You are not the primary care physician who cares for a family, or long-term medical need, and, over time, has developed a strong patient/physician relationship. The pain physician is one more roadblock in a series of frustrations to obtain a desired goal—relief, anxiolysis, and ultimately, a prescription. When their wishes are denied, they threaten you because this is their perceived position of controlling their environment. Your patients will believe that they have certain rights, and will conceive retaliation if they do not obtain their medications, or a desired treatment course.

Vignette

> Patient—"I don't care if I tested positive for marijuana. It is legal in some states, and even the Federal government doesn't care. I know this for a fact. I've been to other places where I've had a positive test for marijuana and they didn't care. I've been on these pain medicines for a long time and just because I went out and smoked a little weed don't mean you won't give me my prescription."

Provider—"That is true. In some states marijuana is legal for various reasons." "However, my DEA certificate is a Federal certificate, and marijuana still remains a schedule 1 drug." "That means there is no legitimate use for it." "Someday this may change, as we discover different forms of marijuana that might have medical use." "I understand you take marijuana to help with your pain but we have other options." "I have to know what you're taking." "Smoking marijuana is not FDA approved, or metered." "What I mean by metered is there is no way to tell the dose or quality of what you are getting." "That is not how I want to practice medicine. I think you can understand that. Let's just clean up, I'll go ahead and continue treating you with other options, but please, understand the policies of our practice and our desire to help you. Let's not use illegal drugs."

Patients often tell you what tests to order, what medications to prescribe, make demands for frequent and immediate access to a physician, and define which medications are the only pharmaceuticals they will accept. "Percs, Roxis, that's all I can take." "I can't take anything with acetaminophen. I'm allergic to everything but Percs." "Nothing else really works." "Why change it if you know what works?" The demanding patient will expect the office staff to bend schedules, break rules, abandon established office protocol, and always accommodate them. They will often threaten the practice. Difficult patients are the bane of many physicians' professional existence and try their professional patience, test their limits, and challenge the core ability to provide care.

Patients may also be exhibiting effects from a true life stressor. This includes job loss, economic crisis, and crushing family responsibilities. This makes compliance with the treatment regimen one more burden, and you are the lightning rod. Because, once again, who is the most powerful person in the room? Not you. It's the *victim*.

Vignette

Patient—"I've been to a lot of doctors, and they usually help me with my problem. As you know I can't work, I've applied for disability, and if that idiot hadn't left that water spot on the floor I wouldn't have slipped and fell. They owe me. My lawyer and I are going to work on this together."

What to do—Physician—"Yeah, sure I understand your frustration. I understand you are getting angry. But let's think. Has anger ever accomplished anything? No. Actually, thoughtful treatment of your problem will probably help you get better. Let's go through that."

The Victim—The Most Powerful Person in the Room

How can we work with those patients who seem "the victim" without compromising the risk of liability? The victim constantly leads to a strain on the patient/physician relationship. Why do these patients persist on misusing or even abusing the patient/physician relationship? Because to them, every day is like the Jerry Springer Show. Chaotic lifestyles might be a problem, and coping skills may be poor. This victim is a poorly defined DSM V diagnosis, but very real. Acquiescence and compromise has been the response prior to an encounter, and out of fear, most providers do not want a confrontation, and patients know this.

The victim demonstrates manipulative behavior and noncompliance. However, noncompliance is not always a poorly understood mystery. Sometimes misunderstanding is born of ignorance and fear. The victim, however, takes a defiant stand. You are expected to bend.

Vignette

Patient—"My medication isn't working, and you keep putting me on ones that don't work. I have to take more, and you don't seem to understand that I am running out of medicine because you're giving me junk. I just need my Percocet®, and everything will be fine."

Provider—"We discussed this. I have other tools, and better medications than that medication that has acetaminophen in it, which might hurt your liver. I'm going to help you understand where I'm going with your benchmarks at 3, 6, 9, and 12 months, because we always have an exit strategy with opioids. That means we don't plan on keeping you on opioids forever, it is just one of the options in our bag, but not a long term interest. Let's stay the course."

The physician is expected to be the compassionate provider, to be predictable, and allow policies to be strained. Some patients may want to do exactly what the physician says, but cannot for various reasons, and communication skills are tested. The physician may need to make concessions or compromises, but a definition is required. Is money an issue? Spouse? Internet? Cultural? Any cultural or religious factors that influence their beliefs about the medical problem and potential treatment can strongly influence the decision-making response and a positive outcome. Determine how the patient understands the problem or disease and their interest and ability to participate in their own care.

Vignette

Provider—"I want you to take your medication four times a day, on a full stomach, and don't forget to take your patch off at three days. Do you understand how that works? That means if you put it on Monday, you will change it on Thursday. Why? Because Monday, Tuesday, and Wednesday are three days, then you change on Thursday ..."

Patient—"What?"

Solution—Make a plan. Have your nurse follow you, because you are in a hurry. Most providers don't realize when they walk out of the room, many of the patients don't understand what you just said, and likely forgot most of it. The pharmacists are another point of the treatment triangle, and they'll have all sorts of medication inserts describing a myriad of side effects that no one discussed in the clinic. The patient will only see a little label on the side of a pill bottle that is so small it is hard to read. This is particularly problematic with the elderly, as they often have no idea how to follow your directions unless they are clear, concise and in a common language. You may not be the one to convey this information. It is not a bad idea you have somebody come behind you with a reinforcement of your instructions.

Ode to the Law

The noncompliant patient's communication disruption may be the reason behind why many treatment discussions are not understood, and why more than 2/3 of patients don't take their medicine correctly [13, 14]. Remember the 9-min rule.

The 9-min rule was taught to me by my father. A defense malpractice attorney, he noticed one thing to be a constant. Somewhere around 9 min the risk of an adverse encounter in the examination room drops. It may be communication; it may be understanding, or just a comfort level. But at about 9 min, the risk of confrontation diminishes. You can use this to your advantage.

Vignette

> Patient—"Young man, my nephew gives me $15 for each one of those pills. That pays for my heart medicine, and helps pay for electricity. You have no right to tell me that what I bought is your business."

Patients may simply not understand their part in the healthcare model. The remaining half of the noncompliant patient population is just noncompliant by choice. A number of patients never fill their original prescription. The chosen medications may be too expensive, or not necessary, but most commonly they don't understand why and what they are taking it for. A common observation is that patients cannot name the medications they are taking, so pharmacy and record checks are mandatory. 40–75 % fail to follow the instructions for taking their medications and 20 % take other people's medication, that is, 1/5 of your patient's sharing pills in the family and community [15, 16].

Diversion

Protecting the community is important. If you suspect misuse, abuse, or diversion in any of your patients, you are concerned about your patient and the community as a whole. With prescription drug overdose deaths currently killing 40 people a day, these drugs require professional vigilance. You are the tip of the pen and as difficult as it is, you must protect the community. Know where your prescribed medications are going and practice robust adherence monitoring.

When patients are noncompliant, the provider is obligated to acknowledge personal and professional limits. You set limits with patients, and strictly adhere to them. It is better to do some things well than to fail by trying to do everything. Know your boundaries and express them.

What Are the Problems? Keeping Your Patients from Becoming "Difficult"

Communication. Your Staff Can Kill You

> *Tomorrow is the most important thing in life. It comes to us very clear at midnight. It's perfect when it arrives and puts itself in our hands. It hopes we learned something from yesterday.*
>
> John Wayne

The most important person in your office is the "go-to" person. Who is that? Often it is the receptionist. A bad interaction with the receptionist, or miscommunication with the receptionist, can result in disastrous consequences. Errors can spill over into the ring of adverse legal considerations. The patient often does not understand the seriousness of their condition. The communication void might be one of vocabulary, denial, or lack of physician emphasis and understanding. The patient often forgets verbal instructions, and tense patients are likely to misunderstand most of the visit and instructions. Others may feel intimidated and fail to ask questions that arise during the discussion. Remember, providers in the environment of care can be intimidating. The reason for failure to take medication might be simple reluctance, such as the World War II generation that doesn't want to "get hooked," or "I can bear the pain" crowd, while others are just plain afraid of the unknown. The receptionist is the first and last person a patient will talk to. Commonly, they will be the telephone voice of reassurance or concern. An untrained front desk person can devolve a repairable conflict to disaster. A good communicator, can, and does, reduce conflict before it starts.

Why Can't Our Patients Be More Responsible?

The No-Show

The no-show does not value the time commitment of a patient encounter and the stretched resources of a physician's office. A purposeful no-show is unacceptable and represents a form of noncompliance to treatment. Therefore, it is incumbent upon the provider to understand if the patient did not remember, if they got what they wanted by phone, or if you and/or your staff just made them mad and they are acting out. It is best to have a policy about the no-show, such as charging for a no-show. All fees are laid out and understood in a document at the initiation of such a policy, with no barrier to communication. No shows are complex.

Vignette

> Patient—"Why are you discharging me just because I've missed a couple of appointments? I called the office, I've talked to everybody, and I know you can't do this to me. I need my medicine, you can't just drop me."

Physician—"You've missed three appointments in a row, and we have no record that you called to let us know your whereabouts or the reason you missed the appointment. This is an enormous drain of clinic resources, and we have no other alternative."

Patient—"I'll Sue You."

What to do—Policies need to be in place to explain to the patient, with no barrier to communication that no shows can't be tolerated. Certainly calling ahead, with 24-h notice, should be documented in the care plan. Confirming appointments 24 h in advance by staff is also recommended, but is labor intensive and not always practical. If it is not and there is no record that the patient called in, you have to use your professional judgment. It also is about your relationship with the patient. The disease state may matter. Be cautious at discharge, particularly for now shows. Beware of abandonment. Understand the patient's personality and communicate clearly. Document your decisions. Discuss this with an attorney, your medical society, even your medical board.

Most likely, the difficult patient is angry at, or depressed about, the chronic condition that necessitates a visit or treatment. The patient may not feel comfortable with the physician or the treatment plan of action. Those with chronic illness often long to be "normal." They tire of treatment that reminds them of weakness, failing health, the stigma of a condition, or even mortality. A patient who feels that you are a disengaged provider is unlikely to share his or her concerns. Those that explain little, exhibit no interest or empathy, or belittle complaints are often the reason behind treatment failure. Refusal to follow a course of care may be as simple as denial, or it might be as complex as a death wish.

Secondary gain is always consideration with a noncompliant patient, conscious or not. It is fueled by an external motivator and seen in many diseases, not just chronic pain. Most frequently, however, blatant noncompliance is about miscommunication. The patient and the physician have differing expectations or goals for prescribed treatment, the action step of the encounter. The physician may simply want improvement, whereas the patient expects a cure. The result is divergent thoughts and a course of care that leads to an unlikely growth and understanding on both sides.

Why Don't They Take My Medicine Correctly?

Most often, the patient finds a drug or treatment regimen too complex. Understanding a complex treatment regimen is not as intuitive as we might think. Patients often take multiple medications, at different hours. Directions are daunting, some require an empty stomach, and others required to be accompanied by food, and the ever-present risk of drug interactions spelled out in microwords given to them by pharmacists that don't truly reflect reality. The insert for a well-known sleep aid states "may cause drowsiness." All medicines cause "headaches." Some just cannot afford that pill and ask for generics—"just give me my Lorcet plus." With many prescriptions now costing over $100, patients are at risk to avoid the medications they need.

Vignette

> Patient—"I know what's right for my body, and you don't know the pain that I have. If you understood you wouldn't be saying these things. I know I have rights and I have a patient advocate. That's me!"

> Well the problem is, I didn't understand what you said last visit. You said I take my what how many times a day and the other one with food or what? I didn't understand. I found that I was sleepy all day long, and I am glad that you helped me understand why I shouldn't be taking my Diazepam with my Gabapentin and Hydrocodone, but I do need my migraine medicine, that one I call the Barbie doll pill (barbiturate).

Others just forget. Patients who are tense in a physician's office are likely to forget most of what is said. This is where written instructions are so important. Clearly written instructions, in simple language, are recommended to accompany oral instructions.

There are cultural influences as well. People may also have religious and cultural beliefs that prohibit a certain treatment or medication. We all know that some religious belief systems refuse blood or blood products, such as Jehovah's Witness. Others reject immunizations. A few refuse antibiotics. Usually, everybody, however, loves oxycodone. The list goes on. These beliefs are not mere adjuncts to a person's life, and they often lie at the person's very sole. If treatment is to be successful, these beliefs need to be explored, understood, and to the extent possible accommodated.

Benchmarks

Clinicians also have to know where they are now in a natural history of disease, and where the direction will be in the future. These are benchmarks, or a proficient forward timeline of management. Often, pain management consists of repetitive visits for reevaluation and medication renewal, with no clear understanding of a plan. It is important to know these benchmarks at 3, 6, 9, and 12 months. If benchmarks fail, understand why these benchmarks were not obtained and respond accordingly.

Vignette

> Physician—"So let's try this. I want you to write down 10 goals for me, put it on your refrigerator, and make them reasonable. We will look at them at 3, 6, 9, and 12 months. We will probably amend them as you reach your benchmark, but think like this."

Patient—"I know I can walk 200 yards three times a week, and I bet I can get up to ¼ mile at the high school's track by 3 months. I can also cut my calories by at least desserts and pizzas. I think I can do this."

Non-payment of Bills

Difficult patients who expect free care may need to be terminated from the practice. Before taking this step, however, the practice needs to consider the underlying issue regarding this noncompliance, and determine whether there are extenuating circumstances that make it difficult for a patient to meet his or her financial responsibilities. Some of the factors that may cause a patient not to pay a medical bill are job layoff, termination of unemployment benefits, illness, death of a family member, and even depression.

Vignette

> Patient—"I don't know how to tell you any differently. I just don't like what I'm doing. I don't want an injection, and I don't think these medicines are helping me. The only thing that seems to help is my Oxycodone, and I've never misused or abused it. I am just being honest." (The patient is behind on your bill.)

Risk Management Suggestions

Set up a payment schedule that is workable for the patient and ensures the payment of a certain amount of money on a regular basis. Patients who do not pay anything for a service devalue that service, while some form of payment ensures patient "buy in" to your treatment. From a risk management perspective, the physician would be wise to post billing practices in a visible location and let patients know at the time of the first visit how they are expected to handle bills, including co-payments. Continue to see the patient who is making good-faith efforts to pay a bill, or who has a reasonable excuse for not doing so, at least temporarily. Consider referring the patient who makes no effort to pay to a collection agency. These solutions, however, are inefficient and expensive options. If the contracted collection agency's policies are not known by you and deemed unscrupulous, the provider will carry the burden. Consider terminating the professional relationship with the patient who is a chronic or persistent non-payer.

Vignette

> Physician—"I'm not going to be able to see you if we don't resolve the financial issues here. This will be our last visit. I don't think you should have a prescription until you pay your bill, and I think you should be more responsible. You are taking time out of my schedule, and I know you don't get your milk and bread for free. Your car had gasoline put

in it, and I see that pack of cigarettes. Can't you make proper choices?" (Communication disaster!)

An office manager, or someone from the billing department, would be the person that suggests, in a positive manner, that they will work with the patient and try to find out if there is an underlying reason and examine financial stressors. Threatening to withhold care based on financial concerns is construed as a form of abandonment [17].

Managed Care Adds Complications—Discharging the Patient Part 1

Some contracts make it difficult to discharge patients, even troublesome ones. An insurance panel may limit a physician's ability to act unilaterally. You could be in violation of your contract, unless you check with the plan and its protocol for discharging troubled patients. In order to determine whether you are able to discharge assigned patients, someone in your organization must read the contract carefully. For example, what form of notice you must give to the patient, and what in-office discharge policies do you have. In most cases, a patient can break the contract at will, simply by not returning to the doctor's office. Unfortunately, it isn't as easy for a physician to show a patient to the door. Care must be utilized when you discharge a patient from your practice to avoid accusations of abandonment or discrimination, which can lead to a complicated legal fight. All said, no doctor has to subject themselves to abusive or threatening behavior by patients. With traditional fees for service and governmental insurance, a physician can dismiss almost any patient as long as he/she provides [18] adequate notice [1] helps the patient find another physician and [2] doesn't stop caring for that person in the midst of a medical crisis. Most plans require that a physician accept all patients who choose him/her from the plan, and many want to be contacted before a doctor dismisses them or does not accept a patient. Try to limit the problem. Patients may be overwhelmed by a multitasked treatment regimen. Let the difficult patient know the professional relationship will be terminated if unacceptable behavior persists. Consider terminating the professional relationship with the patient who disregards the physician's advice and/or abuses the professional relationship. Help the patient solve the problem. However, tempting, but not helpful, is offering an immediate solution to the problem identified by the patient. Don't just give in. Patients who assume an active role in their healthcare planning are more invested in the treatment plan and have better outcomes than those who are simply told what to do. In the case of a very challenging patient, you may want to follow a standard risk management protocol for terminating a professional relationship. It is wise to ask your medical board or medical society how to proceed, apply appropriate recommendations, or even obtain legal counsel. Most importantly, if you do decide to discharge a patient, document it in the record with a letter that has been sent by certified mail. Document any refusal to accept the certified letter as well.

Beware of Abandonment

Document all indications of noncompliance on the part of the patient. Establishing a pattern of "contributory negligence" can be extremely important in a malpractice or abandonment claim. Explain why you cannot care for him/her. Give him/her 30 days to find a new physician and provide resources for finding an appropriate specialty physician of patient need, such as an addictionologist. Suggest you will send his/her records to the new provider with a properly executed release and meet any emergency needs he/she might develop during that time. Remember, chronic pain is not necessariily an emergency. Proper recognition of the potential for withdrawal should be considered, but if a patient is misusing or abusing medications, particularly when diversion is identified, the physician has no obligation to continue medications. Referral to services for withdrawal or developing a medication protocol to limit withdrawal symptoms is recommended. Suggest that he/she go to an emergency department if, after one month, he/she has not found a new physician. Remember, once again, chronic pain is not an emergency.

Vignette

> Patient—"You aren't giving me what I need. I want the Oxycodone because that's the only thing that works, you are my doctor and you should take the responsibility to see that your patients get what they need. I shouldn't have to go through this, and you're abusing me. I am going to turn you over to the Better Business Bureau, the Medical Board, and tell my doctor that you have a terrible bedside manner. If I don't get these medicines, I'm going to go through withdrawal and if I have a problem I'm going to sue you for damage."

Solution—Empathize with the situation. Try to reason, explain your position and educate the patient. It is always about communication. Do not be intimidated by the threat of a law suit. Do document what is medically justified. Termination should be reserved for patients who are not at a critical point in their treatment and beware of the protected class.

Discrimination—Discharging the Patient Part 2

A physician's office is a place of public accommodation and subject to state and educate the patient. It is always about communication. Do not be intimidated by the threat of a law suit. Do document what is medically justified. Termination should be reserved for patients who are not at a critical point in their treatment and beware of the protected class.

Discrimination—Discharging the Patient Part 2

A physician's office is a place of public accommodation and subject to state and federal civil rights laws. The American Medical Association's position is that a physician may not decline to accept patients because of sex, color, creed, race, religion, disability, ethnic origin, national origin, sexual orientation, age, or any other basis that would constitute *invidious discrimination* [19]. Physicians cannot refuse to see a patient who is protected by law against discrimination.

Violence in the Workplace

Patient—"Pain medicines are our right. I'm in pain"

Response—Incorrect. Do not enter into an argument with the patient or family. If a patient becomes threatening, suggesting physical violence. Try to calm him/her and try to reason with them. Attempt to isolate the individual (it may be someone other than the patient) to prevent injury to staff and other patients. Do not hesitate to summon police when necessary.

Boundaries

Your office should have in place appropriate documentation of what boundaries are. This avoids potential for law suits relating to harassment, patient boundary violations, and misunderstandings among staff and patients. Education is mandatory, and policies are defined in the employee handbook.

Vignette

Patient—Medical board complaint. "He was in the room and when examining me, he touched me there. I was horrified. I was so scared I didn't move."

Even the implied boundary violation requires an immediate investigation and response. Take these very seriously as it is not always possible that a nurse accompanies the provider into the room, and if a patient has an agenda, this type of complaint is bound to register a response. Your quick response and documentation can reduce, but maybe not eliminate, the potential for a media circus, an investigation, or even legal concerns. It is protective, however. Obtain immediate legal advice.

How to Handle a Complaint

Complaints come with the territory. We are dealing with controlled substances, and people that act on emotion, and not logic. People come to us with problems, are the victim, and captivated by their class. This is a perfect environment for complaints. There is a right way and a wrong way to handle complaints. Remember, you are in control, do not let the environment control you.

The Board Complaint

A board complaint is a process. It is not an indictment of your personal and professional existence. It is the board's responsibility to protect the community and maintain knowledge that a practitioner is providing care within standard. It is not personal. It may seem like it, but it is not. Most states allow a period of time for you to respond to these board complaints and take that seriously. A timely response is a reflection of confidence. If you are practicing within the community standard, you have nothing to worry about. You don't necessarily have to go talk to a lawyer. Develop an organized approach to resolution. Keep it simple. They just want the facts. So, make sure the medical record is complete and tells the right story. This does not mean you change one word in the medical record. If an addendum needs to be made, it is done with an explanation. Altering the medical record with this scenario will implicate you. There is no need to do it. Most medical boards just want to see the story, follow your medical decision-making, and that's it. Your records should be neat and well organized. You might place them in a 3-ring binder with tabs to each section, emphasizing your progress notes as your clinical story. Occasionally, it is worthwhile to have another member of the staff, such as your nurse, or someone in the know, to include a paragraph with their interpretation of the complaint. Ironically, very good pain doctors have quite a few board complaints. They are doing the right things for the right reasons, and patients, reacting out of emotion and not logic, retaliate.

The Digital Environment

Nowhere is it easier to complain about a provider than on the Internet. These complaints are anonymous, and the companies that claim to be responsible rating services are relying on drama to get the advertising revenue. Under certain circumstances, with great effort, the complaint can be managed, but it's not nec-essarily bad that you have complaints on the Internet. Most people that read these reports can see through those complaints as retaliatory, anonymous, faceless, and inappropriate. You may have to, from time to time, discuss a complaint with a patient. Rarely is it so that a new or existing patient will drop you because of complaints on the Internet. They know you. Be consistent, professional, and predictable.

I Am Going to Sue You

Patients want perfect care, infallible, and the right to sue. It is a one-way street, and we carry insurance for this. If you are threatened, and you believe a patient will truly initiate a legal challenge, notify your insurance carrier. Let them handle it from there and do not engage the patient. This is what insurance companies are for; this is what you pay them for.

Conclusion

We chose pain medicine as a profession because it is rewarding, a progressive specialty in a rapidly changing medical landscape. Pain medicine requires vigilance, patience, and strong communication skills. A good pain medicine provider con-vinces the patient that the light at the end of the tunnel isn't a truck. We all have our issues, and during our professional existence, it is the rare individual that remains unscathed, with a smile on their face and a song in their heart saying "I enjoyed every minute of it." Most all of us will agree, we have encountered many chal-lenging work and patient problems and didn't always know how to respond to them. It's not a perfect world.

You need a tough skin to practice pain medicine these days. If you have a problem, a board complaint, or you get greedy and just don't see why you're doing this, think again. If you are at the depths of frustration, despair, even depression, reflect on what you are. You are of value to society, and this is a high-quality career choice. Whatever the challenge or obstacle, get over it. Whatever it was, get over it. If you need help, get help, but they will tell you the same thing. Get over it. Move on and continue to be the valued member of the society that you are.

Remember, challenging patients and people want to pull you into their world. It is your professional responsibility to maintain your world, predictable, and pro-fessional. Finally, you can fix about anything by remembering these three words: Bless her heart. No matter what it was, the problem will roll off your shoulder when you look at these difficult people and you love them where they're at. Set your boundaries, balance your life, and let difficult people live their life without intruding on yours. Don't forget those that love you. Pet your dog. Get a hobby. Take care of your health. Medicine is a job. It's not a life. Bless their hearts.

References

1. ADA: Q and A—Public Accommodations—EEOC. www.eeoc.gov.
2. Why Do Doctors Commit Suicide? www.NYtimes.com/why-do-doctors-commit-suicide.
3. Hall DE. et al. Informed consent for clinical treatment. CMAJ. 2012 March 20; 184(5):533–540.
4. Four Temperaments—Wikipedia. https://en.wikipedia.org/wiki/four_temperaments.
5. Galen's Personality Theory. https://sites.google.com/psychologyofpersonalityperiod8/type/gal.
6. Narcissistic Personality Disorder. https://en.wikipedia.org/wiki/Narcissistic_personality_disorder.
7. Personality Disorders Fact Sheet DSM-5. www.dsm5.org.
8. Relational Dialectics. https://en.wikipedia.org.
9. Reflective listening. https://en.wikipedia.org.
10. Cognitive Behavioral Therapy. https://en.wikipedia/wiki/cognitive_behavioral_therapy.
11. Baron E. et al. Early transference interventions with male patients in psychotherapy. J Psychother Pract Res. 2001;10(2): 79–92.
12. Transference. https://wikipedia.org.
13. Kleinsinger F. Working with the noncompliant patient. MD Perm J. 2010;14(1):54–60
14. Medication Nonadherence. www.medscape.com/viewarticle/409940.
15. Salzman C. Medication compliance in the elderly. J Clin Psychiatry. 1995;56(1):18–22
16. ASIPP Opioid Guidelines 2012; 15; 51-566 5-67-5116. American Society of Interventional Pain Physicians Guidelines for Responsible Opioid Prescribing In Chronic Non-Cancer Pain Part 1 and 2.
17. Abandoning Patients—Medical and Public Health Law site biotech.law.edu/Books/lbb/x266.htm.
18. Adinoff B. Neurobiologic processes in drug reward and addiction. Harvard Rev Psychiatry. 2004;12(6):305–320.
19. Invidious Discrimination definitions.uslegal.com > legal definitions.

Chapter 14
Controlled Substance Management: Exit Strategies for the Pain Practitioner

Sanford M. Silverman

Opioids: Therapeutic Use and Misuse [1]

Opium has been widely used from ancient times in Sumeria through the present day and was freely available and utilized in its unprocessed form for many centuries. In 1811, a German pharmacist, Frederick Serturner, isolated the active compound and noted that it caused a deep slumber. He named this new compound after Morpheus, the God of dreams, or Morphine. After morphine was isolated, it largely replaced the therapeutic uses of opium. Decades later, a variety of semisynthetic and synthetic derivatives were developed, which include the common prescription opioid analgesics utilized today.

The problem of opioid-related problems has been recognized for centuries. Opium was probably brought to the USA by Chinese immigrants. Opium dens were noted throughout the west and were touted as a cure for alcoholism. The global problem of opioid abuse became well-recognized in the nineteenth century. Opioid use was common broadly in the USA and among various nineteenth-century authors such as Keats and Browning, among many historical figures.

The present-day prescription opioid epidemic parallels a public health problem which was ultimately addressed in the USA in the early twentieth century. Prior to 1914, opioids were freely available and physicians could utilize them to treat opioid addiction. In 1914, the Harrison Controlled Substances Act was passed which attempted to control the sale, distribution, and prescription of controlled substances.

S.M. Silverman
Clinical Biomedical Science, Charles E. Schmidt College of Medicine, Florida Atlantic University, Boca Raton, FL, USA

S.M. Silverman (✉)
Comprehensive Pain Medicine, 100 E Sample Road, Suite 200, Pompano Beach, FL 33064, USA
e-mail: sanfordsilverman@cpmedicine.com

© Springer International Publishing Switzerland 2016   251
P.S. Staats and S.M. Silverman (eds.), *Controlled Substance Management in Chronic Pain*, DOI 10.1007/978-3-319-30964-4_14

Immediately following World War I, there was a significant increase in the incidence of opiate addiction in various large American cities. The Bayer Corporation developed a new drug that they thought would be the savior, or heroine, of society. This new compound was called heroin. In New York City, there were efforts to engage the treatment of more than 8000 heroin addicts through its public health department.

In 1919, the US Supreme Court ruled that the Harrison Narcotic Act (previously passed in 1914) prevented the use of maintenance opioids to treat opioid dependence. From that time forward through the 1970s, opioid addiction was considered criminal behavior rather than a medical problem. In 1970, the Controlled Substances Act (CSA) was passed by Congress which scheduled the use of opioids and other controlled substances for medicinal uses. In 1972, methadone was addressed at the federal level with regulations (21 CFR part 291). In 1974, the Narcotic Addict Treatment Act was passed which created federal and state-licensed methadone clinics in order to treat heroin dependence. In the 1970s, however, prescription drug abuse was relatively rare, at least by today's standards.

Between 1974 and 2000, a patient who required treatment for opioid addiction had to rely on care administered through methadone clinics. A physician who desired to treat patients with opioid addiction needed to obtain additional registration from state and federal authorities. There was thus an intimidating bureaucratic gauntlet that few physicians were willing to negotiate.

In 2000, Congress passed the Drug Addiction Treatment Act (DATA 2000) which was an amendment to the original CSA of 1970. This allowed certified physicians to prescribe and dispense schedule III, IV, and V drugs that had been approved by the Food and Drug Administration (FDA) for use in the treatment of addiction (i.e., maintenance or medical withdrawal/detoxification). The FDA approved schedule III sublingual buprenorphine for the treatment of opioid dependence in October 2002.

Prior to the availability of sublingual buprenorphine, only methadone or levo-a-acetyl methanol (LAAM) was approved for the treatment of opioid dependence. Eventually, LAAM was replaced by methadone and outpatient clinics were restricted to methadone as the sole opioid agonist for the treatment of opioid dependence.

The therapeutic use of opioids has dramatically increased in this country despite prior legislative actions and a lack of evidence regarding the effectiveness, long-term efficacy, and safety data in chronic non-cancer pain [2, 3]. The Institute of Medicine (IOM) [4] reported that the cost of chronic pain in the USA was approximately $635 billion and recognized a "moral duty" of healthcare professionals to provide effective pain management. While recognizing that the problem of diversion and abuse of opioids is serious, the IOM report stated that opioids can be used effectively for postoperative pain, procedural pain, and palliative care, but did not support the indiscriminate use in chronic non-cancer pain. Therefore, there appears to be some disagreement between the proponents of opioid use for chronic non-cancer pain and the authors of the IOM report.

Undertreatment and Overtreatment of Pain

The alleged undertreatment of chronic non-cancer pain has led to numerous initiatives to address barriers to the responsible treatment. The Federation of State Medical Boards (FSMB) is probably one of the most notable organizations, which has created national standards established for the treatment of chronic pain [5]. While other entities have proposed guidelines for the use of opioids in non-cancer pain, the evidence for such is either lacking or fair at best [2, 3].

It has been reported that as many as 90 % of patients who are treated in pain management centers are receiving opioids for chronic pain [6, 7]. One prospective study showed that 90 % of patients were utilizing opioids and 42 % utilizing benzodiazepines prior to presenting to an interventional pain management center, and more than one type of opioid was utilized by many patients [6]. The overutilization of opioids is further documented by increased retail sales and consumption of these medications (Table 14.1; Fig. 14.1).

Table 14.1 Increases in retails sales of prescription opioids

	1997	2004	Percentage of change (%)
Methadone	518,737	4,730,157	812
Oxycodone	4,449,562	29,177,530	556
Fentanyl base	74,086	370,739	400
Morphine	5,922,872	14,319,243	142
Hydrocodone	8,669,311	24,081,900	178
Hydromorphone	241,078	655,395	172
Meperidine	5,765,954	4,856,644	−16
Codeine	25,071,410	20,264,555	−19

From Manchikanti [8]

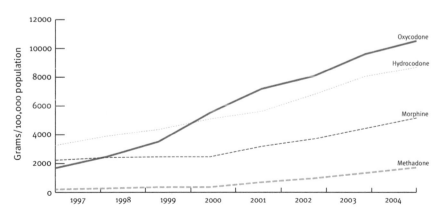

Fig. 14.1 Increased use of therapeutic opioid use in the USA. From Manchikanti [8]

As the number of chronic pain patients in the USA using controlled substances has increased, so have the problems associated with their use. Clearly, not all patients do well with chronic opioid management and many require detoxification, or titration of the opioids. It is therefore essential for the pain practitioner to develop an "exit strategy" when initiating and maintaining chronic controlled substance therapy and always to consider the aviation rule of thumb "don't take off unless you can land."

State and federal laws also contribute to the problems the pain practitioner faces when he/she is forced to discharge abusers of prescribed medication for violating a controlled substance agreement. This puts the practitioner between the proverbial "rock and a hard place." Continuing to treat the patient who has violated an agreement may result in sanctions from state medical boards or legal action from law enforcement. This could result in fines, criminal charges, or revocation of a medical license [9]. We advocate taking positive steps for patients who appear to have an addiction disorder. These acts should be documented in the medical record and may include entries such as "referral given for substance abuse, or medically supervised withdrawal from medications" rather than "discharged from practice for violation of our controlled substance agreement."

The majority of patients are not "abusers," hence are not included in this scenario, with a minority suffering from substance abuse and addiction [10]. Taking this into consideration with certain exceptions, such as illegal diversion of prescribed medications, the suffering of the abuser and addict is often ostensibly worse than that of the appropriate user of medications for pain management. Exit strategies exist to not merely help the practitioner, but offer options to dumping patients which merely results in "kicking the can down the road."

The strategies employed to reduce opioid and sedative/hypnotic consumption have historically been developed to treat substance dependence and addiction. These time-tested strategies are relied upon by substance abuse clinics and treatment facilities alike. Pain practitioners should consider employing similar strategies to treat complications associated with controlled substance therapy.

Abuse and Overdose Associated with Prescription Opioids

In 2011, over 41,340 people died from drug poisonings in the USA and nearly 17,000 from prescription opioid overdoses. For every death, there were approximately 10 treatment admissions for abuse, 32 emergency department visits for misuse or abuse, 130 persons who abuse or were addicted, and 825 non-medical users [11–13] (Fig. 14.2).

For many years, chronic pain has been undertreated. In 1999, the Joint Commission on hospital accreditation and other organizations highlighted the importance of managing patients with chronic pain. The financial, moral, and ethical basis has been covered in numerous venues. All of the approaches emphasized medication management in the treatment of uncontrolled pain. This led

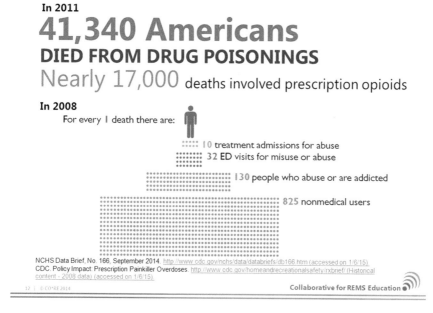

Fig. 14.2 Prescription drug deaths and associated complications in the USA. For references, visit: http://www.cdc.gov/homeandrecreationalsafety/rxbrief

to the explosion of prescription opioid use and unfortunately abuse [2]. The sales of opioid analgesics quadrupled between 1999 and 2010 with hydrocodone sales increasing by 280 % from 1997 to 2007. In 2009, the estimated number of prescriptions filled for opioid analgesics in the USA exceeded 256 million.

Hydrocodone in combination with acetaminophen was the number one prescription medication in the USA from 2006 to 2011 which was followed by L-thyroxine, simvastatin, and lisinopril, respectively [14]. The population of the USA is approximately 4.6 % of the overall world's population, yet we consume approximately 83 % of the world's oxycodone and 99 % of the hydrocodone [14].

Benzodiazepines are also associated with misuse, abuse, and dependence [15]. Benzodiazepines can enhance or boost the effects of opioids [16]. Emergency department and substance abuse treatment data show that the combined use of benzodiazepines and opioid pain relievers is common and that people who co-abuse these drugs have been described as a high-need, treatment-resistant population [17–19]. This is partly because people who abuse both benzodiazepines and opioids report more severe withdrawal symptoms than patients withdrawing from opioid pain relievers alone, resulting in higher treatment attrition rates [20].

The number of annual benzodiazepine and opioid combination admissions increased 569.7 percent from 5032 admissions in 2000 to 33,701 admissions in 2010 (Fig. 14.3) [21].

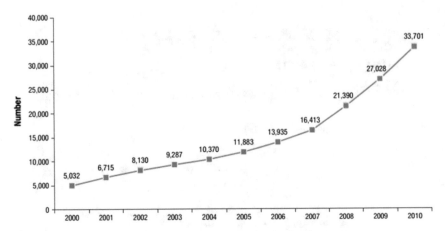

Fig. 14.3 Number of benzodiazepine and narcotic pain reliever combination admissions: 2000–2010. From Substance Abuse and Mental Health Services Administration, Center for Behavioral Health Statistics and Quality [21]

Opioid Use Disorder

In making the determination to discontinue opioid prescribing, it is important to distinguish between opioid misuse and diversion. The Diagnostic and Statistical Manual of Mental Disorders Fifth Edition (DSM-V) [22] definition for opioid use disorder replaces the prior DSM-IV definition for opioid dependence as follows.

Diagnostic Criteria

A problematic pattern of opioid use leading to clinically significant impairment or distress, as manifested by at least **two** of the following, occurring within a 12-month period:

- Opioids are often taken in larger amounts or over a longer period than was intended.
- There is a persistent desire or unsuccessful efforts to cut down or control opioid use.
- A great deal of time is spent in activities necessary to obtain the opioid, use the opioid, or recover from its effects.
- Craving, or a strong desire or urge to use opioids.
- Recurrent opioid use resulting in a failure to fulfill major role obligations at work, school, or home.
- Continued opioid use despite having persistent or recurrent social or interpersonal problems caused or exacerbated by the effects of opioids.
- Important social, occupational, or recreational activities are given up or reduced because of opioid use.

- Recurrent opioid use in situations in which it is physically hazardous.
- Continued opioid use despite knowledge of having a persistent or recurrent physical or psychological problem that is likely to have been caused or exacerbated by the substance.
- Tolerance, as defined by either of the following:

  - A need for markedly increased amounts of opioids to achieve intoxication or desired effect.
  - A markedly diminished effect with continued use of the same amount of an opioid.
  - *Note: These criteria are not considered to be met for those taking opioids solely under appropriate medical supervision.*

- Withdrawal, as manifested by either of the following:

  - The characteristic opioid withdrawal syndrome (see Opioid Withdrawal section).
  - Opioids (or a closely related substance) are taken to relieve or avoid withdrawal symptoms.
  - *Note: These criteria are not considered to be met for those individuals taking opioids solely under appropriate medical supervision.*

The DSM-V definition "opioid use disorder" was an improvement over the previous (DSM-IV) definition of "opioid dependence" because many chronic pain patients who appropriately utilize opioids often display both tolerance and withdrawal within a 12-month period, thus creating a bias against this population. The original DSM-IV definition was developed for populations abusing illicit drugs and was never intended for those who were receiving chronic opioid therapy for medicinal purposes.

The definition of addiction (abridged) per the American Society of Addiction Medicine (ASAM) is as follows[23]:

- Addiction is a primary, chronic disease of brain reward, motivation, memory, and related circuitry.
- Dysfunction in these circuits leads to characteristic biological, psychological, social, and spiritual manifestations.
- This is reflected in an individual pathologically pursuing reward and/or relief by substance use and other behaviors.
- Addiction is characterized by inability to consistently abstain, impairment in behavioral control, and craving, diminished recognition of significant problems with one's behaviors and interpersonal relationships, and a dysfunctional emotional response.
- Like other chronic diseases, addiction often involves cycles of relapse and remission.
- Without treatment or engagement in recovery activities, addiction is progressive and can result in disability or premature death.

This action is a brain disease characterized by loss of *control*, *compulsive* use, impaired *control* over use, *craving*, and continued use despite harm.

Opioid Withdrawal

Withdrawal or abstinence is a normal physiologic phenomenon which occurs with physical dependence. This can occur with any medication. For example, it is common to experience headache and fatigue with cessation of caffeinated beverages. Discontinuation of certain selective serotonin reuptake inhibitors (paroxetine) can result in serious withdrawal. Withdrawal from opioids can be variable with some patients exhibiting only one symptom and for others the entire spectrum.

Opioid withdrawal is characterized by the following (DSM-V) [22]:

1. Dysphoric mood,
2. Nausea or vomiting,
3. Muscle aches,
4. Lacrimation or rhinorrhea,
5. Pupillary dilation, piloerection, or sweating,
6. Diarrhea,
7. Yawning,
8. Fever, and
9. Insomnia.

Opioid withdrawal can be further categorized by the neurotransmitters that modulate the symptoms, most notably norepinephrine and dopamine. The *autonomic* signs and symptoms of withdrawal are mediated by norepinephrine activity in the locus coeruleus. During acute opioid use, there is reduction of central norepinephrine levels and activity. With chronic opioid use, there is upregulation of central norepinephrine and noradrenergic activity. During withdrawal, there is increased noradrenergic activity, resulting in autonomic changes such as elevations in blood pressure, heart rate, peristalsis, diaphoresis, myalgias, sweating, piloerection, and increased CNS irritability.

The *affective* component of opioid withdrawal is mediated by dopamine via the mesolimbic pathway [24], in particular the ascending limb from the ventral tegmental area to the nucleus accumbens (Fig. 14.4). During acute opioid use, there is a concomitant elevation of dopamine, resulting in euphoria and elevated mood. With chronic opioid use, tolerance develops and there is downregulation of mesolimbic dopamine levels and activity. During withdrawal, there are affective symptoms such as anhedonia, dysphoria, and depression due to chronically depressed dopamine levels.

Medically Supervised Withdrawal

When deciding to implement an exit strategy from opioid therapy, the physician may discuss the reduction or cessation of opioid medications. The patients will almost always respond with "but doctor, what about my pain?" The concept of opioid-induced hyperalgesia (OIH) is not easy to explain to a clinician, let alone a

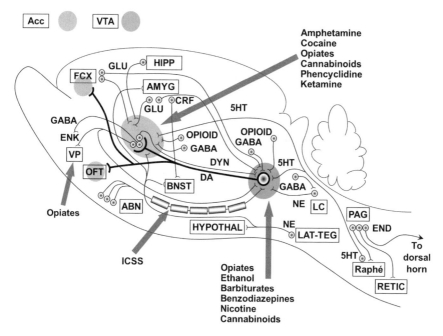

Fig. 14.4 The mesolimbic pathway of reward. From Gardner [24]

patient. Analogies such as "resetting a thermostat" or "rebooting a computer" are often useful to explain that the medications used to treat pain are in fact causing more pain. In the case of addiction, misuse, or abuse, the concept is somewhat easier to comprehend. Imparting these concepts to patients is crucial to ensure "buy in" to an exit strategy.

Medically supervised withdrawal involves targeting both the adrenergic and dopaminergic components with pharmacologic interventions. Medications that reduce central adrenergic activity are often utilized. Opioids which are potent yet less euphorigenic (methadone, buprenorphine) may be substituted for the abused or prescribed medication. Symptomatic treatment of other withdrawal symptoms can be accomplished with antidiarrheals, antiemetics, and anxiolytics such as antidepressants without the use of benzodiazepines. Opioid antagonists (naloxone, naltrexone) can be utilized to reduce craving and maintain abstinence. Antidepressants that may increase dopamine levels, such as bupropion, can be effective.

Clonidine

Clonidine is an alpha-2 adrenergic agonist which selectively binds to be presynaptic receptors on adrenergic neurons. These neurons are located in the locus coeruleus and possibly in the A1 and A2 cell groups of the medulla that project to the extended amygdala. Clonidine is FDA approved for the treatment of hypertension. The major limiting side effect of clonidine is hypotension.

Clonidine has been demonstrated to be significantly better than placebo and nearly comparable to a slow methadone taper [25]. It is widely used by physicians to treat opioid withdrawal and does not require specific credentialing and licensing, as with methadone or buprenorphine.

Clonidine may be dosed 0.1–0.4 mg every 4–6 h as needed for withdrawal symptoms. The dose is typically increased until the patient experiences orthostatic hypotension or a diastolic blood pressure below 60 mm. The other autonomic symptoms of opioid withdrawal may be treated symptomatically with antiemetics (ondansetron, antihistamines) and antidiarrheals (loperamide).

Naltrexone

Naltrexone is an orally administered opioid mu receptor antagonist. When naltrexone is given, all clinical effects of mu receptor agonists are blocked, thus reducing the cravings associated with opioid use disorder. Therefore, the patient will not experience euphoria, craving, and mood enhancement (elevation of hedonic tone). The patient must be free of all mu receptor agonists prior to the use of naltrexone to avoid withdrawal (approximately 5–7 days for short-acting opioids; 7–10 days for extended-release long-acting opioids). A challenge dose of naltrexone is usually given to determine whether withdrawal occurs. If not, then naltrexone may be initiated at 25 mg per day and increased to a maximum of 100 mg. An intramuscular formulation of extended-release naltrexone was approved in 2010 (Vivitrol® Alkermes Inc., Dublin Ireland) which is administered on a monthly basis.

This technique occasionally demonstrates poor patient compliance due to the fact that dopaminergic activity is not enhanced, which is often desired by patients. However, it can be quite effective in certain selected patient populations, such as professionals (physicians, attorneys, etc.) for whom the consequences of relapse are quite high. These groups can be maintained on naltrexone for extended periods of time and may represent the best alternative for treatment.

Ultra-Rapid Opioid Withdrawal

Ultra-rapid opioid withdrawal involves the administration of an opioid antagonist intravenously (naloxone) to provoke withdrawal usually under anesthesia. Upon emergence, the other symptoms of withdrawal are treated with clonidine, antiemetics, antidiarrheals, or benzodiazepines. There is resolution of withdrawal usually within 2–3 days with the concomitant use of naltrexone. This is a controversial technique with few well-designed clinical studies to support its use.

However, it may be appropriate in certain patient populations who cannot undergo long-term detoxification based on logistical concerns [26].

Opioid Agonist Therapy (OAT)

Physicians treating opioid dependency must be familiar with the basic pharmacology of opioids and physiologic manifestations of withdrawal. There is variability between opioid agonists for the treatment of pain as well as addiction. This variability extends to the patient population as well, which is complex, and requires a comprehensive evaluation prior to the treatment. There is a significant overlap of this population with those who have chronic pain [10].

These patients present a tremendous challenge to the healthcare system. Evidence-based studies have shown that OAT with methadone, and now with buprenorphine, combined with behavioral therapy can improve the success in the treatment of opioid dependence [27–30].

Methadone

Methadone has been the gold standard for treating opioid addiction for decades. It is given in its liquid or tablet form once or twice daily either observed or with take-home doses. The goal is to suppress withdrawal and cravings with maintenance dosing that can be maintained indefinitely.

Methadone is very inexpensive. It is metabolized primarily by the 3A4 and secondarily by the 2D6 cytochrome P450 system. Analgesia and sedative effects are mediated by the L-isomer, while D-isomer is an N-methyl-D-aspartate (NMDA) antagonist. It is the NMDA antagonism which may provide a certain niche treatment for difficult chronic pain conditions, such as neuropathic pain.

Liquid methadone has a slow onset of action but is rapidly absorbed. The half-life of methadone is quite variable and may range from 24 to 150 h depending on the dose. In the USA, the average daily dose of methadone for the treatment of opioid dependence is 80–120 mg. For the treatment of opioid addiction, methadone requires special licensing and credentialing, but not for the treatment of chronic pain. Although the overall plasma half-life of methadone is quite long, the analgesic half-life is relatively short. Experience treating chronic pain demonstrates that the analgesic half-life is approximately 6–8 h. This requires methadone to be dosed three to four times daily to treat chronic pain. Methadone also demonstrates incomplete cross-tolerance with respect to other opioid mu receptor agonist. Specifically, the conversion dose of methadone (with respect to morphine equivalents) is not linear but varies with dose [31] (Table 14.2).

Metabolism of methadone may be affected by certain inhibitors and inducers of the CYP450 (Table 14.3).

Table 14.2 Incomplete cross-tolerance of methadone

Morphine equivalents (mg)	Ratio of morphine/methadone
30–90	4:1
90–300	8:1
>300	12:1

Modified from Ripamonti et al. [31]

Table 14.3 Inhibitors and inducers of CYP2D6 and CYP3A4

Enzyme	Substrates	Inhibitors	Inducers
CYP2D6	Amitriptyline, bupropion, clomipramine, clozapine, clonazepam, codeine, clonazepam, codeine, desipramine, dextromethorphan, doxepin, fluoxetine, haloperidol, hydrocodone, imipramine, methadone, modafinil, morphine, nortriptyline, olanzapine, oxycodone, paroxetine, sertraline, tiagabine, tramadol, venlafaxine	Citalopram (weak), desipramine, fluoxetine, olanzapine (weak), paroxetine, sertraline, venlafaxine (weak)	Carbamazepine, phenobarbital, phenytoin
CYP3A4	Alfentanil, alprazolam, amitriptyline, bupropion, citalopram, clozapine, cyclosporin, dexamethasone, dextromethorphan, etoposide, fentanyl, fluoxetine, ifosfamide, imipramine, ketamine, lidocaine, meperidine, modafinil, paclitaxel, prednisone, sertraline, tamoxifen, tiagabine, venlafaxine, vincristine	Dexamethasone, dextromethorphan, fluoxetine, paroxetine (weak), sertraline, venlafaxine	Carbamazepine, dexamethasone, erythromycin, modafinil, phenobarbital, phenytoin

In addition to respiratory depression, another potentially lethal side effect of methadone has been reported. This involves prolongation of the QT interval which is a dose-dependent phenomenon. Severe ventricular arrhythmias such as Torsades de pointes have been reported (Fig. 14.5). The long plasma half-life of methadone predisposes its accumulation with multiple doses. Furthermore, the use of a CYP3A4 inhibitor may increase the risk of such an arrhythmia. In addition, there may be certain factors that predispose patients to torsades de pointes which may include bradycardia, congenital QT prolongation, hypokalemia, and concomitant

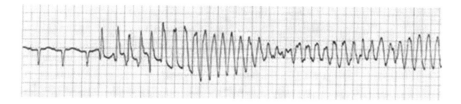

Fig. 14.5 Torsades de pointes

use of medications which may prolong the QT interval. Treatment includes magnesium, atrial pacing, isoproterenol, overdrive pacing, and, in extremis, the use of defibrillation. Cardioversion is contraindicated.

Buprenorphine

Naturally occurring opiates from the poppy include morphine, codeine, and thebaine. Buprenorphine is a synthetic thebaine derivative which has certain unique properties which make it ideal for the treatment of opioid dependence. It is potent and has a very high affinity for the mu opioid receptor, binding more tightly and competitively than other mu agonists and antagonists. This results in a slow dissociation from the mu receptor, with milder withdrawal symptoms, as well as a prolonged half-life. It is also a kappa receptor *antagonist*, which is unique in comparison with other partial agonists/mixed antagonist–agonists [32] (Table 14.4).

Buprenorphine is highly lipophilic and has a rapid onset of action after both sublingual and intravenous administration, approximately 30–60 min and 5–15 min, respectively. This also allows buprenorphine to penetrate the blood–brain barrier more easily than morphine. The peak effect for sublingual administration occurs around 100 min, and the duration is dose related.

There is an extensive first-pass effect with buprenorphine which results in poor absorption via the oral route. However, buprenorphine's bioavailability improves markedly with sublingual, buccal, and transdermal administration (Fig. 14.6).

Buprenorphine has a relatively long elimination half-life of approximately 37 h, which is felt to be secondary to its slow dissociation from the mu receptor. It is highly bound to plasma proteins and has a relatively high volume of distribution. The metabolism is via the cytochrome P450 system into the active metabolite norbuprenorphine (25 % the potency of buprenorphine). Both buprenorphine and norbuprenorphine are conjugated with glucuronic acid and excreted through the bile, with approximately 15 % of buprenorphine excreted unchanged in the urine. Despite this, there is relatively little effect on buprenorphine metabolism in renal failure.

Buprenorphine is a partial agonist and therefore has *less* activity at the mu receptor. This results in a ceiling effect with respect to analgesia, respiratory

Table 14.4 Properties of partial agonists, antagonists

	Buprenorphine	Pentazocine	Nalbuphine	Butorphanol
Mu receptor activity	Partial agonist	Partial agonist	Antagonist	Partial agonist
Kappa receptor activity	Antagonist	Agonist	Agonist	Strong agonist
Schedule	III	IV	Unscheduled (schedule IV in KY)	IV

Modified from Johnson et al. [32]

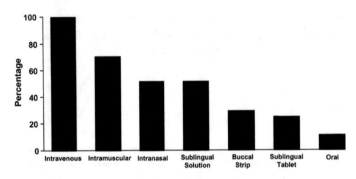

Fig. 14.6 Bioavailability of buprenorphine. From Johnson et al. [32]

depression, and other opioid side effects to include withdrawal. The kappa receptor is associated with spinal analgesia, sedation, miosis, and dysphoric effects. At the kappa receptor, buprenorphine is an *antagonist*, which may provide a unique role in treating OIH and opioid tolerance [33].

Buprenorphine is FDA approved for the treatment of opioid dependence in its sublingual form (generic and Subutex® [Reckitt Benckiser Group, UK]) and in a 4:1 (buprenorphine: naloxone) combination product (generic and Suboxone® [Reckitt Benckiser Group, UK]). Other combination products include Zubsolv® (OrexoAB, Sweden) tablets and Bunavail® (Biodelivery Systems, NC, USA). Buprenorphine is also commercially available to treat pain in a parenteral formulation (Buprenex® [Reckitt Benckiser Group, UK]) and as a transdermal formulation (Butrans® [Purdue Pharma L.P., CT, USA]).

For the treatment of opioid dependence, both the medication and the practitioner must meet certain requirements. Requirements for the practitioner include the following:

1. The physician holds a subspecialty board certification in addiction psychiatry from the American Board of Medical Specialties.
2. The physician holds an addiction certification from the ASAM.
3. The physician holds a subspecialty board certification in addiction medicine from the American Osteopathic Association.

4. The physician has completed not less than 8 h of training with respect to the treatment and management of opioid-addicted patients. This training can be provided through classroom situations, seminars at professional society meetings, electronic communications, or otherwise. The training must be sponsored by one of five organizations authorized in the DATA 2000 legislation to sponsor such training, or by any other organization that the secretary of the Department of Health and Human Services (the secretary) determines to be appropriate.
5. The physician has participated as an investigator in one or more clinical trials leading to the approval of a narcotic drug in Schedule III, IV, or V for maintenance or detoxification treatment, as demonstrated by a statement submitted to the secretary by the sponsor of such approved drug.
6. The physician has other training or experience, considered by the state medical licensing board (of the state in which the physician will provide maintenance or detoxification treatment) to demonstrate the ability of the physician to treat and manage opioid-addicted patients.
7. The physician has other training or experience the secretary considers demonstrates the ability of the physician to treat and manage opioid-addicted patients.

Once one of these criteria is met, the physician may apply to obtain a waiver from the Drug Enforcement Administration (DEA) and the Substance Abuse and Mental Health Services Administration/Center for Substance Abuse Treatment (SAMHSA/CSAT). Upon submission [notification of intent to use Schedule III, IV, or V Drugs For Maintenance and Detoxification Treatment Of Opiate Addiction; Under 21 USC 823(g)(2)], SAMHSA/CSAT has 45 days to determine whether the physician meets the requirements. The DEA then assigns an "X number" to the physician, in addition to their standard DEA number, which allows them to prescribe controlled substances for the treatment of opioid dependence established by DATA 2000. Initially, physicians may treat up to 30 patients for opioid dependence with sublingual buprenorphine. As of 2007, a physician can treat up to 100 patients with secondary notification to SAMHSA/CSAT.

Only specific formulations of buprenorphine can be utilized under DATA 2000. It is illegal to use the parenteral formulation of buprenorphine to treat opioid dependence. Sublingual buprenorphine is the *only* Schedule III drug currently approved by the FDA to treat opioid dependence established by law under DATA 2000.

Prior to its use in the USA, buprenorphine in its sublingual form was used very successfully in Europe for the treatment of opioid addiction. Unfortunately, the single component formulation was also widely abused, intravenously in Europe, in particular France and the UK, which prompted the combination product with naloxone, (which deters abuse) widely utilized in the USA.

The combination product contains buprenorphine: naloxone in a 4:1 ratio. Both entities are poorly absorbed via the oral route. Buprenorphine is absorbed very well via the sublingual route, whereas naloxone is less than 10 % absorbed. If abused via the parenteral route, both are absorbed very well and the naloxone antagonizes the effect of the buprenorphine at the mu receptor. In opioid-dependent individuals, this reduces the euphoria caused by buprenorphine and also results in precipitated

Table 14.5 Therapeutic indices for morphine and buprenorphine

Opioid	LD_{50}, acute (mg/kg)	ED_{50}, tail pressure (mg/kg)	Therapeutic index LD_{50}/ED_{50}
Morphine	306 [237, 395]	0.66 [0.26, 1.6]	464
Buprenorphine	197 [145, 277]	0.016 [0.011, 0.024]	12,313

Modified from Johnson et al. [32]

withdrawal. The purpose of the combination product is to deter parenteral abuse. However, the combination product can be abused and has street value for diversion, when commonly utilized by addicts to manage withdrawal between binges [34].

Buprenorphine and its combination with naloxone have been validated as an alternative to methadone [35–39]. The therapeutic index of buprenorphine is relatively high (Table 14.5) which in part is due to its ceiling effect on respiratory depression.

The safety of buprenorphine has been studied in the treatment of opioid dependence. Heroin addicts were treated with sublingual buprenorphine daily (8 mg) for up to 36 days with no significant morbidity [37]. Buprenorphine was studied in a maintenance therapy program during an observational study [39]. The mortality rate was 4 % (3 of 77). The successful retention rate with respect to treatment was felt to be secondary to the use of buprenorphine. However, comorbidities of cocaine and other opiate dependence may have contributed to morbidity and mortality.

Buprenorphine was found to have less morbidity and better retention in a study of heroin addicts when it was continued for up to 350 days as opposed to rapidly withdrawn [39]. A randomized controlled study found that buprenorphine had similar efficacy to methadone in a maintenance program for opioid dependence [36].

Buprenorphine and Precipitated Withdrawal

Buprenorphine has a very high affinity for the mu receptor and will displace opioid agonists and antagonists from the mu receptor. Since it is a partial agonist, it has a lower intrinsic activity at the mu receptor than a pure agonist. When administered to a patient who is physically dependent on a pure mu agonist, this reduced receptor activity results in withdrawal. Therefore, if a patient is currently taking a full mu agonist and is *not* in withdrawal, the administration of buprenorphine will *precipitate* withdrawal. Hence, patients must be in some degree of opioid withdrawal in order to be treated with buprenorphine for opioid dependence (Fig. 14.7).

Fig. 14.7 Precipitated withdrawal. The net decrease in activity at the mu receptor results in withdrawal symptoms

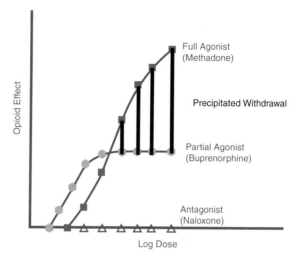

Patient Selection

Some patients may present a challenge to providing office-based buprenorphine treatment. For example, relative contraindications to its use in this setting include polysubstance abuse, history of multiple relapses, poor compliance, poor psychosocial functioning, and medical instability. Absolute contraindications to the use of buprenorphine include severe side effects from the previous exposure or hypersensitivity to buprenorphine and/or naloxone.

Induction

Induction is the process by which the patient presents for the initial administration of buprenorphine for medically supervised withdrawal. The clinician must determine how and when the patient should discontinue their opioids to ensure adequate (but not severe) withdrawal.

In general, extended-release opioids should be discontinued 24 h prior to induction and short-acting opioids approximately 12 h. The physician should also ascertain whether the patient has experienced withdrawal in the past and how soon these symptoms occur after stopping opioids.

The Clinical Opiate Withdrawal Scale (COWS) [40] can be utilized to objectively quantify withdrawal status. The induction should not proceed until the patient is an adequate withdrawal (COWS = 8–11; Fig. 14.8).

Typical inductions are performed in a supervised office setting. Dosing typically begins at 2–4 mg, and a repeat assessment of COWS should be done approximately 1 h later. The dose may then be repeated and titrated to the severity of withdrawal

Patient's Name:_____ Date: _____
Buprenorphine induction:
Enter scores at time zero, 30 min after fist dose, 2 h after fist dose, etc.
Times: _____ _____ _____ _____
Resting Pulse Rate: (record beats per minute)
Measured after patient is sitting or lying for one minute
0 pulse rate 80 or below
1 pulse rate 81–100
2 pulse rate 101–120
4 pulse rate greater than 120
Sweating: *over past ½ hour not accounted for by room*
temperature or patient activity.
0 no report of chills or flushing
1 subjective report of chills or flushing
2 flushed or observable moistness on face
3 beads of sweat on brow or face
4 sweat streaming off face
Restlessness *Observation during assessment*
0 able to sit still
1 reports difficulty sitting still, but is able to do so
3 frequent shifting or extraneous movements of legs/arms
5 Unable to sit still for more than a few seconds
Pupil size
0 pupils pinned or normal size for room light
1 pupils possibly larger than normal for room light
2 pupils moderately dilated
5 pupils so dilated that only the rim of the iris is visible
Bone or Joint aches *If patient was having pain previously,*
only the additional component attributed to opiates
withdrawal is scored
0 not present
1 mild diffuse discomfort
2 patient reports severe diffuse aching of joints/ muscles
4 patient is rubbing joints or muscles and is unable to sit still
because of discomfort
Runny nose or tearing *Not accounted for by cold symptoms*
or allergies
0 not present
1 nasal stuffiess or unusually moist eyes
2 nose running or tearing
4 nose constantly running or tears streaming down cheeks
GI Upset: *over last ½ hour*
0 no GI symptoms
1 stomach cramps
2 nausea or loose stool
3 vomiting or diarrhea
5 Multiple episodes of diarrhea or vomiting

Fig. 14.8 The Clinical Opiate Withdrawal Scale. From Wesson et al. [40]

Tremor *observation of outstretched hands*
0 No tremor
1 tremor can be felt, but not observed
2 slight tremor observable
4 gross tremor or muscle twitching
Yawning *Observation during assessment*
0 no yawning
1 yawning once or twice during assessment
2 yawning three or more times during assessment
4 yawning several times/min
Anxiety or Irritability
0 none
1 patient reports increasing irritability or anxiousness
2 patient obviously irritable anxious
4 patient so irritable or anxious that participation in the
assessment is difficult
Gooseflesh skin
0 skin is smooth
3 piloerection of skin can be felt or hairs standing up on arms
5 prominent piloerection
Total scores
Score: 5–12 = mild
13–24 = moderate
25–36 = moderately severe
More than 36 = severe withdrawal

Fig. 14.8   (continued)

symptoms. At 16 mg, 75–95 % of the brain's mu receptors are blocked by buprenorphine [41]. Therefore, most patients will respond to 16 mg of sublingual buprenorphine during induction.

If precipitated withdrawal should occur, repeated doses of buprenorphine should be given until withdrawal symptoms abate (up to 32 mg).

Maintenance

Most patients can be stabilized on once daily sublingual dosing with average doses quite variable (8–16 mg). As the patient is weaned from the initial induction dose, administration may shift to every other day to facilitate complete discontinuation of buprenorphine.

The dosing may also be given 2–3 times daily, which is often effective in patients experiencing chronic pain, since the analgesic half-life of buprenorphine, like methadone, is relatively short (approximately 6–8 h). Sublingual buprenorphine is ideal for treating patients who suffer from both opioid use disorder and chronic pain.

Use in Pregnancy

The gold standard during pregnancy has always been methadone maintenance therapy and then treatment of newborn for neonatal withdrawal. Medical detoxification during pregnancy may cause irreparable harm to the fetus and/or miscarriage.

Sublingual buprenorphine *without* naloxone can be utilized for maintenance therapy during pregnancy. Due to the unknown effects of naloxone on the fetus, it is a category C teratogen.

Buprenorphine was compared to methadone for the treatment of opioid dependence during pregnancy with similar outcomes. However, the newborns in the buprenorphine group required less morphine to treat neonatal abstinence syndrome, displaying less withdrawal symptoms [42].

Buprenorphine for Pain

Once the patient has been successfully withdrawn from pure mu receptor agonists, buprenorphine can be utilized to manage *both* chronic pain and opioid dependence. The patient can be successfully maintained on sublingual buprenorphine to provide both analgesia and prevent relapse of addiction. Buprenorphine has been shown to be intermediate in its ability to induce pain sensitivity in patients maintained on methadone and control patients not taking opioids [43]. Buprenorphine showed an enhanced ability to treat hyperalgesia experimentally induced in volunteers compared to fentanyl [44]. Spinal dynorphin, a kappa receptor agonist, increases during opioid administration, thus contributing to OIH. Buprenorphine is a kappa receptor antagonist. For these reasons, buprenorphine may be unique in its ability to treat chronic pain and possibly OIH, thus having a niche role in the treatment of complex chronic pain patients [33].

Buprenorphine provides good analgesia without significant respiratory depression via epidural administration [45, 46]. It has been shown to provide more prolonged pain relief in postoperative Cesarean section patients compared with controls who did not utilize buprenorphine [47]. Buprenorphine can be given subcutaneously to provide postoperative pain control at approximately 30 mcg per hour [48]. It has also been shown to significantly reduce analgesic requirements after knee arthroscopy when intra-articular injection is provided during surgery [49]. The addition of buprenorphine to the local anesthetic in axillary brachial plexus blockade provided significant postoperative analgesia [50].

Transdermal buprenorphine is indicated for the treatment of chronic pain. It was studied in a moderate quality, open-label, parallel-group randomized trial which compared it to extended-release tramadol for the management of osteoarthritis of the hip and knee, yielding indeterminate results [51]. In the USA, it is available in 5, 7.5, 10, 15, and 20 mcg per hour patches (Butrans®), which provide seven days of therapy. Due to its ceiling effect on analgesia, it is not recommended for patients who have daily requirements greater than 80 mg morphine equivalents. It should not be used for the treatment of opioid dependence because even at the maximum dose (20 mcg per hour), it corresponds to a mere 0.48 mg daily of buprenorphine. For opioid addiction, dosing of sublingual buprenorphine varies from 2 to 24 mg per day. Therefore, the use of buprenorphine to treat opioid addiction corresponds to a relative *overdose* compared to that for chronic pain. At 16 mg, 75–95 % of the brain's mu receptors are blocked by buprenorphine [41]. Therefore, very low doses of buprenorphine are required for analgesia.

Sublingual buprenorphine is FDA approved for the treatment of opioid dependence requiring a waiver from the DEA and SAMHSA/CSAT. However, it is a schedule III medication and can be used to treat pain, which does *not* require a waiver [52, 53].

Sedatives and Hypnotics

Sedatives and hypnotics in combination with opioids can result in accidental overdose and death [17]. Exit strategies regarding the use of these medications typically involve the weaning, conversion to a less euphorigenic benzodiazepine, or conversion to phenobarbital with subsequent weaning.

Gamma-aminobutyric acid (GABA) is the major inhibitory neurotransmitter in the CNS. Benzodiazepines modulate the effect of GABA via binding to a specific site on the GABA-A receptor in the CNS. This effect results in enhanced chloride conductance, hyperpolarization, and depressed neuronal activity. Barbiturates and, in particular, in combination with ethanol, prolong the opening of the chloride channel, while benzodiazepines increase the frequency of channel opening.

Barbiturates

Carisoprodol is widely used to treat muscle spasm and is metabolized to meprobamate, a barbiturate. This may result in physical dependence or addiction. This medication has been linked to increased emergency department visits and deaths, often in combination with opioids, and has largely been abandoned by the pain management community [54]. Carisoprodol can be weaned in a schedule manner.

Butalbital is used in combination with caffeine and acetaminophen or aspirin (Fioricet or Fiorinal) for the abortive treatment of migraine. Physical dependence can occur with the use of this medication, and overuse frequently results in medication overuse headache and rebound [55].

Benzodiazepines

Benzodiazepines were introduced to replace barbiturates in the late 1950s. In the 1970s, benzodiazepines (diazepam) virtually replaced barbiturates largely because of their higher therapeutic index and perceived improved safety. Many physicians routinely use benzodiazepines for acute anxiety, insomnia muscle spasm, back pain, and other psychiatric problems such as post-traumatic stress disorder, panic disorder, and generalized anxiety disorder. While they may have some use in treating acute anxiety and stress reactions, the evidence for their chronic use is lacking [56].

Approximately 30 % of patients with chronic non-cancer pain are concurrently prescribed benzodiazepines and opioids [7] and approximately 40–60 % of those with chronic pain abuse benzodiazepines [57].

Withdrawal

When discontinuing benzodiazepines, a rebound in anxiety symptoms occurs, followed by withdrawal symptoms. Withdrawal symptoms are unique time-dependent signs and symptoms which may ultimately lead to grand mal seizures and death (Table 14.6).

The severity of benzodiazepine rebound symptoms and withdrawal depends not only on the specific drug, but the patient as well. A concomitant diagnosis of panic disorder, preexisting high levels of anxiety, concomitant substance use disorder, or psychopathology (neurosis, personality disorder) will increase the difficulty of tapering medications increasing severity of rebound [58].

The most severe withdrawal symptoms are seen with drugs that have short elimination half-lives, rapid onset of action, and high potency. The time course of benzodiazepine withdrawal will also depend upon the dose, elimination half-life, and the existence of active metabolites. For example, the effect of diazepam is greatly prolonged by its active metabolite, desmethyldiazepam, which has a half-life

Table 14.6 Benzodiazepine rebound anxiety and withdrawal symptoms

Anxiety	Withdrawal
Irritability	Depression
Hyperhidrosis	Nausea
Impaired concentration	Anorexia
Headache	Depersonalization
Insomnia	Increased sensory perceptions
Fatigue	Abnormal sensory perceptions
Myalgias	Delirium
Dizziness	Grand mal seizures
Tremor	Death

Table 14.7 Benzodiazepine pharmacology and relative potency

Drug	Potency	Onset	Half-life (h)	Active metabolite
Clonazepam	0.25	Intermediate	18–50	None
Alprazolam	0.5	Fast	6–20	None
Lorazepam	1.0	Intermediate	10–20	None
Diazepam	5.0	intermediate	50–100	Desmethyldiazepam
Chlorazepate	7.5	Fast	30–100	Desmethyldiazepam
Chlordiazepoxide	1.0	Intermediate	5–100	Desmethyldiazepam
Oxazepam	15	Slow	5–12	None

of about 51 h (at about age 20), and is markedly prolonged in the elderly (up to 150 h at age 90).

Management of Dependence

When treating benzodiazepine and sedative dependence, there are essentially two avenues: tapering or conversion and tapering. As with the use of buprenorphine and methadone in opioid-dependent patients, conversion to a less potent, less euphorigenic, and longer acting benzodiazepine may facilitate tapering [59]. Unlike opioids, benzodiazepines do not appear to exhibit incomplete cross-tolerance (Table 14.7). Therefore, conversion among benzodiazepines is relatively straightforward.

The tapering of the first 50 % of the drug may be accomplished rapidly. The remaining 50 % is often more challenging, requiring a more controlled and slower reduction with each successive 25 % due to rebound symptoms. Conversion to clonazepam has been shown to be effective for weaning from more euphorigenic benzodiazepines [59]. The concomitant use of antiepileptic medications such as carbamazepine, valproic acid, and gabapentin may also be used for seizure prophylaxis.

Conversion to phenobarbital has been employed as well to prevent withdrawal seizures. Phenobarbital has little effect on anxiety and other behaviors, but is advantageous in managing withdrawal from most sedative/hypnotics, and may be more advantageous for the polysubstance abuser in a medically monitored setting [60]. Cognitive–behavioral therapy (CBT) may be helpful to increase the success rate of weaning. But most importantly, one must obtain "buy in" from the patient and family support to ensure success as an outpatient.

If patients are on multiple substances or present with extreme challenges, inpatient medically supervised withdrawal is recommended.

Behavioral Therapies

Chronic pain patients often are plagued by not only the physical, but the psychological stressors of their disease. CBT has been successfully utilized to treat both chronic pain patients and those suffering from substance dependence. The CBT approach to chronic pain is based on the premise that the disease becomes established as part of the patient's cognitions and beliefs, often unconsciously, which creates an impression that has a profound impact on the short- and long-term adjustment to pain [61]. The therapy focuses on the cognitive processes underlying the patient's assumptions and beliefs of pain, the behaviors that need to be extinguished and those that should be reinforced to cope with the pain. In this manner, CBT can reduce the use of analgesics and opioids by improving the functionality and mood.

CBT is one of several behavioral models of multidisciplinary pain management that has been developed over the past 3 decades [62]. Behavioral therapy has been successful in treating opioid-dependent patients with buprenorphine, with 53 % of patients completing treatment utilizing behavioral therapy v. 20 % who did not receive behavioral therapy [63]. Motivational Enhancement Therapy (MET) has been used to engage patients to accept opioid weaning or detoxification as part of their treatment plan. MET often is used in conjunction with CBT. Behavioral assessments are strongly recommended for chronic pain patients, especially if the clinician suspects significant psychiatric comorbidities and or substance use disorders. The assessment of pain attitudes, locus of self-control, and catastrophic thinking are all required components to implement CBT.

When developing an exit strategy from controlled substance management, it is essential that the clinician has access to a therapist who can assist the strategy. Patients are often reluctant to change even though they may not be improving functionally. Behavioral therapy utilized in conjunction with medically supervised withdrawal is an integral part of any exit strategy from controlled substance use.

The Exit Algorithm

There are several of scenarios in which the clinician should consider the cessation of controlled substance therapy. Figure 14.9 illustrates these scenarios and actions.

Overdose Prevention

The prescription opioid epidemic requires all physicians who prescribe controlled substances for the management of pain to engage in the utmost care to avoid accidental overdose by their patients. Opioid overdoses can occur after deliberate

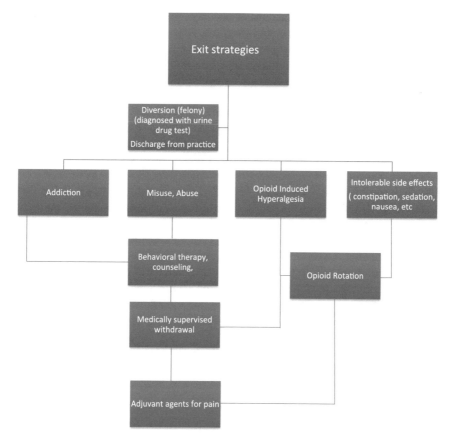

Fig. 14.9 Exit algorithm

abuse of prescription opioids and heroin. However, accidental overdoses are much more insidious, in that they are unanticipated. They frequently involve patients who are receiving polypharmacy, such as benzodiazepines and opioids. Alcohol and over-the-counter medications such as antihistamines, in combination with prescribed opioids, can further depress respiration. Chronic opioid use can cause central sleep apnea [64]. Patients may overuse their pain medications secondary to chemical-coping behaviors related to stress and other factors. Chemical coping is maladaptive behavior where patients will use prescribed opioids (or other medications) to treat different symptoms, such as anxiety, insomnia, or fatigue. Patients who have psychiatric comorbidities are at increased risk of substance use disorders and therefore overdose.

The overdose rate is directly proportional to the amount of opioid prescribed. Several studies have documented increased morbidity and mortality associated with increasing morphine equivalent dosing [65–68].

This has prompted substance abuse treatment programs to consider the distribution of naloxone to prevent opioid overdose. A systematic review was conducted of community-based opioid overdose prevention programs [69]. The review found that take-home naloxone was utilized by relatives or bystanders to treat witnessed opioid overdose. Naloxone was used successfully by participants in all but one reviewed study, for a total of 1949 recorded naloxone administrations across 18 programs. Eleven of these programs reported 100 % survival rate post-naloxone administration. The remaining articles reported a range of 83–96 % survival. The review also cited increasing non-medical bystander knowledge of prevention, risk factors, and recognition of opioid overdose. Limitations of the review included that it was not a randomized controlled study, and the overall quality of evidence was fair. However, the study population was somewhat challenging in that it involved heroin addicts. The demographics in a chronic pain population may be quite different however.

Using intranasal naloxone, the state of Massachusetts studied opioid overdose rates and implementation of overdose education [70]. The program trained 2912 potential bystanders who reported 327 rescues. There was a significantly reduced adjusted rate ratio of overdose compared with communities with no implementation. This observational study demonstrated that opioid overdose death rates were reduced in communities where overdose education and nasal naloxone distribution programs were implemented.

SAMHSA recently released an overdose toolkit [71] in which it recommends prescribing naloxone along with the patient's initial opioid prescription. Patients who are potential candidates for such overdose kits include those:

- taking high doses of opioids for long-term management of chronic malignant or non-malignant pain;
- receiving a rotating opioid medication regimen and are at risk of incomplete cross-tolerance;
- discharged from emergency medical care following opioid intoxication or poisoning;
- at high risk of overdose because of legitimate medical need for analgesia, coupled with a suspected or confirmed history of substance abuse, dependence, or non-medical use of prescription or illicit opioids;
- on certain opioid preparations that may increase risk of opioid overdose such as extended-release/long-acting preparations;
- completing mandatory opioid detoxification or abstinence programs; and
- recently released from incarceration and a past user or of abuser of opioids (and presumably with reduced opioid tolerance and high risk of relapse to opioid use).

This reduced tolerance often leads to overdose. SAMHSA also recommends providing an overdose plan to share with the patient's friends and family.

Recently, the FDA approved a prescription treatment for opioid overdose consisting of an autoinjector of naloxone, Evzio® (Kaleo, Richmond Virginia). The injector is a device which combined with audio directions, administers 0.4 mg of naloxone intramuscularly. The state of Massachusetts, department of public health, has developed an opioid overdose prevention and reversal program utilizing intranasal naloxone. Overdose naloxone toolkits may be required by other states and mandated as part of an integrated adherence monitoring program utilized by a pain practice.

Summary

Patients receiving controlled substances for the management of chronic pain should have risk mitigation strategies in place to include but not limited to the following:

1. Opioid treatment agreement;
2. Random urine drug testing;
3. Assessment of risk factors for substance abuse to include psychiatric comorbidities (anxiety disorders, depression, bipolar disorder, PTSD);
4. Family history or actual history of substance use disorder;
5. Risk stratification tools such as the Opioid Risk Tool (ORT) or the Screener and Opioid Assessment in Pain Patients-Revised (SOAPP-R); and
6. An exit strategy regarding controlled substance therapy.

However, if things go awry, the physician must have an exit strategy. Discharging problem patients merely transfers the problem elsewhere. Offering patients a solution to iatrogenic dependence on controlled substances is a viable and compassionate path for the both the patient and the practitioner.

References

1. Silverman SM. Medically supervised withdrawal for opioid dependence. In: Kaye DA, Vadivelu N, Urman RD, editors. Substance abuse, inpatient and outpatient management for every clinician. Springer: New York; 2015. p. 549–66.
2. Manchikanti L, et al. American Society of Interventional Pain Physicians (ASIPP) guidelines for responsible opioid prescribing in chronic non-cancer pain: parts 1–2. Pain Phys. 2012;15:S1–116.
3. Chou R, et al. American Pain Society-American Academy of Pain Medicine Opioids Guidelines Panel. Clinical guidelines for the use of chronic opioid therapy in chronic non-cancer pain. J Pain. 2009;10:113–30.
4. Institute of Medicine. Relieving pain in america: a blueprint for transforming prevention, care, education, and research. Washington, DC: The National Academies Press; 2011.
5. Model Policy for the Use of Controlled Substances for the Treatment of Pain. The Federation of State Medical Boards of the United States. Inc., May 2004.
6. Manchikanti L, et al. Prospective evaluation of patients with increasing opiate needs: prescription opiate abuse and illicit drug use. Pain Phys. 2004;7:339–44.
7. Manchikanti L, et al. Patterns of illicit drug use and opioid abuse in patients with chronic pain at initial evaluation: a prospective, observational study. Pain Phys. 2004;7:431–7.

8. Manchikanti L. Prescription drug abuse: what is being done to address this new drug epidemic? Testimony before the subcommittee on criminal justice, drug. policy and human resources. Pain Phys. 2006;9:287–321. ISSN 1533-3159.
9. CS/CS/HB 7095: Prescription Drugs; Florida Senate; Chapter No. 2011-141.
10. Webster LR, Webster RM. Predicting aberrant behaviors in opioid-treated patients: preliminary validation of the opioid risk tool. Pain Med. 2005;6(6):432–42.
11. Kochanek K et al. National Vital Statistics Report 2011: 60:1-117. CDC Vital Signs. Prescription Painkiller Overdoses. Use and abuse of methadone as a painkiller. 2012.
12. Warner M, et al. Drug poisoning deaths in the United States, 1980–2008. NCHS data brief: 81. Hyattsville, MD: National Center for Health Statistics. 2011.
13. National Center for Injury Prevention and Control. Division of Unintentional Injury Prevention. Policy Impact. Prescription Painkiller Overdoses: Nov 2011.
14. IMS Institute for Healthcare Informatics. The use of medicines in the United States: Review of 2011: April 2012.
15. Substance Abuse and Mental Health Services Administration, Office of Applied Studies. The DAWN Report: Benzodiazepines in drug abuse-related emergency department visits: 1995–2002. Rockville, MD; 2004.
16. Ghitza UE, et al. Self-report illicit benzodiazepine use on the addiction severity index predicts treatment outcome. Drug Alcohol Depend. 97(1–2):150–157.
17. Manchikanti L, et al. Opioid epidemic in the United States. Pain Physician. 2012;15:ES9–ES38.
18. O'Brien CP. Benzodiazepine use, misuse and dependence. J Clin Psychiatry. 2005;66(Suppl. 2):28–33.
19. Lintzeris N, et al. Pharmacodynamics of diazepam co-administered with methadone or buprenorphine under high dose conditions in opioid dependent patients. Drug Alcohol Depend. 91(2–3):187–94.
20. De Wet C, et al. Benzodiazepine co-dependence exacerbates the opiate withdrawal syndrome. Drug Alcohol Depend. 76(1):31–5.
21. Substance Abuse and Mental Health Services Administration, Center for Behavioral Health Statistics and Quality. (December 13, 2012). The TEDS Report: Admissions Reporting Benzodiazepine and Narcotic Pain Reliever Abuse at Treatment Entry. Rockville, MD.
22. Diagnostic and Statistical Manual of Mental Disorders (5th ed.) American Psychiatric Association 2014:1000 Wilson Boulevard, Suite 1825, Arlington, Va. 22209–3901.
23. Adopted by the ASAM Board of Directors. American Society of Addiction Medicine 4601 North Parke Avenue, Upper Arcade, Suite 101 Chevy Chase, MD 20815-4520. 19 April 2011.
24. Gardner E. The mesolimbic pathway of reward. Brain Reward Mechanisms. In Lowinson JH, et al, editors. Substance abuse: a comprehensive textbook. Philadelphia: Lippincott; 1997. pp. 51–8.
25. Gold M, et al. Clonidine blocks acute opioid withdrawal symptoms. Lancet. 1978;1:929–30.
26. Tetrault J, O'Connor P. Management of opioid intoxication and withdrawal (Vol. 12). In Ries R, et al, editors. Principles of addiction medicine. 4th ed. Philadelphia: Lippincott Williams and Wilkins: 2009. pp. 679–84.
27. Mattick RP, et al. Buprenorphine versus methadone maintenance therapy: a randomized double-blind trial with 405 opioid-dependent patients. Addiction. 2003;98:441–52.
28. Ling W, et al. A multi-center randomized trial of buprenorphine-naloxone versus clonidine for opioid detoxification: findings from the National Institute on Drug Abuse Clinical Trials Network. Addiction. 2005;100:1090–100.
29. Ahmadi J, et al. Controlled, randomized trial in maintenance treatment of intravenous buprenorphine dependence with naltrexone, methadone or buprenorphine: a novel study. Eur J Clin Invest. 2003;33:824–9.
30. Ling W, et al. Buprenorphine maintenance treatment of opiate dependence: a multicenter, randomized clinical trial. Addiction. 1998;93:475–86.
31. Ripamonti C, et al. An update on the clinical use of methadone for cancer pain. Pain. 1997;70 (2–3):109–15.

32. Johnson RE, Fudala PJ, Payne R. Buprenorphine: considerations for pain management. J Pain Symptom Manage. 2005;29(3):297–326.
33. Silverman SM. Opioid induced hyperalgesia: clinical implications for the pain practitioner. Pain Phys. 2009;12:679–84.
34. Yokel Michael A, et al. Buprenorphine and buprenorphine/naloxone diversion, misuse, and illicit use: an international review. Curr Drug Abuse Rev. 2011;4(1):28–41.
35. Ling W, et al. A clinical trial of buprenorphine: comparison with methadone in the detoxification of heroin addicts. A controlled trial of buprenorphine treatment for opioid dependence. Am J Psychiatry. 1994;151:1025–30.
36. Kakko, et al. A stepped care strategy using buprenorphine and methadone versus conventional methadone maintenance in heroin dependence: a randomized controlled trial. Am J Psychiatry. 2007;164:797–803.
37. Lange RW, et al. Safety and side-effects of buprenorphine in the clinical management of heroin addiction. Drug Alcohol Depend. 1990;26:19–28.
38. Fareed A, et al. Safety and efficacy of long-term buprenorphine maintenance treatment. Addict Dis Treat. 2011;10(3):123–30.
39. Kakko, et al. Buprenorphine Improved Treatment Retention in patients with Heroin Dependence. Lancet. 2003;361:662–8.
40. Wesson DR, et al. The clinical opioid withdrawal scale. J Psychoactive Drugs. 2003;35:253–9.
41. Zubieta JK, et al. Buprenorphine-induced changes in mu-opioid receptor availability in male heroin dependent volunteers: a preliminary study. Neuropsychopharmacology. 2000;23(3):326–34.
42. Jones HE, et al. Neonatal abstinence syndrome after methadone or buprenorphine exposure. N Engl J Med. 2010;363:2320–31.
43. Compton P, et al. Pain intolerance in opioid-maintained former opiate addicts: Effect of long acting maintenance agent. Drug Alcohol Depend. 2001;63:139–46.
44. Koppert W, et al. Different profiles of buprenorphine induced analgesia and antihyperalgesia in a human pain model. Pain. 2005;118:15–22.
45. Scherer R, et al. Complications related to thoracic epidural analgesia: a prospective study in1071 surgical patients. Acta Anaesthesiol Scand. 1993;37(4):370–4.
46. Inagaki Y, et al. Mode and site of analgesic action of epidural buprenorphine in humans. Anesth Analg. 1996;83(3):530–6.
47. Celleno D, et al. Spinal buprenorphine for postoperative analgesia after caesarean section. Acta Anaesthesiol Scand. 1989;33(3):236–8.
48. Matsumoto S, et al. The effect of subcutaneous administration of buprenorphine with patient controlled analgesia system for post-operative pain relief. Masui. Jpn J Anesthesiol. 1994;43(11):1709–13 (in Japanese).
49. Varrassi G, et al. Intra-articular buprenorphine after knee arthroscopy. A randomized, prospective, double-blind study. Acta Anaesthesiol Scand. 1999;43(1):51–5.
50. Candido K, et al. Buprenorphine added to the local anesthetic for axillary brachial plexus block prolongs postoperative analgesia. Reg Anesth Pain Med. 2002;27(2):162–7.
51. Karlsson M, et al. Efficacy and safety of low-dose transdermal buprenorphine patches (5, 10, and 20 micrograms/h) versus prolonged-release tramadol tablets (75, 100, 150, and 200 mg) in patients with chronic osteoarthritis pain: a 12-week, randomized, open-label, controlled, parallel-group non inferiority study. Clin Ther. 2009;31:503–13.
52. Heit H, et al. Dear DEA. Pain Med. 2004;5:306–7.
53. Malinoff HL, et al. Sublingual buprenorphine is effective in the treatment of chronic pain syndrome. Am J Ther. 2005;12:379–84.
54. Substance Abuse and Mental Health Services Administration, Center for Behavioral Health Statistics and Quality. The DAWN Report: ED Visits Involving the Muscle Relaxant Carisoprodol. Rockville, MD, 27 October 2011.
55. Paemeleire et al. Practical management of medication-overuse headache. Acta Neurol. Belg. 2006;106:43–51

56. Baldwin DS, et al. Evidence-based guidelines for the pharmacological treatment of anxiety disorders: recommendations from the British Association for Psychopharmacology. J Psychopharmacol. 2005;19(6):567–96.
57. Kouyanou K et al. Medication misuse, abuse and dependence in chronic pain patients. J Psychosom Res 1997: 43:497–504.
58. Rickels K, et al. Long- term therapeutic use of benzodiazepines. 1. Effects of abrupt discontinuation. Arch of General. Psychiatry. 1990;47:899–907.
59. Lader M, Tylee A, Donoghue J. Withdrawing benzodiazepines in primary care. CNS Drugs. 2009;23(1):19–34.
60. Smith DE, et al. Benzodiazepine dependency discontinuation: focus on the chemical dependency detoxification setting and benzodiazepine—poly drug abuse. J Psychiatric Res. 1990;24(Suppl 2):145–56.
61. Coupland M. CBT for pain management. Int Assoc Ind Accid Boards Comm (IAIABC). 2009;6(2):77–91.
62. Fordyce WE. Behavioral methods for chronic pain and illness. USA: St. Louis Mosby; 1976.
63. Bickel W, et al. Effects of adding behavioral treatment to opioid detoxification with buprenorphine. J Consult Clin Psychol. 1997;65(5):803–10.
64. Shahrokh J. Opioid-induced central sleep apnea: mechanisms and therapies. Sleep Med Clin. 2014;9(1):49–56.
65. Dunn KM, et al. Opioid prescriptions for chronic pain and overdose: a cohort study. Ann Int Med. 2010;152(2):85–92.
66. Gomes T, et al. Opioid dose and drug-related mortality in patients with nonmalignant pain. Arch Int Med. 2011;171:686–91.
67. Bohnert AS, et al. Association between opioid prescribing patterns and opioid overdose-related deaths. JAMA. 2011;305:1315–21.
68. Von Korff M, et al. Long-term opioid therapy reconsidered. Ann Int Med. 2011;155:325–8.
69. Clark AK, et al. A systematic review of community opioid overdose prevention and naloxone distribution programs. J Addict Med. 2014;8(3):153–163.
70. Walley AY, et al. Opioid overdose rates and implementation of overdose education and nasal naloxone distribution in Massachusetts: interrupted time series analysis. Br Med J. 2013;346: f174.
71. Substance Abuse and Mental Health Services Administration. SAMHSA Opioid Overdose Prevention Toolkit. HHS Publication No. (SMA) 1 4-4742. Rockville, MD: Substance Abuse and Mental Health Services Administration, 2014.

Chapter 15
Alternatives to Opiates in the Management of Non-cancer-related Pain

Peter S. Staats, Sean Li and Sanford M. Silverman

Introduction

Chronic pain is one of the greatest healthcare issues affecting Americans today. With an aging population, this trend is likely to continue. Unfortunately, chronic pain, as a major healthcare crisis, will be with industrialized and developing countries for years to come. It is unlikely that any single approach or medication will revolutionize the treatment of chronic pain to a point that we will not require comprehensive strategies to address this problem. No vaccine, simple pharmaceutical, or medical device will eliminate the problem of chronic pain.

The use of opiates is undoubtedly a major treatment strategy that can be effective in the management of pain. While the focus of this book is on the appropriate use of opioids, it is just as important to understand that opiates are not indicated for everyone and that they are not a panacea for all problems. As such, it is important to understand when *not* to use an opiate and when alternative strategies may be beneficial. While the opioid class of medication is most definitely effective in certain

P.S. Staats (✉)
Department of Anesthesiology and Critical Care, Department of Oncology,
Johns Hopkins University, and Premier Pain Centers, 167 Avenue at the Common,
Shrewsbury, NJ 07702, USA
e-mail: peterstaats@hotmail.com

S. Li
Premier Pain Centers, LLC, 170 Avenue at the Common, Suite 6,
Shrewsbury, NJ 07702, USA

S.M. Silverman
Department of Integrated Medical Science, Charles E. Schmidt College of Medicine,
Florida Atlantic University, Boca Raton, FL, USA

S.M. Silverman
Department of Surgery, Boca Raton Regional Hospital, Broward North Medical Center,
100 E Sample Road, Suite 200, PO Box 50607, Pompano Beach, FL 33064, USA

© Springer International Publishing Switzerland 2016
P.S. Staats and S.M. Silverman (eds.), *Controlled Substance
Management in Chronic Pain*, DOI 10.1007/978-3-319-30964-4_15

settings, in other settings they carry untoward risks. It is important to remember that the opiates are only one class of many medications and one of many therapeutic strategies employed in treating patients with non-cancer-related pain.

Recognizing that pain was undertreated, physician, patient advocate groups, governmental organizations, and pharmaceutical companies pressed for improved pain control. In the 1990s, many stakeholders believed that patients were undertreated for their pain and pushed for increased availability for the use of opioids. Citing the World Health Organization guidelines on cancer pain, and the belief that addiction was markedly overstated, consumer advocacy groups, physicians, pharmaceutical companies, and societies pushed for the liberalization of opiates in non-cancer pain. In a 100 word letter to the editor in the NEJM, it was reported that less than one percent of patients admitted to Boston University Medical Center who were placed on an opiate became addicted [1]. Taking into account the incidence of addictive disorders roughly 10 % in the general population, this result of this study seems inaccurate. A second study in the journal Pain concluded that patients with non-cancer pain "can be safely and effectively prescribed to selected patients with relatively little risk of producing the maladaptive behaviors that define opiate abuse" [2]. Weissman and Haddox [3] opined that the concerns of addiction were overstated and that when a patient was frequently requesting more medications, or running out early, they were not addicted, but rather undertreated. They coined this phenomenon pseudoaddiction and suggested that the physicians were *under* treating patients with opiates for their severe pain. However, they were all mistaken.

In spite of the lack of peer-reviewed data, it was believed that opioids were uniformly effective in non-cancer pain as well as cancer pain. Numerous guidelines were created that incorporated the use of opioids in the management of non-cancer- and cancer-related pain [4]. In 1999, the agency for healthcare quality and research began to discuss pain as the fifth vital sign and indicated that pain management was a right of all patients. The American Pain Society and the Academy of Pain Medicine issued a joint position statement, indicating that opioids were appropriate in the management of non-cancer-related pain [5]. While well intentioned, physicians and providers may not have been adequately instructed to prescribe opioids safely and, most importantly, when to consider alternative strategies. They were given an oversimplified three step (WHO ladder) ladder that was intended for cancer patients in developing countries, and told to apply this to the non-cancer population within a modern healthcare system. Many underestimated the risks of opiates, believing that this was a uniformly safe approach to managing most pains. Others have been more critical of widely advocating the use of opiates and have called for a more balanced approach.

As healthcare providers increased their opioid prescribing, with it came a large increase in opioid-related complications including iatrogenic addiction, overdose resulting in ER admissions, and even deaths. The pendulum has thus swung from underprescribing with needless suffering, to overprescribing (in certain settings) to patients who should not be receiving chronic high-dose opiate therapy.

We need to recognize that chronic pain remains a great problem in society. However, the problem of drug abuse, diversion, and addiction needs to be taken seriously, as well. Thus in revisiting the balance, one needs to understand the wealth of options available to patients with chronic pain. This begins with establishing an accurate diagnosis. From here, a treatment plan can be developed that is individualized, safe, and effective.[1] When physicians and caregivers do not know how to make an accurate diagnosis, they tend to label the disorder in a very non-specific manner. For example, the diagnosis may be "chronic pain syndrome" or "back pain." This is simply inadequate in defining the appropriate therapeutic plan. This lack of understanding leads to administering inappropriate drugs while failing to define the problem and establishing the most appropriate strategy.

What Is Pain?

Pain is defined by the International Association for the Study of Pain as "an unpleasant sensory and emotional experience associated with actual or potential tissue damage, or defined in such terms" [6]. As such, there is typically an emotional component as well as a biologic component underpinning the experience of pain [7]. Pain has also been defined as "whatever the patient says it is."

The challenge for the treating physician is to assess the patient from both a psychosocial and biologic perspective in order to establish the most appropriate therapeutic plan.

Physicians need to treat pain from the biological, psychological, and social perspectives. For most physicians who are trained primarily in the biological approach, it can be challenging to evaluate a patient with severe chronic pain who has comorbid psychiatric disorders. Likewise, many psychiatrists and psychologists who are expert pain clinicians may lack the expertise to diagnose and manage the biological underpinnings. Patients with similar injuries can present with dramatically different experiences of pain. This can occur for a variety of reasons that are not always evident. For example, some patients with psychological disorders including severe depression, anxiety, and other psychiatric disorders will frequently present with increased pain beyond what would be expected based on the injury or objective findings. Patients with negative thoughts will experience more pain with neutral and positive thoughts [8]. On the other hand, there may be biologic factors that influence pain sensitivity that and experience. Patients can have genetic disorders that lead to the absence of pain fibers and experience no pain following an otherwise traumatic injury. These patients with "congenital insensitivity to pain" truly feel no pain [9]. Patients with coexisting substance use disorders often experience increased sensitivity to pain or hyperalgesia.

Most patients we see in clinical practice have an identifiable biologic basis for their pain but also have an emotional component that leads to suffering. The job of

---

[1]Conservative options can include interventional therapies, including surgery. In some settings, starting patients on opioids may be considered riskier and with a higher morbidity and lower chance of success than alternative invasive options.

the pain physician is to not only determine source of pain, but also to apportion the component of pain that emanates from the biological underpinnings, as well as the emotional suffering. This evaluation can be complex and may involve a more comprehensive evaluation with psychology. In the more acute setting, however, this evaluation can be relatively straightforward.

Diagnostic Workup

This chapter certainly does not attempt to make the reader expert in all of the different disorders that cause pain. There are entire treatises devoted to the diagnosis and management of chronic pain [10, 11]. Physicians should, on the other hand, do their best to establish a diagnosis and come up with the most appropriate therapeutic plan. This is achieved by taking a thorough history and physical examination, followed by performing the appropriate diagnostic workup. The expectation is that one understands that not all pain patients have a "chronic pain syndrome," a nondescript entity that deserves an opiate prescription. Rather in most cases, specific biologic correlates, or underpinnings, can be identified in a manner that may explain a patient's pain. While most patients do have some component of an emotional overlay, psychological morbidity is rarely the primary pathology.

Whenever possible, prior to starting opiate therapy, the source of the pain should be identified and a presumptive diagnosis should be made. Once a diagnosis has been made, a care plan should be established that may or may not include opiate therapy. The complete history and physical examination for all painful disorders is beyond the scope of this chapter; however, the concept of establishing a presumptive diagnosis before embarking on therapy cannot be overstated.

The Visit

The initial consultation begins with a comprehensive history and physical examination. Prior to considering implementation of a long-term strategy for chronic intractable pain, the physician should establish a diagnosis, or at least a presumptive diagnosis. With a diagnosis, one can establish the most appropriate therapeutic plan. The visit should include a careful history of substance abuse, a family history of substance abuse, and risk factors for abuse if opioid management is being considered.

Chief Complaint

Why is the patient here to see you? What is the primary pain problem?

Table 15.1 Features of a pain history	The location of pain (body part)
	The severity of pain (0–10, faces, mild, moderate, severe)
	Quality of pain (sharp, lancinating, shooting or burning, dull or achy)
	Time course of pain (When is it bad? Does it wax and wane throughout the day, week, or month?)
	Alleviating factors (what makes it better?)
	Aggravating factors (what makes it worse?)
	Changes or limitations in functional status caused by pain
	Review of diagnostic workup (previous EMG, MRI, laboratory tests)
	Review of previous treatment (previous surgery, rehabilitation strategies, medication strategies)

History

During an initial intake, one needs to take a history and understand the inciting events, the time course and character, and severity of the pain (Table 15.1). What makes the pain better or worse? Verbal descriptors of pain can help determine whether the pain is neuropathic or nociceptive.

Past Medical History

Obtaining a past medical history is part of comprehensive evaluation for pain. Comorbid diseases can be central in defining a differential diagnosis. Patients with a history of many disorders (including diseases such as cancer or diabetes) develop painful disorders as result of the disease or its treatment. A complete understanding of the patient's history thus can be helpful when trying to establish a diagnosis. For example, patients with uncontrolled diabetes may develop peripheral neuropathies that can be quite painful. The practitioner should understand that part of the treatment of the pain is to work with the primary care physician/endocrinologist to get diabetes under control.

Previous Treatment

As part of the comprehensive evaluation, one should understand what treatments have been tried to date and what the outcome has been of previous treatments. Has a patient previously tried medications, injections, physical medicine modalities, or surgical interventions?

Physical Examination

The pain practitioner typically takes a history and follows with a focused physical examination that is determined by the history. This helps the physician narrow the differential, or presumptive, diagnosis. This typically involves inspection, palpation, provocative maneuvers, and a neurologic examination.

Laboratory Workup

Laboratory workup can be used to help make a diagnosis or determine whether it is safe to proceed with a planned course of therapy. In addition with the use of some pharmacologic agents, some laboratory testing may help identify complications that can occur with the treatment strategies. Urine drug testing is employed to establish patient compliance with controlled substance therapy. More commonly, laboratory workup may be used to determine whether it is safe to proceed with interventional pain procedures.

The reason to obtain additional studies is to establish a diagnosis and to help guide therapy. One should only perform the additional studies below if it is going to guide therapy.

Imaging Studies

Plain X-ray: Plain X-rays use X-ray radiation to take a still picture of a body structure including the spine. Differences in densities of hard and soft tissues are then illustrated in varying shades in resulting film. These can be helpful in arthritic disorders and evaluating other connective tissues. Flexion extension films of the spine are taken with patients in multiple positions to assess stability of the spine if a spondylolisthesis is suspected. This test helps determine whether there is spinal instability. In addition by carefully orienting the patient in the correct plane, fractures, and foraminal compromise can be identified and correlated with a patient's symptoms.

MRI: Magnetic resonance imaging utilizes strong magnetic fields to assess soft tissues. The detailed images captured allow insight to the nature of the internal soft tissues being evaluated. They are frequently used to evaluate soft tissues, such as nervous tissue, or herniated disks in the spine. In the spine, MRI often provides superior definition of spinal cord, surrounding CSF, and extradural structures, such as intervertebral disks. Moreover, architecture of the disks and the level of disk dehydration can be assessed by the changes in signal intensity within the spine. MRI with and without contrasts may help distinguish malignancy and inflammatory or scar tissues from a reherniation.

CT: Computed tomography utilized a series of X-ray-generated images formatted into two-dimensional and now three-dimensional images of both soft and hard tissues. Scans can help identify hard tissue abnormalities. Cancer as well as additional spinal pathologies can be identified with CT scans.

Ultrasound: Ultrasound establishes and image in of internal structures by measuring their capacity to transmit and reflect high-frequency sound waves. They can be used to evaluate soft tissue abnormalities. Because of the refractive elements of bony structures, they cannot be used to visualize structures deep to bony tissue. In soft tissue, patterns of tears can be seen in muscles, and abnormal activity can be seen in soft tissue. It is frequently used to evaluate muscle and ligamentous tears as well as soft tissue structures such as cysts. The relative low cost, portability, and safety profile of ultrasound allows for higher utilization. Ultrasound is also widely used for image guidance for many office-based diagnostic procedures and therapeutic injections.

EMG/NCV: EMG, or electromyography, measures electrical activity within muscles. Various patterns of altered activity can indicate both primary muscle pathology and denervation. Nerve conduction velocity (NCV) tests help determine whether there is damage along the path of specific nerves. The pattern of abnormalities identified can help distinguish between radiculopathies, plexopathies, and primary nerve injuries. These patterns can be used to guide therapy.

Biopsy: Tissue diagnosis can be helpful with some neurologic and rheumatologic pain states, visceral pains, as well as with cancer diagnosis.

Consultation with other specialties: If the practitioner is not clear on the diagnosis, it is appropriate to obtain consultation with pain physicians or members of other specialties.

Treatment Strategies

All too often, practitioners may have not established a clear diagnosis or have an inaccurate diagnosis. The treatment strategy chosen should be determined after one has a diagnosis and treatment plan. Broadly speaking, there are several general approaches to treating patients with chronic pain: medical approaches, anatomic or surgical approaches, neuromodulatory approaches, psychological approaches, alternative approaches, and interventional approaches. Opiates should *not* be the mainstay of every patient with chronic pain. Generally, one should consider conservative approaches prior to the more invasive approaches. One should generally have a clinical matrix, understanding the risks of the therapies being recommended, the likelihood of *curing* or *managing* the problem, the risks of the proposed therapy for any given patient, and indeed the costs of the therapies over both the short- and long-term strategies. If a patient presents with back pain, it is important to understand the pathology, as well as the patient's comorbid medical disorders prior to making decisions on the appropriate strategy. A young patient with new onset neurologic deficit, herniated disk, and classic radicular findings may benefit from a micro-discectomy early in the treatment algorithm. Alternatively, an elderly patient with comorbid medical disorders and back pain may benefit from early treatment with physical therapy. There is quite a bit of judgement that the practitioner must exercise in making this decision.

Medication Management

There are several classes of medications frequently used in the treatment of pain. They can be used for a variety of indications. Table 15.2 lists several types of medications. Within each class of medication, there are multiple medications that are commonly used. Within each class of medication, there are numerous side effects and risks. The class of medication chosen is determined by the patient's disorder, and side effect profile of the agents chosen. For example, neuropathic pain can be most effectively treated with anti-epileptic medications and antidepressant medications. If a patient were to present with chronic burning pain and a comorbid depression, the physician may choose an antidepressant class of medication. Severe lancinating pain is more commonly treated with anti-seizure medications (Table 15.3).

Alternatively, if a patient has a primary inflammatory process, an anti-inflammatory agent may be considered. However, if the patient has significant kidney dysfunction, one may shy away from this class of medication.

Physical Medicine Modalities

Physical modalities include all modalities designed to modify the muscular or painful tendinous insertions. Examples of such conventional therapies include chiropractic care with manipulation, physical therapy deep tissue include massage, exercise heat cooling tens units etc. All of these approaches can be effective for many types of pain.

Cognitive Behavioral and Psychologic Approaches

Many patients with chronic pain can benefit from a comprehensive psychological evaluation. The degree of suffering and comorbid psychologic disorders can be dampened. Biofeedback can decrease arousal of pain and provide additional pain relief. Relaxation techniques such as biofeedback, guided visual imagery, and hypnosis are few of the coping mechanism that contribute to the multimodal pain treatment strategy. The restoration of sleep in the activity rest cycle is a key element in the psychosocial component of chronic pain. Treatment is often maintained

Table 15.2 Common medications and their routes of administration for pain

Class of medication	Mechanism of action	Route	Concerns	Notes
Nonsteroidal anti-inflammatory	Inhibits prostaglandin synthesis	Oral and IV	GI bleeding/platelet dysfunction Renal dysfunction Cardiovascular risk	Acute chronic and cancer
Acetaminophen	Central	Oral and IV	Hepatotoxicity in higher doses or chronic use	Hidden in many other combo medications and OTC formulations
Steroids	Potent anti-inflammatory	Oral IV topical	Bone Immune depression Hyperglycemia associated with GI bleeding Autologous steroid depression	Not a long-term option
Anti-seizure medications	Multiple mechanisms	Oral	Hematologic abnormalities Drug–drug interactions	Neuropathic pain
Antidepressant medications	Can alter reuptake of serotonin and norepinephrine	Oral	Serotonin syndrome a rare side effect Anticholinergic effects	Neuropathic pain
Opiates	Bind opiate receptor	Oral IV, IM, intrathecal	Respiratory depression Endocrine Addiction and constipation Death	Neuropathic Nociceptive pain (limited)
Cytokine modulators	Affects TNF-alpha	Oral Intravenous	Immune suppression	Rheumatoid arthritis
Local anesthetics	Blocks Na channels	Topical Epidural and intrathecal	Seizures Tachyphylaxis	Less common oral or IV
NMDA receptor antagonists	Blocks N Methyl D Aspartate receptor	Topical Intravenous	Hallucination Sialorrhea	May affect tolerance
Alpha 2 agonists	Binds the alpha 2 receptor centrally and peripherally	Topical/intrathecal	Hypotension	Sympathetically maintained pain
Bisphosphonates	Inhibit pyrophosphate metabolism	Oral Intravenous	Jaw disease	Used in clinical trial for CRPS type 1 osteoporosis

Table 15.3 Anti-seizure medications

Drug	Mechanism of action	Starting dose	Typical daily dose	Primary clinical use	Special considerations
Gabapentin	Binds to voltage-gated calcium channels	300 mg	1800–3600 mg	Post-herpetic neuralgia (general neuropathic pain)	Start at low dose and slow titration upward
Pregabalin	Binds to voltage-gated calcium channels	50 mg	150–600 mg	Diabetic peripheral neuropathy, fibromyalgia, spinal cord injury	Start at low dose and slow titration upward
Topiramate	(1) Blocks voltage-gated Na channels (2) Augments GABA A receptors (3) Antagonizes AMPA/Kainate receptors (4) Inhibits carbonic anhydrase (Isozyme II and IV)	50 mg per day	100–200 mg	Primary indication seizure disorder Effective in migraine prophylaxis	(1) Side effect is weight loss (2) Used in bipolar disorder (3) Effective with headaches
Gabapentin enacarbil (Horizant)	Extended release gabapentin	600 mg	1200 mg	Restless leg syndrome and neuropathic pain	Different pharmacokinetic profile than gabapentin
Gabapentin (Gralise)	Extended release gabapentin	300 mg	1800 g once daily in the evening	Post-herpetic peripheral neuropathy and neuropathic pain	Different pharmacokinetic profile than gabapentin
Phenytoin	Voltage-dependent block of voltage-gated sodium channels Class 1b antiarrhythmic	100 mg tid	200 mg tid	Treatment of trigeminal neuralgia (second choice to carbamazepine)	Narrow therapeutic index

through self-management interventions that may comprise of scheduled group sessions utilizing the social support and peer.

An important aspect of treating chronic pain is bridging the gap between patient's expectations of the treatment plan and the reality of what is actually achieved. Utilizing cognitive behavioral therapy, the focus of pain relief is redirected from "the pain" itself to goal-oriented improvement of function. Negative mechanisms such as catastrophizing are replaced with adaptive more constructive mechanisms such as self-reassurance. This cognitive restructuring focuses on the value of attitudes, beliefs, and emotional responses to pain and allows the sufferer to resume pleasurable activities and activities of daily living.

Interventional Pain Management

Interventional pain management techniques are minimally invasive procedures, including percutaneous precision needle placement, with the placement of drugs in the targeted areas or ablation of targeted nerves, and some surgical techniques, such as laser or endoscopic discectomy, intrathecal infusion pumps, and spinal cord stimulators, for the diagnosis and management of chronic, persistent, or intractable pain [12]. Lack of knowledge, or fear of the risks of some of these techniques, has led to overprescribing of opiate analgesics. Some primary care physicians hesitate to refer out for these procedures, considering them risky or may not know of their efficacy. However, when used judiciously, it is possible to decrease the amount of opiates and complications related to opiates, improve the quality of life, and some instances improve life expectancy [13, 14].

Epidural Steroid Injections

One of the classic interventional or minimally invasive approaches is epidural steroids or the application of small amounts of steroids to specific sites within the epidural space [15]. It is thought to decrease inflammation reduce nociceptive input from neural structures, resulting in improved pain scores, function and decrease opiate consumption in patients with acute radiculopathies secondary to disk herniations.

Vertebroplasty and Kyphoplasty

This therapy is indicated for patients with focal pain due to a spinal compression fracture. These are minimally invasive, fluoroscopically guided technique to restore the structural instability of a fractured vertebral body by placing a small amount of bone cement either directly through a cannula. The compressed vertebral body height may be restored during a kyphoplasty by first placing a pneumatic balloon into the crushed vertebrae. This newly created cavity is then filled with bone cement to stabilize the augmented vertebral body. Both of these procedures have been demonstrated to improve pain and decrease opiate consumption in patients with semi-acute and acute vertebral compression fractures [16].

Minimally Invasive Lumbar Decompression

The minimally invasive lumbar decompression has been recently developed to treat lumbar spinal stenosis as a result of ligamentum flavum hypertrophy. Patients with spinal stenosis present with progressive neurogenic claudication where low back and/or lower extremity pain is exacerbated with standing or walking. This is a minimally invasive, fluoroscopically guided technique for decompressing the narrowed spinal canal by removing portions of the ligamentum flavum through 5-mm trocar sites. This procedure may help chronic pain patients obtain pain relief with less risk than open spinal surgery. Numerous well-controlled trials have been performed with the level one evidence pending [17].

Neuromodulation

Neuromodulation is the field of medicine that targets electrical stimulation or intraspinal medication to the nervous system to treat symptoms or modify disease.

Spinal Cord Stimulation

Spinal cord stimulation involves implanting electrodes into the epidural space to modify pain or disease. The therapy has been demonstrated to be more effective than repeat back surgery and medication management in the control of pain [18, 19]. Traditional or tonic stimulation has been used since the 1960s and is a widely accepted approach to managing neuropathic pains. Traditional stimulation would layer a sensation of buzzing or tingling over an area of pain, effectively masking the painful sensation with a gentle buzzing sensation. In order to experience pain relief with traditional stimulation parameters, there was a requirement of stimulating the area of pain. Both rechargeable and non-rechargeable power sources have been used to control pain. These therapies have been traditionally most effective for neuropathic pain in the trunk and limbs.

Newer stimulation targets or approaches may even improve on the success of traditional spinal cord stimulation. Dorsal root ganglion (DRG) stimulation, for example, involves placing the electrodes directly on the DRG and stimulating the DRG that is presumed to be involved in the processing of painful stimuli. It appears to be superior to traditional spinal cord stimulation in certain settings [20]. Electrodes are also placed on peripheral nerves in the head and neck to modulate headaches. A novel approach approved in Europe and Australia stimulates the vagus nerve noninvasively as a prophylaxis and treatment for cluster headaches and migraines [21].

New frequencies are also improving the efficacy of spinal cord stimulation. High-frequency spinal cord stimulation involves utilization of frequencies in the 10,000 hertz range and requires a larger energy requirement. It is typically set subthreshold, so the patient feels no paresthesias as they typically do with traditional or tonic stimulation. High-frequency spinal cord stimulation was recently compared to traditional or tonic stimulation in a FDA clinical trial. In a non-inferiority study design, high-frequency stimulation demonstrated superior pain control for both back and leg over traditional or tonic stimulation [22]. Burst stimulation involves utilizing novel frequencies that have *bursts* of electrical activity followed by a quiescent period. It is also widely used in Europe and Australia and is the subject of FDA-approved clinical trials in the USA [23].

Intrathecal Therapy

Intrathecal therapy has been relegated to a salvage approach for most patients with severe cancer- and non-cancer-related pains [24]. Intrathecal therapy involves placing a catheter into the intrathecal space and connecting it to an implantable pump to deliver analgesics including opioids. This approach has been demonstrated to be effective in both cancer and non-cancer populations. In the cancer population, intrathecal opiates have been shown to improve pain control side effects and possibly improve life expectancy when compared to medical management alone [25]. In addition, when compared to the costs of systemic opiates, intrathecal therapy becomes cost-effective after 28 months. The high upfront costs of the device are offset by the lower costs of maintenance of intrathecal opiates. Moreover, with over 16,000 deaths attributed each year to prescription systemic opiates, the overall higher safety profile of controlled delivery is favorable on multiple fronts [26].

In addition, the use of non-narcotics in the intrathecal space to manage severe pain is quite common. Novel agents, including intrathecal ziconotide, have been demonstrated to be effective in patients with severe pain related to cancer and aids, and in non-cancer-related pain [27, 28]. Algorithms have been developed that guide physicians through various medications [29]. The therapy is widely considered a safe therapy and is used for patients with chronic severe pain who have failed an adequate response to other conservative therapies including low-dose opiate therapy.

Summary

There are multiple treatment strategies that are effective in the management of cancer- and non-cancer-related pain. While opiates remain an important tool for physicians, they should not be considered the only tool that physicians have in managing chronic pain. Whichever treatment strategy the physician chooses, he/she should begin with a thorough history and physical examination. After a history and physical examination is performed, a presumptive diagnosis should be established. This diagnosis, thus, should lead the physician to create an individualized treatment algorithm. Understanding the treatment options, and relative risks, will facilitate appropriate treatment with the safest and most conservative option.

References

1. Porter J, Jick H. Addiction rare in patients treated with narcotics. N Engl J Med. 1980;302 (2):123.
2. Portenoy RK, Foley KM. Chronic use of opioid analgesics in non-malignant pain: report of 38 cases. Pain. 1986;25(2):171–86.
3. Weissman DE, Haddox JD. Opioid pseudoaddiction–an iatrogenic syndrome. Pain. 1989;36 (3):363–6.
4. Manchikanti L, et al. American society of interventional pain physicians (ASIPP) guidelines for responsible opioid prescribing in chronic non-cancer pain: Part I-evidence assessment. Pain Physician. 2012;15:S1–66.
5. Chou R, et al. Clinical guidelines for the use of chronic opioid therapy in chronic noncancer pain. J Pain. 2009;10(2):113–30.
6. Merskey H, Bodguk N. Classification of chronic pain: descriptions of chronic pain syndromes and definition of pain terms. 2nd ed. Seattle: IASP Press; 1994.
7. Staats PS, Hekmat H, Staats AW. Psychological behaviorism theory of pain: a basis for unity. Pain Forum. 1996;5:194–207.
8. Staats PS, Staats A, Hekmat H. The additive impact of anxiety and a placebo on pain. Pain Med. 2001;2:267–79.
9. Cox JJ, Reimann F, Nicholas AK, Thornton G, Roberts E, Springell K, Karbani G, Jafri H, Mannan J, Raashid Y, Al-Gazali L, Hamamy H, Valente EM, Gorman S, Williams R, McHale DP, Wood JN, Gribble FM, Woods CG. An SCN9A channelopathy causes congenital inability to experience pain. Nature. 2006;444(7121):894–8.
10. Staats PS, Wallace MS. Pain medicine: just the facts. 2nd ed. New York: McGraw Hill; 2015.
11. Diwan S, Staats PS. The Diwan Staats atlas pain medicine procedures. New York: McGraw Hill; 2015.
12. Medicare Payment Advisory Commission. Report to the congress: paying for interventional pain services in ambulatory settings. Washington, DC: MedPAC, Dec 2001. http://www. medpac.gov/publications/congressional_reports/dec2001PainManagement.pdf.
13. Staats PS. The effect of pain on survival. In: Staats PS, editor. Interventional pain management anesthesiology clinics of North America Guest, vol. 21, No. 4, Dec 2003.
14. Staats PS. Pain, depression and survival. Am. Fam. Physician. 1999;60:42–4.
15. Manchikanti L, Staats PS, Nampiaparampil DE. What is the role of epidural injections in the treatment of lumbar discogenic pain: a system 4/2015. Korean J Pain. doi:10.3344/kjp.2015. 28.2.75.

16. Anselmetti, et al. Percutaneous vertebroplasty in osteoporotic patients: an institutional experience of 1,634 patients with long-term follow-up. J Vasc Interv Radiol. 2011;22 (12):1714–20.

17. Benyamin R, Staats PS, Davis K et al. Midas encore. Pain Physician 2015.

18. North RB, Kidd DH, Shipley et al. Spinal cord stimulation versus reoperation for failed back surgery syndrome: a cost effectiveness and cost utility analysis based on a randomized controlled clinical trial. Neurosurgery 2007;61:361.

19. Kumar K et al. The effects of spinal cord stimulation in neuropathic pain are sustained: a 24 month follow up of the prospective randomized controlled multicenter trial of effectiveness of spinal cord stimulation. Neurosurgery 2008;63:762–70.

20. Kramer, Draper, Deer et al. Dorsal root ganglion stimulation: anatomy physiology and potential for therapeutic targeting in chronic pain. In: Diwan S, editor. The Diwan Staats atlas of pain medicine procedures. New York: McGraw Hill; 2015. pp. 626–31.

21. Deer TR, Mekhail N, Petersen E, Krames E, Staats P, Pope J, Saweris Y, Lad SP, Diwan S, Falowski S, Feler C, Slavin K, Narouze S, Merabet L, Buvanendran A, Fregni F, Wellington J, Levy RM. The appropriate use of neurostimulation: stimulation of the intracranial and extracranial space and head for chronic pain. Neuromodulation. 2014;17:551–70.

22. Buyten Van, et al. High-frequency spinal cord stimulation for the treatment of chronic back pain patients: results of a prospective multicenter european clinical study. Neuromodulation. 2013;16(1):59–66.

23. DeRidder D et al. Burst stimulation for back and limb pain. World Neurosurg 2013 Nov;80 (5):642–9. doi:10.1016/j.wneu.2013.01.040. Epub 2013 Jan 12.

24. Pope J, Deer T, McRoberts WP. Intrathecal therapy: the burden of being positioned as a salvage therapy. Pain Med 2015;16(10):2036–8.

25. Smith TJ, Coyne PJ, Staats PS, Deer T, Stearns LJ, Rauck RL, Boortz-Marx RL, Buchser E, Català E, Bryce DA, Cousins M, Pool GE. An implantable drug delivery system (IDDS) for refractory cancer pain provides sustained pain control, less drug-related toxicity, and possibly better survival compared with comprehensive medical management (CMM). Ann Oncol. 2005;16(5):825–33 Epub 2005 Apr 7.

26. Kumar Hunter Demeria. Treatment of chronic pain by using a intrathecal drug delivery compared to conventional treatments. A cost effectiveness analysis. J Neurosurg. 2002;97 (4):803–10.

27. Staats PS Et al. Intrathecal Ziconotide in the Treatment of Refractory Pain in Patients With Cancer or AIDS: a randomized controlled clinical trial. JAMA. 2004 Jan 7;291(1).

28. Wallace MS, Charapata S, Fisher R, Staats PS, et al. The ziconotide nonmalignant pain study group. Intrathecal Ziconotide in the treatment of chronic nonmalignant pain: a randomized double blind placebo controlled trial. Neuromodulation. 2006;9:75–86.

29. Deer TR, Prager J, Levy R, Rathmell J, Buchser E, Burton A, Caraway D, Cousins M, De Andrés J, Diwan S, Erdek M, Grigsby E, Huntoon M, Jacobs MS, Kim P, Kumar K, Leong M, Liem L, McDowell GC II, Panchal S, Rauck R, Saulino M, Sitzman BT, Staats P, Stanton-Hicks M, Stearns L, Wallace M, Willis KD, Witt W, Yaksh T, Mekhail N. Polyanalgesic consensus conference 2012: recommendations for the management of pain by intrathecal (intraspinal) drug delivery: report of an interdisciplinary expert panel. Neuromodul Technol Neural Interface. 2012;15:436–66. doi:10.1111/j.1525-1403.2012.00476.x.

Appendix A
American Society of Interventional Pain Physicians (ASIPP) Guidelines for Responsible Opioid Prescribing in Chronic Non-cancer Pain

Part 1: http://painphysicianjournal.com/2012/july/2012;15;S1-S66.pdf
Part 2: http://painphysicianjournal.com/2012/july/2012;%2015;S67-S116.pdf

© Springer International Publishing Switzerland 2016
P.S. Staats and S.M. Silverman (eds.), *Controlled Substance Management in Chronic Pain*, DOI 10.1007/978-3-319-30964-4

Appendix B
Sample Opioid Agreement/Informed Consent

PATIENT:

DATE:

PHYSICIAN/PATIENT INFORMED CONSENT AND AGREEMENT FOR LONG-TERM OPIOID/CONTROLLED SUBSTANCE THERAPY FOR TREATMENT OF PAIN

You have agreed to receive opioid/controlled substance therapy for the treatment of pain. The goal(s) of this treatment is to:

(a) Reduce your pain.

(b) Improve your level of function at home and at work.

Alternative therapies and medications have been explained and offered to you. You have elected a trial of opioid/controlled substance therapy as one component of treatment.

The use of cigarettes demonstrates a dependence on nicotine. This complicates opiate therapy and makes it ineffective. **Therefore, you must agree to stop smoking**.

You must be aware of the potential risks and side effects of these medications. They are explained below.

Side Effects

Side effects are normal physical reactions to medications. Common side effects of opioid/controlled substances include mood changes, drowsiness, dizziness, constipation, nausea, and confusion. Many of these side effects will resolve over days or weeks. Constipation often persists and may require additional medication. If other side effects persist, different opioids may be tried or they may be discontinued.

You should **NOT**:

(a) Operate a vehicle or machinery if the medication makes you drowsy.

(b) Consume **any** alcohol while taking opioid/controlled substances.

(c) Take any other non-prescribed sedative medication while taking narcotics.

If you hold a commercial driver's license (CDL) and or a commercial pilot's license (CPL) or are regulated by the Department of Transportation (DOT) in safety sensitive positions, you may not be able to continue these duties due to safety concerns. If you hold a CDL or CPL, you cannot take methadone per DOT regulations.

The effects of alcohol and sedatives are additive with those of opioid/controlled substances. If you take these substances with opioid/controlled substances, a dangerous situation could result such as coma, organ damage, or even death.

If you develop a respiratory infection (pneumonia, bronchitis) which can impair your breathing, you may have to reduce your pain medication dose until it resolves. Please contact the office if you develop a respiratory infection.

Driving while taking opioid/controlled substances for chronic pain is considered medically acceptable, as long as you do not have side effects such as sedation or altered mental status. These side effects usually do not occur while taking opioids chronically. However, it is **possible** that you could be considered DUI if stopped by law enforcement while driving.

Opioids have also been known to cause decreased sexual function and libido. This is due to their effects on suppression of certain hormones such as testosterone and DHEA which can cause these side effects. If these side effects occur, we can treat them with supplemental testosterone and DHEA (for women).

*INITIAL-*_____

Constipation is a well-known side effect of opioid therapy and can usually be treated with stool softeners or gentle laxatives. Constipation is a side effect that usually does not go away and requires treatment.

Dependence
Physical dependence is an expected side effect of long-term opioid/controlled substances therapy. This means that if you take opioid/narcotics continuously and then stop them abruptly, you will experience a withdrawal syndrome. This syndrome often includes sweating, diarrhea, irritability, sleeplessness, runny nose, tearing, muscle and bone aching, gooseflesh, and dilated pupils. Withdrawal is not life-threatening. To prevent these symptoms, the opioid/controlled substances should be taken regularly or, if discontinued, done gradually under the supervision of your physician.

Tolerance
Tolerance to the pain-relieving effect of opioid/controlled substances is possible with continued use. This means that more medication is required to achieve the same level of pain control experienced when the opioid was initiated. This may occur even though there has been no change in your underlying painful condition. When tolerance does occur, sometimes it requires tapering or discontinuation of the opioid/narcotic. Sometimes tolerance can be treated by substituting a different opioid/narcotic. When initiated, doses of medications must be adjusted to achieve a therapeutic pain-relieving effect; upward adjustments during this period are not viewed as tolerance.

Increased Pain (HYPERALGESIA)

The long-term effects of opiates on the body's own pain-fighting systems are unknown. Some evidence suggests that opiates may interfere with pain modulation, resulting in an **increased** sensitivity to pain. Sometimes individuals who have been on long-term opioids, but who continue to have pain, actually note decreased pain after several weeks off the medications.

Addiction

… a primary, chronic, neurobiological disease, with genetic, psychosocial, and environmental factors influencing the development and manifestations. It is characterized by behaviors that include one or more of the following:

- Impaired control over drug use.
- Compulsive use.
- Continued use despite harm.
- Craving.

Most patients with chronic pain, who use long-term opioids are able to take medications on a scheduled basis as prescribed, do not seek other drugs when their pain is controlled and experience improvement in their quality of life as the result of opioid therapy. Therefore, they are **NOT** addicted. **Physical dependence** is **NOT** the same as addiction.

INITIAL-_____

Risk to Unborn Children

Children born to women who are taking opioid/controlled substances on a regular basis will likely be physically dependent at birth. Women of childbearing age should maintain safe and effective birth control while on opioid therapy. Should you become pregnant, immediately contact your physician and the medication will be tapered and stopped.

Long-Term Side Effects

The long-term effect of opioid/controlled substances therapy is not truly known. Most of the long-term effects have been listed above. In some patients, testosterone levels may decrease over time resulting in decreased sexual activity. This can be monitored and treated. See above section.

PRESCRIPTION AND USE OF MEDICATIONS

Your medication will be prescribed on an around-the-clock, regular basis for the continuous control of pain. You will be provided enough medication on a monthly basis. New injuries or pain problems will require reevaluation.

   You agree to fill opioid prescriptions at one pharmacy.

   This pharmacy is _____Tel._____.

   You agree secure your pain medications in safe locked source to prevent loss or theft. You are responsible for any loss of theft.

   Lost, stolen or destroyed prescriptions or drugs **will not** be replaced and may result in discontinuation of treatment.

You agree to obtain opioid medication from one prescribing physician, _____, or his substitute if not available.

You agree to be evaluated initially and on a monthly (or regular not more than 3 months) basis and thereafter as your physician believes are needed.

You agree to necessary blood and/or urine testing to monitor the levels of medication or other drugs and any organ side effects. You also agree that other doctors and law enforcement may be notified of the results.

You agree NOT to call the physician for refills or replacement medications during evening hours or on weekends/holidays. Medication refills and or replacements will be handled during regular business hours. You also **understand** and **agree** that if you lose your medication or run out early due to overuse, you may experience and go through withdrawal from opioids.

You agree to bring all prescription medication in their bottles or containers to the office during regularly scheduled visits.

You agree to provide a list from your pharmacy detailing all medications received from that pharmacy and to provide updated lists as requested by your physician.

INITIAL-_____

FOR PATIENTS TAKING METHADONE

Methadone has significant interactions with many other medications. Some of these medications may reduce your body's ability to metabolize methadone, thus **INCREASING** the methadone in your body, which could be dangerous. Therefore, you **MUST** notify this office of **ALL** medications prescribed for **ANY** condition while taking methadone.

OPIOID/CONTROLLED SUBSTANCES THERAPY MAY BE DISCONTINUED IF YOU:

- develop progressive tolerance which cannot be managed by changing medications,
- experience unacceptable side effects which cannot be controlled,
- experience diminishing function or poor pain control,
- develop signs of addiction,
- abuse any other controlled substance (this may be determined by random blood/urine testing),
- obtain and or use street drugs (this may be determined by random blood/urine testing),
- increase your medication without the consent of your physician,
- refuse to stop or resume smoking,
- obtain opiates from other physicians or sources,
- fill prescriptions at other pharmacies without explanation,
- sell, give away, or lose medications AND.

<u>Call for refills during evenings, weekends, or holidays</u>

Medication replacement will be handled during **regular business hours only!** After hour refills are not allowed. Our office hours are adequate to ensure that these requests are handled efficiently by our staff. <u>**YOU**</u> are responsible for ensuring that you have enough medication!

Therefore, you must see the physician every 28–30 days for medication refill.

I have read the above and understand fully the Physician/Patient Informed Consent Form for long-term opioid/controlled substances therapy for the treatment of chronic pain. I have been given the opportunity to ask questions about the proposed treatment (including no treatment), potential risks, complications, and benefits. I accept the risks and terms of the proposed treatment as presented.

Patient's signature _____ **Date** _____

Physician signature _____ **Date** _____

Witness signature _____ **Date** _____

Spouse signature _____ **Date** _____

Appendix C

Date _____

Patient Name _____

OPIOID RISK TOOL

		Mark each box that applies	Item Score If Female	Item Score If Male
1. Family History of Substance Abuse	Alcohol	[ ]	1	3
	Illegal Drugs	[ ]	2	3
	Prescription Drugs	[ ]	4	4
2. Personal History of Substance Abuse	Alcohol	[ ]	3	3
	Illegal Drugs	[ ]	4	4
	Prescription Drugs	[ ]	5	5
3. Age (Mark box if 16 – 45)		[ ]	1	1
4. History of Preadolescent Sexual Abuse		[ ]	3	0
5. Psychological Disease	Attention Deficit Disorder, Obsessive Compulsive Disorder, Bipolar, Schizophrenia	[ ]	2	2
	Depression	[ ]	1	1
	TOTAL		_____	_____

Total Score Risk Category
Low Risk 0 – 3
Moderate Risk 4 – 7
High Risk ≥ 8

Reference: Webster LR. Predicting aberrant behaviors in opioid-treated patients: Preliminary validation of the opioid risk tool. *Pain Medicine*. 2005;6(6):432-442. Used with permission.

© Springer International Publishing Switzerland 2016
P.S. Staats and S.M. Silverman (eds.), *Controlled Substance Management in Chronic Pain*, DOI 10.1007/978-3-319-30964-4

Appendix D

Screener and Opioid Assessment for Patients with Pain-Revised (SOAPP®-R)

The following are some questions given to patients who are on or being considered for medication for their pain. Please answer each question as honestly as possible. There are no right or wrong answers.

	Never	Seldom	Sometimes	Often	Very often
	0	1	2	3	4
1. How often do you have mood swings?	○	○	○	○	○
2. How often have you felt a need for higher doses of medication to treat your pain?	○	○	○	○	○
3. How often have you felt impatient with your doctors?	○	○	○	○	○
4. How often have you felt that things are just too overwhelming that you can't handle them?	○	○	○	○	○
5. How often is there tension in the home?	○	○	○	○	○
6. How often have you counted pain pills to see how many are remaining?	○	○	○	○	○
7. How often have you been concerned that people will judge you for taking pain medication?	○	○	○	○	○
8. How often do you feel bored?	○	○	○	○	○
9. How often have you taken more pain medication than you were supposed to?	○	○	○	○	○

(continued)

© Springer International Publishing Switzerland 2016
P.S. Staats and S.M. Silverman (eds.), *Controlled Substance Management in Chronic Pain*, DOI 10.1007/978-3-319-30964-4

(continued)

	Never	Seldom	Sometimes	Often	Very often
	0	1	2	3	4
10. How often have you worried about being left alone?	○	○	○	○	○
11. How often have you felt a craving for medication?	○	○	○	○	○
12. How often have others expressed concern over your use of medication?	○	○	○	○	○
13. How often have any of your close friends had a problem with alcohol or drugs?	○	○	○	○	○
14. How often have others told you that you had a bad temper?	○	○	○	○	○
15. How often have you felt consumed by the need to get pain medication?	○	○	○	○	○
16. How often have you run out of pain medication early?	○	○	○	○	○
17. How often have others kept you from getting what you deserve?	○	○	○	○	○
18. How often, in your lifetime, have you had legal problems or been arrested?	○	○	○	○	○
19. How often have you attended an AA or NA meeting?	○	○	○	○	○
20. How often have you been in an argument that was so out of control that someone got hurt?	○	○	○	○	○
21. How often have you been sexually abused?	○	○	○	○	○
22. How often have others suggested that you have a drug or alcohol problem?	○	○	○	○	○
23. How often have you had to borrow pain medications from your family or friends?	○	○	○	○	○
24. How often have you been treated for an alcohol or drug problem?	○	○	○	○	○

Please include any additional information you wish about the above answers. Thank you.

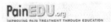

Appendix E

McGILL PAIN QUESTIONNAIRE

RONALD MELZACK

Patient's Name _____ Date _____ Time _____ am/pm

PRI: S _____ A _____ E _____ M _____ PRI(T) _____ PPI _____
    (1–10)   (11–15)   (16)   (17–20)   (1–20)

1 FLICKERING QUIVERING PULSING THROBBING BEATING POUNDING	11 TIRING EXHAUSTING
2 JUMPING FLASHING SHOOTING	12 SICKENING SUFFOCATING
3 PRICKING BORING DRILLING STABBING LANCINATING	13 FEARFUL FRIGHTFUL TERRIFYING
4 SHARP CUTTING LACERATING	14 PUNISHING GRUELLING CRUEL VICIOUS KILLING
5 PINCHING PRESSING GNAWING CRAMPING CRUSHING	15 WRETCHED BLINDING
6 TUGGING PULLING WRENCHING	16 ANNOYING TROUBLESOME MISERABLE INTENSE UNBEARABLE
7 HOT BURNING SCALDING SEARING	17 SPREADING RADIATING PENETRATING PIERCING
8 TINGLING ITCHY SMARTING STINGING	18 TIGHT NUMB DRAWING SQUEEZING TEARING
9 DULL SORE HURTING ACHING HEAVY	19 COOL COLD FREEZING
10 TENDER TAUT RASPING SPLITTING	20 NAGGING NAUSEATING AGONIZING DREADFUL TORTURING

BRIEF MOMENTARY TRANSIENT	RHYTHMIC PERIODIC INTERMITTENT	CONTINUOUS STEADY CONSTANT

E = EXTERNAL
I = INTERNAL

PPI
0 NO PAIN
1 MILD
2 DISCOMFORTING
3 DISTRESSING
4 HORRIBLE
5 EXCRUCIATING

COMMENTS:

© Springer International Publishing Switzerland 2016
P.S. Staats and S.M. Silverman (eds.), *Controlled Substance
Management in Chronic Pain*, DOI 10.1007/978-3-319-30964-4

Appendix F

CDC RECOMMENDATIONS FOR PRESCRIBING
OPIOIDS FOR CHRONIC PAIN—UNITED STATES, 2016

The Centers for Disease Control and Prevention (CDC) has issued guidelines with recommendations for primary care clinicians who prescribe opioids for chronic pain outside of active cancer treatment, palliative care, and end-of-life care. Specifically, the recommendations cover when to initiate or continue opioid treatment, which opioids should be used, duration of treatment, and how to address potential harms associated with treatment.

For each recommendation statement, the CDC provides a category:

Category A recommendation: Applies to all persons; most patients should receive the recommended course of action.

Category B recommendation: Individual decision making needed; different choices will be appropriate for different patients. Clinicians help patients arrive at a decision consistent with patient values and preferences and specific clinical situations.

Evidence type, which is based on study design as well as a function of limitations in study design or implementation, imprecision of estimates, variability in findings, indirectness of evidence, publication bias, magnitude of treatment effects, dose-response gradient, and constellation of plausible biases that could change effects, is also provided for each statement.

Type 1 evidence: Randomized clinical trials or overwhelming evidence from observational studies.

Type 2 evidence: Randomized clinical trials with important limitations, or exceptionally strong evidence from observational studies.

Type 3 evidence: Observational studies or randomized clinical trials with notable limitations.

Type 4 evidence: Clinical experience and observations, observational studies with important limitations, or randomized clinical trials with several major limitations.

© Springer International Publishing Switzerland 2016
P.S. Staats and S.M. Silverman (eds.), *Controlled Substance
Management in Chronic Pain*, DOI 10.1007/978-3-319-30964-4

DETERMINING WHEN TO INITIATE OR CONTINUE OPIOIDS FOR CHRONIC PAIN

1. Nonpharmacologic therapy and nonopioid pharmacologic therapy are preferred for chronic pain. Clinicians should consider opioid therapy only if expected benefits for both pain and function are anticipated to outweigh risks to the patient. If opioids are used, they should be combined with nonpharmacologic therapy and nonopioid pharmacologic therapy, as appropriate. **(Recommendation, category: A, evidence type: 3)**.

2. Before starting opioid therapy for chronic pain, clinicians should establish treatment goals with all patients, including realistic goals for pain and function, and should consider how therapy will be discontinued if benefits do not outweigh risks. Clinicians should continue opioid therapy only if there is clinically meaningful improvement in pain and function that outweighs risks to patient safety. **(Recommendation, category: A, evidence type: 4)**

3. Before starting and periodically during opioid therapy, clinicians should discuss with patients known risks and realistic benefits of opioid therapy and patient and clinician responsibilities for managing therapy. **(Recommendation, category: A, evidence type: 3)**

OPIOID SELECTION, DOSAGE, DURATION, FOLLOW-UP, AND DISCONTINUATION

4. When starting opioid therapy for chronic pain, clinicians should prescribe immediate-release opioids instead of extended-release/long-acting (ER/LA) opioids. **(Recommendation, category: A, evidence type: 4)**

5. When opioids are started, clinicians should prescribe the lowest effective dosage. Clinicians should use caution when prescribing opioids at any dosage, should carefully reassess evidence of individual benefits and risks when increasing dosage to ≥50 morphine milligram equivalents (MME)/day, and should avoid increasing dosage to ≥90 MME/day or carefully justify a decision to titrate dosage to ≥90 MME/day. **(Recommendation, category: A, evidence type: 3)**

6. Long-term opioid use often begins with treatment of acute pain. When opioids are used for acute pain, clinicians should prescribe the lowest effective dose of immediate-release opioids and should prescribe no greater quantity than needed for the expected duration of pain severe enough to require opioids. Three days or less will often be sufficient; more than seven days will rarely be needed. (Recommendation, category: A, evidence type: 4)

7. Clinicians should evaluate benefits and harms with patients within 1 to 4 weeks of starting opioid therapy for chronic pain or of dose escalation. Clinicians should evaluate benefits and harms of continued therapy with patients every 3 months or more frequently. If benefits do not outweigh harms of continued opioid therapy, clinicians should optimize other therapies and work with patients to taper opioids to lower dosages or to taper and discontinue opioids. **(Recommendation, category: A, evidence type: 4)**

ASSESSING RISK AND ADDRESSING HARMS OF OPIOID USE

8. Before starting and periodically during continuation of opioid therapy, clinicians should evaluate risk factors for opioid-related harms. Clinicians should incorporate into the management plan strategies to mitigate risk, including considering offering naloxone when factors that increase risk for opioid overdose, such as history of overdose, history of substance use disorder, higher opioid dosages (≥50 MME/day), or concurrent benzodiazepine use, are present. **(Recommendation, category: A, evidence type: 4)**

9. Clinicians should review the patient's history of controlled substance prescriptions using state prescription drug monitoring program (PDMP) data to determine whether the patient is receiving opioid dosages or dangerous combinations that put him or her at high risk for overdose. Clinicians should review PDMP data when starting opioid therapy for chronic pain and periodically during opioid therapy for chronic pain, ranging from every prescription to every 3 months. **(Recommendation, category: A, evidence type: 4)**

10. When prescribing opioids for chronic pain, clinicians should use urine drug testing before starting opioid therapy and consider urine drug testing at least annually to assess for prescribed medications as well as other controlled prescription drugs and illicit drugs. **(Recommendation, category: B, evidence type: 4)**

11. Clinicians should avoid prescribing opioid pain medication and benzodiazepines concurrently whenever possible. **(Recommendation, category: A, evidence type: 3)**

12. Clinicians should offer or arrange evidence-based treatment (usually medication-assisted treatment with buprenorphine or methadone in combination with behavioral therapies) for patients with opioid use disorder. **(Recommendation, category: A, evidence type: 2)**
    LINK TO CDC GUIDELINES:http://www.cdc.gov/mmwr/volumes/65/rr/rr6501e1er.htm.

Index

© Springer International Publishing Switzerland 2016
P.S. Staats and S.M. Silverman (eds.), *Controlled Substance*
Management in Chronic Pain, DOI 10.1007/978-3-319-30964-4

Printed in the United States
By Bookmasters